Design and Development

of Biological, Chemical, Food and Pharmaceutical Products

T0233704

Design and Development

of Biological, Chemical,
Food and
Pharmaceutical
Products

J.A. Wesselingh

*Emeritus Professor of Chemical Engineering,
University of Groningen and Technical University of Denmark*

Søren Kiil

*Associate Professor, Department of Chemical Engineering,
Technical University of Denmark*

Martin E. Vigild

*Associate Professor, Department of Chemical Engineering,
Technical University of Denmark*

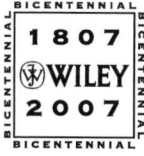

John Wiley & Sons, Ltd

Other Wiley Editorial Offices

John Wiley & Sons Inc., 111 River Street, Hoboken, NJ 07030, USA

Jossey-Bass, 989 Market Street, San Francisco, CA 94103-1741, USA

Wiley-VCH Verlag GmbH, Boschstr. 12, D-69469 Weinheim, Germany

John Wiley & Sons Australia Ltd, 42 McDougall Street, Milton, Queensland 4064, Australia

John Wiley & Sons (Asia) Pte Ltd, 2 Clementi Loop #02-01, Jin Xing Distripark, Singapore 129809

John Wiley & Sons Canada Ltd, 6045 Freemont Blvd, Mississauga, Ontario, L5R 4J3, Canada

Wiley also publishes its books in a variety of electronic formats. Some content that appears in print may not be available in electronic books.

Anniversary Logo Design: Richard J. Pacifico

Library of Congress Cataloging-in-Publication Data

Wesselingh, J. A.
Design and Development of Biological, Chemical, Food and Pharmaceutical Products / J.A Wesselingh, Sören Kiil, Martin E. Vigild.
    p. cm.
Includes bibliographical references and index.
ISBN 978-0-470-06154-1
1.   Biochemical engineering. 2.   New products. 3.   Design, Industrial.   I. Kiil, Sören. II. Vigild, Martin E. III. Title.
  TP248.3.W47 2007
  660.6 – dc22

                     2007014316

British Library Cataloguing in Publication Data

A catalogue record for this book is available from the British Library

ISBN 978-0-470-06154-1 (HB)
ISBN 978-0-470-06155-8 (PB)

Typeset in 10/12 TimesNewRomanPSMT by Laserwords Private Limited, Chennai, India

Contents

continued on the next page

Preface

The twentieth century saw a huge expansion of the chemical industry – and of the career possibilities for industrial chemists and chemical engineers. For example, between 1950 and 1980 the number of cars in many western countries grew about one hundred times. And so did the industry delivering the fuels, lubricants, metals, polymers and paints required. Growth rates of 20% per year were not uncommon. This stopped around 1980 as markets saturated, and since then development in the bulk chemical industries has slowed down markedly as have the numbers of young graduates getting employed there.

Nowadays many chemical engineers are finding work in the development of new products. They work for a much more diverse set of industries – in which chemistry is usually only one of the disciplines that are important. You may find these engineers in electronics, in printing, in medical technology, in the food, car and cosmetic industries ... The skills required in such industries are quite different from those in the (rather sheltered) bulk chemical industry. Development is mostly done in multidisciplinary and multifunctional teams. Young engineers have to learn to work together in projects with people who speak different languages (both literally and metaphorically). Speed and a sense of urgency are more important than in the optimizing of bulk chemical processes. Team members are not only expected to be good engineers, but also to understand why cost, marketing and selling are important.

In this book we introduce major techniques used in designing and developing, roughly in the sequence in which they will be used. We show how techniques have been used (or could have been used) in a variety of products: a laundry detergent, insulated windows, toothpaste, anti-fouling paint, an insulin injector, a powder coating, a box of matches, herbicide capsules, foamed snacks, a pharmaceutical tablet, Rockwool insulation, a ballpoint and a methanol catalyst. The authors have been involved in the development of several of these products.

One can only learn to design and develop a product by doing it – not by reading a book. In our own courses about eighty percent of the time is devoted to project work – we give some examples. This is hard on both students and on us, because we have to follow what the students are doing without telling them what to do. We use the lessons for the other twenty percent: to introduce students to the techniques and to provide a framework for their projects. We hope that you will like them.

Groningen/Lyngby, January 2007
Hans Wesselingh (Johannes in Denmark),
Søren Kiil and Martin E. Vigild

Acknowledgments

This book has a long history. It is the result of two threads: one starting in Delft (and later Groningen) in The Netherlands, and the other in Lyngby in Denmark. Around 1980 at Delft University of Technology, the chemist H.C.A. van Beek† was having a hard time trying to get people to accept that large changes were coming in the chemical industry, and that they should be looking at higher-value (structured) products. He managed to convince a few of his colleagues, among them J.A. Wesselingh (JAW), L.P.B.M. Janssen (LJ) and H. van Bekkum. Together they put a curriculum together for students interested in what was then called 'product engineering'. In 1982 JAW and LJ started a course which gradually evolved into 'learn how a product works by doing experiments and setting up your own theories'. It was very successful.

In 1990 both LJ and JAW had changed universities. By coincidence they were working together in the small department of chemical engineering of Groningen where they continued their course, but otherwise were very busy with other things. In 1996 the board of the university – alarmed by the falling numbers of students in chemistry and chemical engineering – asked JAW to look at the possibility of setting up a study on product engineering. This was to be broader than engineering alone, and they suggested to do it together with people from the group of industrial pharmacy (N.W.F Kossen and later H.W. Frijlink) and to form a co-operation with the technically oriented people from the large department of business administration. The idea was supported by the deans of the Faculty of Sciences (P.C. van der Kruit and later D.A. Wiersma). JAW set up a number of projects in which teams of two to four masters' students worked a year on the development of some product, together with a local industry. The students were given a small budget and had to run their own project organization with help from industry and university. This was all very exciting, although it did conflict with the usual way of doing things in university. (The two big problems were that the university was not used to giving budget and project responsibility to students, and that development projects do not provide scientific research output.) JAW was retired in 2002, but his successor A.A. Broekhuis and R.M Voncken† have carried on the idea. The department has a healthy influx of students once again.

In Lyngby an initiative was started in the year 2000. The head of the chemical engineering department, K. Dam-Johansen, who had been working as a research manager in the paint industry, realised that product development was missing in the chemical engineering curriculum. He started several initiatives involving the young staff members S. Kiil (SK), G. Kontogeorgis (GK), J. Abildskov (JA), M.E. Vigild (MEV) and T. Johannessen (TJ). They were joined by JAW who spent large parts of 2003 and 2004 as a visiting professor in Lyngby.

The first and largest initiative was a 7th semester course called Chemical and Biochemical Product Design. It runs over three months, in which students are expected to spend 16 hours a week. The greater part is in projects which are done in teams of three to five students. In the last project students are to develop their own product (as far as possible in the limited time). This very ambitious course was first organised in 2002 by SZK, GK and JA. In 2003 and 2004 JAW organised a series of some twenty discussions with SZK, GK, JA, KDJ and MEV on how the subject should be structured and taught. With six people involved with different backgrounds (and large numbers of students interfering and contributing) these were hectic and emotional, but we learned greatly. What you see in this book is the course material as it has evolved over these last four years. It will keep on evolving (at least in the coming years), but we do have the feeling that we have found a suitable basic structure.

We have been greatly helped by young engineers from nearby Danish companies (Hempel – marine paints; Novo-Nordisk – insulin; Novozymes – industrial enzymes; Lundbeck – pharmaceuticals; and Coloplast – healthcare products). They gave guest lectures, commented on our ideas, and made it clear to students that this subject was one they were going to encounter in their careers. Some of their topics have found their way into the book. We have also had a lot of help and comment on the different examples by people who were involved at some time. These are acknowledged separately in the different lessons. Matthias Kind has provided us with a more general criticism. Bart Drinkenburg worked carefully through the whole manuscript and provided us with very useful comment and corrections. Then we must thank the hundreds of students that we have had on our courses. They have shaped our ideas with their many projects. The 2005 and 2006 groups have provided extensive comment and helped us to eliminate errors in the text. The staff of Wiley has converted the English of the Dutchman and two Danes into something readable and provided many other improvements. We must mention two other great helps: the books of Karl T. Ulrich and Steven D. Eppinger (*Product Design and Development*, McGraw Hill 1995, 2003) and E.L. Cussler and G.D. Moggridge (*Chemical Product Design*, Cambridge University Press 2001).

The three authors wish to thank their wives Trudi, Jette, and Éva for tolerating all the work outside office hours needed to put the book together. We would not have managed otherwise.

Introduction

Welcome to 'Design and Development'. In this course you are going to find out how new products are conceived, designed, developed, manufactured and sold – and how you may be involved in doing this.

This book is a text where *we* (the three authors) are saying something to *you* (as a member of a design team, so not to you as a single person). The book describes how we run our course – others may do this differently.

We warn you to expect something different from most other courses. You will be learning *how* to do something: how to design and develop a product. The emphasis is not on understanding how the product works (although it can be handy to know that). Here science is a tool, not an end. There are other things that you may find unfamiliar:

(1) After the introduction you will start doing things in teams – not alone.
(2) You are the ones who will have to find the answers, not we as your teachers. We do not know everything, but will try to help you. We are also learning.
(3) The problems are *open*: questions to which there is no single correct answer. You may not like the resulting uncertainty, unless you manage to see this type of work as adventure.
(4) Our course and this book are work in progress. We hope you will help us to improve them.

Projects

The core consists of four projects (Figure 0-1). We have given a few recent examples from our teaching under 'Projects': usually we change these every year. Four or five students work about forty hours each on the first three projects. The final project takes about eighty hours per person. Here each team is to design a new product of its own invention/desire/imagination/creation ... The time teams have available for the final project is perhaps one hundredth of that required for a full industrial development. So you will not be able to do everything perfectly and completely. However, we expect you to gain own working experience from this exercise and a feeling for what designing, developing and project work are like.

The first project uses lessons 1–4; the second, lessons 5–9; the third, lessons 10–15, and the fourth requires everything. Projects are done by teams of four or five students, and end with a presentation or a report.

The first three projects are *learning* projects only. You should try to master the subject; perfect results are not the aim. In the final project you are expected to consider all aspects of design and development and to *sell* your ideas.

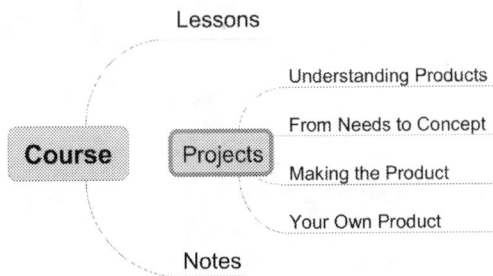

Figure 0-1 Position of the four projects

Lessons

In parallel with the projects is a series of some eighteen short lessons. We only show the four groups in Figure 0-2. The lessons give examples of product development, and introduce what you need to do. The titles of the lessons suggest activities that should be done in a well-defined sequence, but product development is more complicated than that. It is more like a cycle or set of cycles.

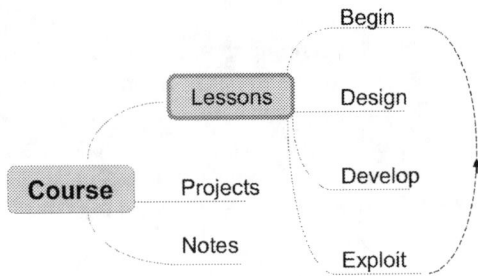

Figure 0-2 The four groups of lessons

Notes

There are notes on some of the many subjects that help you run your projects, but they are not central in the development sequence. Different notes may be relevant to different teams.

Colloids (with T. Johannessen)

There is a part of science that few of our students seem to have encountered, and that is important for the products that we have considered. That is Colloid Science (or Interfacial Engineering). These notes contain the minimum you need on this subject as a novice product developer.

Lessons

Eighteen case studies and a conclusion. We hope these will give you a feeling for how products are designed and developed.

Part 1   Begin

New experiences can bring adventure, but also uncertainty and chaos. That applies to new product development just as well. These first four lessons will help you to get started, and to bring some order in the chaos.

Lesson 1: Look Around

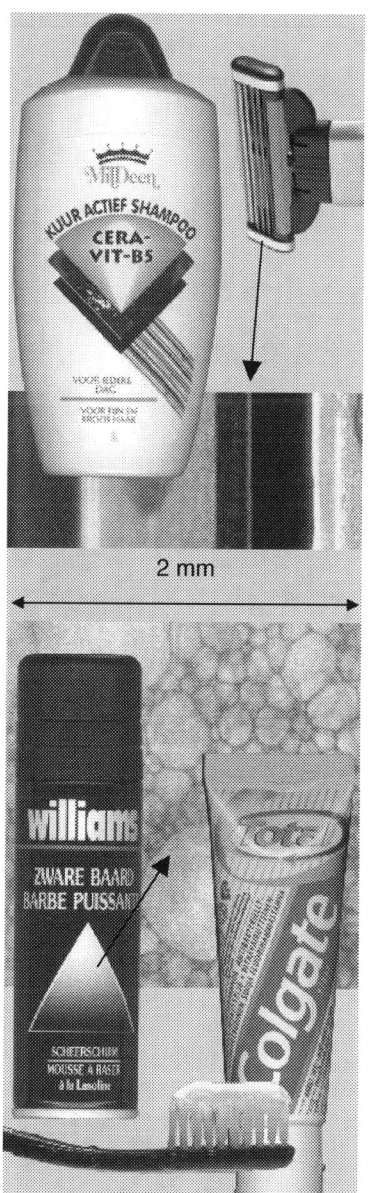

2 mm

To become a product developer, you must develop an interest in products. You must learn to look around, to find out how things work, and to find ways of improving them. We begin by walking around the house of one of the authors (JAW), which is nothing special. Here is what you see.

Products At Home

In the bathroom you find shampoo, a shaving razor with cream, toothbrushes with toothpaste, and a lot of cleaning agents. The shampoo is a translucent, viscous liquid: a concentrated solution of surfactants in water with thickeners, a pH-regulator and perfume. The razor, with three blades, is sharp. It is made such that the user cannot cut himself deeply. The new metal blades are straight and gleaming under the microscope. The edge is not visible; its radius is no more than a few micrometres. The blade is used with shaving cream: a stiff foam with bubbles of around a tenth of a millimetre. No way of improving these you might think. However, you would be surprised how much they have improved in the past 20 years.

The toothpaste is like a solid, but liquid when sheared. It stays on a toothbrush as a little white sausage. It contains a large fraction of fine solid particles, as you find out by diluting with water and vinegar, and letting the mixture settle. The particles (which are mildly abrasive) are smaller than 30 μm. How could you get toothpaste to be effective in the crevices between the teeth where it really is necessary?

The first thing you see in the kitchen is the coffee machine. The coffee is in the cupboard above it, in a vacuum pack of metal foil. It consists of ground particles of about a millimetre of roasted beans. Why not smaller, why not larger? The coffee machine is an intriguing apparatus with a vaporiser that pumps boiling water into a filter where the coffee is extracted. As an engineer you might like to get an understanding of it using two-phase flow theory. Coffee has been around for centuries. Even so, it is still being developed. The companies Philips and Douwe Egberts made the mistake of underestimating the market for their Senseo Crema system which makes coffee using capsules. Good coffee made more quickly than with this machine. The companies have had to refuse customers because of insufficient capacity. There are more ingredients for drinks in this cupboard, but you move on to the next one.

Here you find the pastes. Hazelnut paste is a dispersion of particles in a thick emulsion of two liquids, as is peanut butter. Jam is thickened by natural polymers. Soft cheese, butter and margarine are in the refrigerator; these are complicated structures of fat crystals, oil, water and many other components. All these pastes have a yield stress that is low enough to let them be spread by a knife, but not so low that they run off bread. Users do find the cold butter a bit stiff and the jam a bit thin. As a developer you might want to improve these things. Bread – a solid foam – is a surprising structure when looked at it closely. Fresh bread is often too soft to cut easily.

In the same cupboard you find powders: sugar, salt and powdered sugar. Here you can see a lot under the microscope: the one-millimetre crystals of sugar, the smaller salt crystals (surprisingly battered and not the nice cubes that textbooks would tell you) and the fine, ground particles of powdered sugar. The two coarse powders flow freely, but the powdered one is partly caked and agglomerated. It is also dusty; could that be improved? The package tells that it contains an anti-caking agent E554; you wonder what that is and whether you could not find something with a friendlier name.

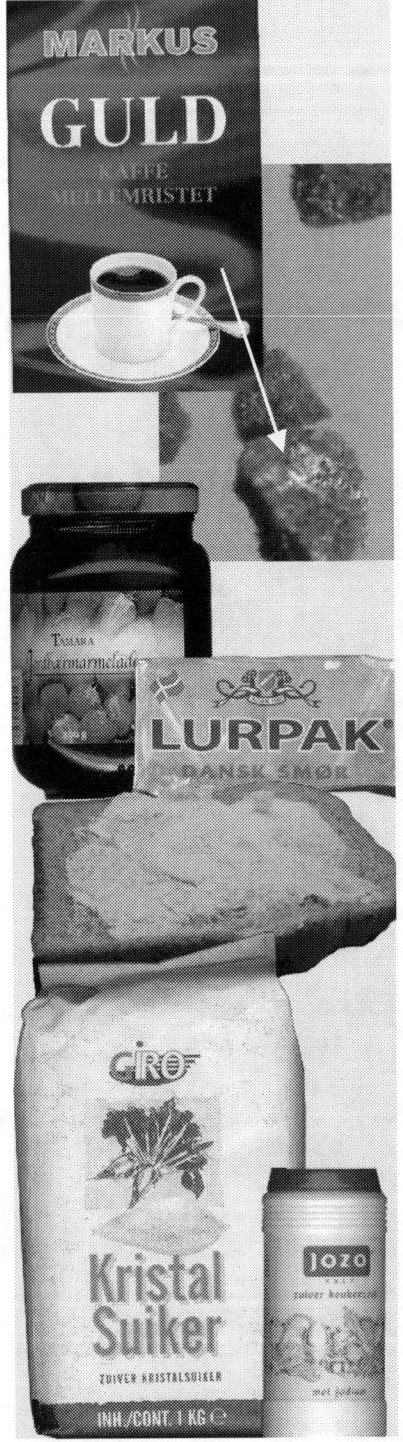

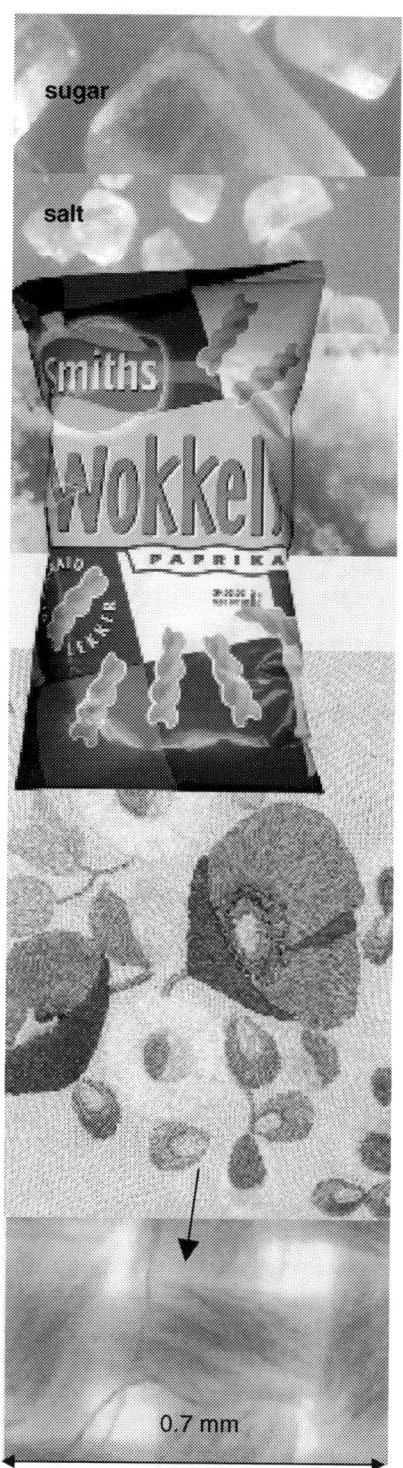

sugar

salt

Smiths

Wokkel

PAPRIKA

0.7 mm

The snacks in the next cupboard are bad for consumers: you get hungry when you see and smell them. The manufacturers may be getting into some trouble because they tempt people to eat too much of these. What could you do about that? The 'Wokkels' have an interesting foamed structure; this lets you wonder how they have been made. Coating nuts with chocolate would not seem that easy either. And how do you bake cookies with bits of chocolate in them? If you were to try the chocolate would melt. There is a lot of packaging and marketing to these products. They seem to be changing all the time. Why would that be?

There is a linen cloth decorated with silk flowers on the kitchen table. It is old, and was embroidered by J's mother, 60 years ago. That was on the island of Tasmania, where the family had got marooned at the beginning of the second world-war. The mother got the silk by telling the shopkeeper that she was alone with two young children, and that her husband had disappeared in the fighting on Java. There was not much silk in Tasmania during the war. Under the microscope you see the double structure of the textile: the yarns with a diameter of about 200 μm, which are twined from fibres of about 10 μm. It is this double structure that provides small pores that allow textile to adsorb moisture and other things.

Textile can take up a lot of moisture, but the paper tissue on the window sill can take up even more: it still feels dry with four times its own weight of water. An estimate of the density of the roll tells you that over 90% of the volume consists of air. It is not easy to make a structure like that. The tissue takes up water rapidly, but the capillary rise is limited to about twelve centimetres as a simple experiment shows. You need to understand capillary flow if you want to improve such products. You do not see much under the microscope, but where two sheets have been torn apart you can see the separate cellulose fibres. They are about 10 μm thick.

When textile gets soiled you have to wash it, in a machine in the scullery. The detergent powder is a clever structure of builder (calcium-removing zeolite particles), anionic and non-ionic surfactants, a chemical bleach and biochemical enzymes. The dosing and temperature-history appear to be quite important, and need good programming of the machine. You might wonder how such a system of textile – detergent – washing machine has evolved. The three parts are made by totally different companies!

Out of the kitchen into the living room, where JAW has his desk. Pens are no longer as important as when he was young, but he still has markers in his drawer. They make a nice picture on a piece of paper. The marks are translucent, and you can see that they have about the same thickness everywhere. It is surprising that you can get that with such a simple technique. You might start looking at the cartridges and ink in the printer, but there is no time for that today.

In one of the drawers JAW has a collection of adhesives. This is a diverse lot. The first is rubber in a solvent. The second is a tri-functional monomer and cross-linker that are stored in separate cylinders, but give a strong, stiff polymer after mixing and setting. The third is a little bottle of stuff that hardens almost immediately with any water: you have to be careful not to glue your fingers together. Then a water-based gel to glue paper, and the tacky polymer-on-tape that gives a connection that you can break and re-form many times. This is a nice picture of the development of polymer technology.

In the next drawer there are batteries for a mouse and battery lamp, and behind the laptop is a lithium-ion battery with its dire warnings that it should never be taken apart. Ah, electrochemistry! There are also candles and matches, just in case .... Candles are now a niche product, but once they were the only reliable source of lighting during the night, and bearers of a great industry.

Back to the bathroom where this began; you had skipped the medicine cupboard. As the owners

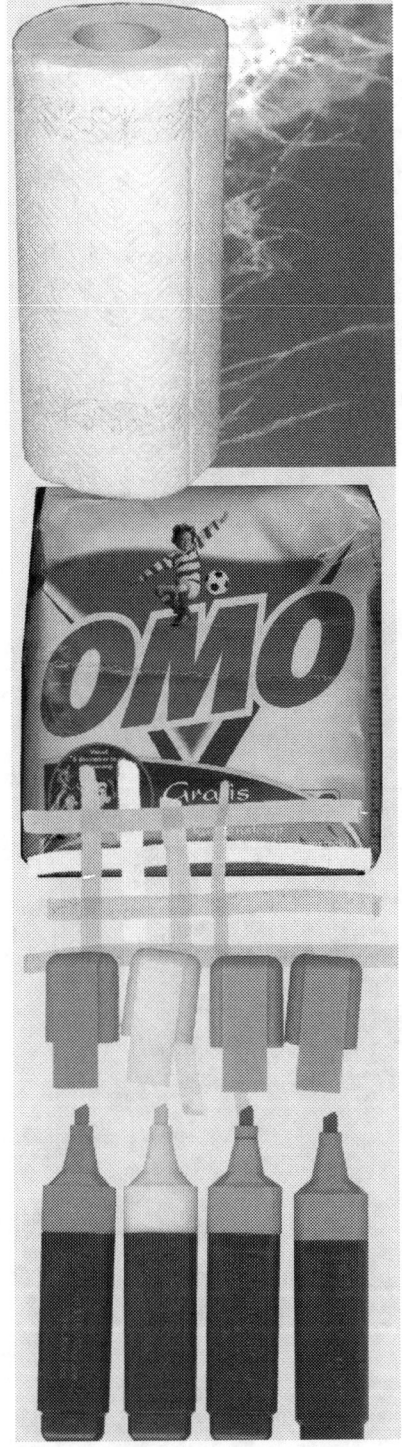

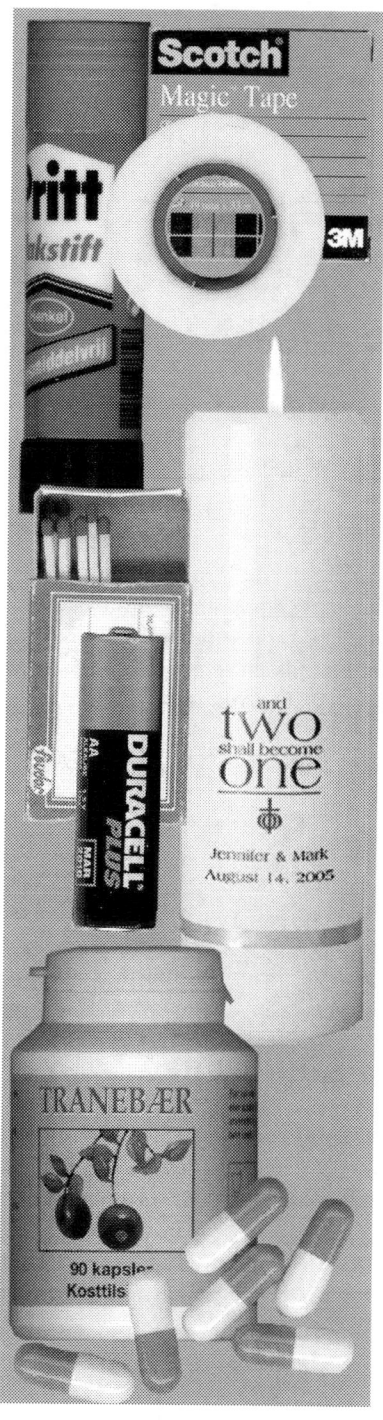

are getting older, this is gradually filling up with remnants of medicine from times when they were ill. (They know they should tidy them up.) There are also pills that are really being used, and pretty complicated ones too as one can read from the slips of paper that accompany them.

You can easily extend this set of examples. Just go to a supermarket, a pharmacy or a do-it-yourself shop. However, we have finished the tour around the house of Johannes and hope to have awakened your interest in the many aspects of product development that normally do not meet the eye.

Common Factors of Products

This was a diverse set of products, coming from a number of industries and using many different technologies. You might wonder whether they have anything in common: they do. They even have a common name: all are *formulated* products. They are not simple chemicals: they have many components, and each has a purpose. Nearly all consist of several phases which are arranged in a *structure*.[1] This micro- and nano-structure is essential for the application. Making a good structure is often the difficult job. The products often *change* during application: controlling this change can be important. Finally they are judged on their performance, not on their composition.

As an engineer you might encounter any of these products in your professional life. You might become involved in development, application, making or selling of new, better products like these. You will see that their methods of development show many similarities and you will explore these during the course.

Product Development

We end with a few remarks on product development. The time between a first idea and the launching of a new product varies, but is often a few years. This is short compared to the time needed

---

[1] We will talk more about product structure in the 'Colloids' section at the end of the book.

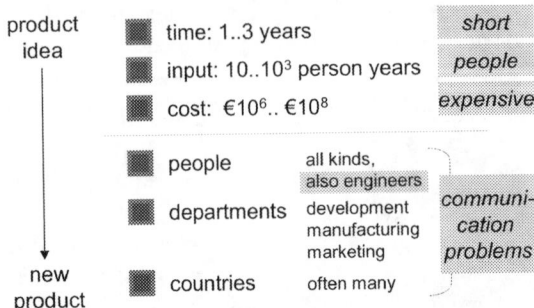

Figure 1-1 Characteristics of product development

for good research. The amount of work to be done is much larger than most beginners realize; this book will show why. It may require tens or hundreds of person-years, so many people have to work in parallel on product development. All these people have to be paid, and that makes product development expensive: a cost of ten million euros is nothing exceptional.

One not only needs engineers in product development, but all kinds of people. These people will be in different departments or even in different companies; they are often located in several countries. This leads to many communication problems. You will have realized that product development is never done by a single person: one needs more people, often large numbers. These characteristics are summarized in Figure 1-1. In the next lesson we consider how people work together on development.

Summary

We will end every lesson with a summary – although this one hardly needs that.

1. You have seen how many formulated products there are around you, and realized how important they are to you as customers and consumers.
2. Formulated products make use of just about every part of chemistry, but they are not simple chemicals. They always consist of several, and often many, components. Each of these has a purpose.
3. Most formulated products have a micro- or nano-structure that is important for their function; obtaining this structure is often the big challenge.
4. You may expect to encounter such products in your career.
5. Developing a new product is quite an undertaking. It usually requires years of work (and large amounts of money to pay for these). You cannot do it alone.

Further Reading

For everything on everyday products: Ben Selinger *Chemistry in the Marketplace*, 5th edition, Harcourt Brace 1998.

Lesson 2: Team Up

You can seldom develop a product alone, so you need an organization. This lesson introduces such organizations, and shows where you might fit in.

Firms, Customers and Personnel

Products are developed to satisfy the *needs* of a *customer*. Most of this development is done by a *firm* (company) or a combination of firms. The firm converts inputs such as the needs, materials, parts, services and knowledge into products or other services (Figure 2-1). It also produces waste. In addition, the firm uses means such as capital, personnel and resources from the community. The firm can only work if it provides sufficient benefits to its *personnel*, the owners, suppliers and the community. And again: if it manages to please the customer.

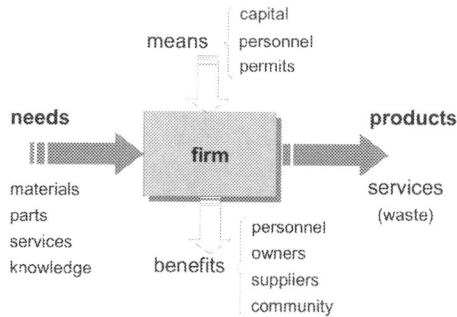

Figure 2-1 A firm with its surroundings

A firm is run by people like you; for most firms these are the most important asset.[1] How people behave and work depends on how they are organized: in which function, how they are linked to other people, how they get on with their boss, and by many other things, including the content of the work.

Functional Organizations

Most firms have a *functional organization*, at least in part (Figure 2-2). People are organized by *function*. Important functions in a product firm are design, manufacturing and marketing. The firm also needs other functions, but these are not so important in this book. Functional organizations are usually hierarchical: each person reports to his boss. The highest level in the daily hierarchy is the management of the firm. The board oversees management in a broad manner.

---

[1] You might not always think so, but in good firms people are taken seriously.

Design and Development of Biological, Chemical, Food and Pharmaceutical Products   J.A. Wesselingh,
S. Kiil and M.E. Vigild
© 2007 John Wiley & Sons, Ltd

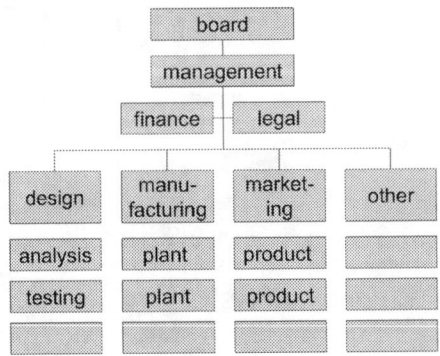

Figure 2-2 A functional organization

Many functions in a firm play some role in product development. Marketing chooses the market segments for the firm; it helps to find customer needs and competing products. Designing creates new concepts to please the customers; it also does part of the testing of these concepts. Manufacturing finds out whether a product can really be made and helps to estimate the production cost. Finance may do the economic analysis and Legal may help with patent issues.

A functional organization focuses on activities that are done continuously – long term functions. It is good for repetitive work, such as in manufacturing. In such an organization people are grouped as marketers in a marketing department, as manufacturing engineers in manufacturing, as designers in a design department, and so on. This allows people to learn specialist knowledge from each other, and to become experts in their field. A manufacturing plant such as an oil refinery will be largely organized by function. Universities are organized by scientific function. Most governments are solely organized by function (in ministries). A functional organization is stable, but it tends to *stagnation*. People see themselves as part of their function – not of the firm as a whole. As a result, personnel are not flexible, and there can be many boundary problems between functions.

Project Organizations

The opposite of the functional organization is a project organization (Figure 2-3). Here, every activity is regarded as temporary. Every project is run by a team with the required people in house.

A project organization focuses on temporary activities: it is aimed at the short term. Project organizations are good for new things, for change. People in project teams learn to be flexible. Building corporations and engineering contractors are mostly project organizations. Also project organizations have their problems: projects do not always follow each other in a neat sequence and there can be gaps or overlap in the work. This causes many people to be uncertain or even anxious. It is not so easy to build up expertise in a project organization: experts can easily move out of a firm when a project is finished. Finally, because each project is seen as an end in itself, the overall objectives of the organization may be lost. This can result in chaos and anarchy.

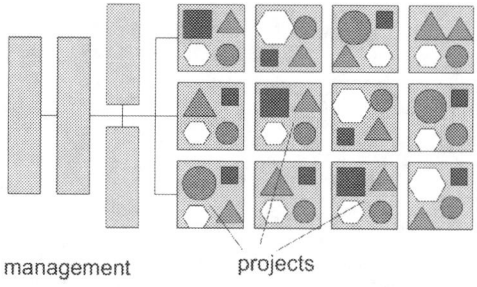

management   projects

each project has 'everything'

Figure 2-3 A project organization

Matrix Organizations

Most firms try to obtain the advantages of both functional and project organizations. They have a mixed or *matrix* organization (Figure 2-4). In one form, projects are assigned to temporary *teams* recruited from the functions. This is the most common way of organizing development. A firm can also be mainly project-oriented, but try to develop specialists by forming expertise groups outside the projects.

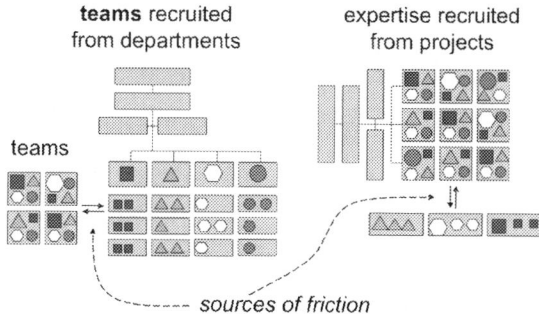

Figure 2-4 Two kinds of matrix organization

In both types of matrix organization, assignment of personnel to temporary jobs is a source of friction. There can be friction between departments and teams, and between team leaders who compete for people and other resources. The organization easily reverts to either of the organization extremes – active management is required to maintain a balance.

Project Teams

Product development is nowadays done in *project teams* (Figure 2-5). Small projects are done in a single team, with four to eight members. With larger numbers co-ordination becomes difficult. In larger projects one needs *sub-teams*, with the efforts being co-ordinated by a *core team*. Teams must have people with different types of knowledge: they are multi*disciplinary*.

As noted, teams are also used in functional organizations. All important functions have to take part there: the team is multi*functional*. In teams you will be working with people with

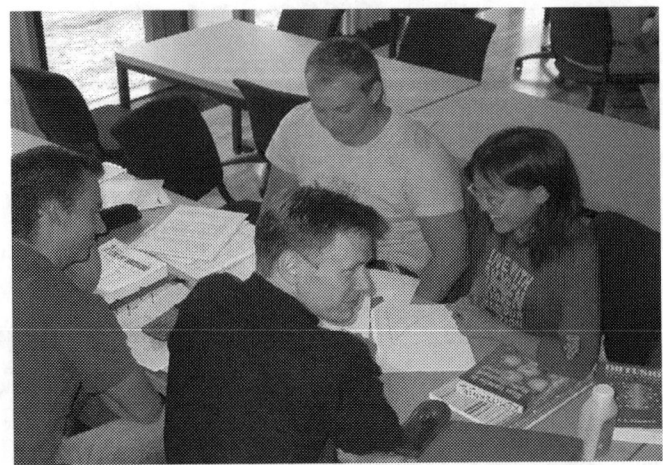

Figure 2-5 Project team around the table

backgrounds different from yours. You will bring in your expertise such as biochemistry, chemistry or engineering, but must learn to appreciate others, and to help each other when necessary.

The composition of the team is important. Teams with *no* 'bright' members do not produce bright results. What is less well known is that teams with only bright members are no better: they waste their time on arguing and cannot reach decisions. A good team has a mix of skills and personalities.

In describing methods of product development, we will assume that the team members have been well chosen, and that the team is functioning properly. This is not always so. Some of the problems you may run into are that others (higher in rank) interfere too much in the doings of the team. A second, more common problem is that team members put their functional position ahead of the project. They regard themselves more as 'the chemical engineer', than as 'one of the developers of a new kind of paint'. A third problem can be when team members are required for urgent tasks outside the project. A source of bad feelings can be inadequate resources. These are often because the team does not have representatives from important parts of the company, and so fails to get its needs known.

One of the purposes of this course is to train your capabilities in team work. There is much more to be said about the subject than we can do here.[2]

Your Position

In a matrix organization, part of your work will be in a function such as chemistry, engineering or production. The other part will be in project teams – getting new things done. You will

[2] There is more on teamwork in Note 2 'Plan Your Project'.

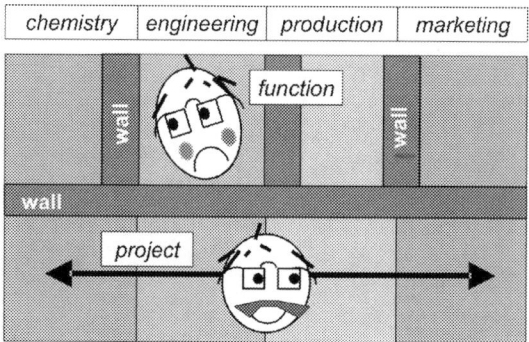

Figure 2-6 Having two bosses

have two or more bosses (Figure 2-6): one or more project leaders, and a functional boss. This can be difficult, as your bosses often do not see each other enough to know what you are doing. There are walls between departments!

In all modern organizations, you are the one who is responsible for your own development. You must fight for time and facilities to develop yourself, but your bosses may help. Things have to be done together with other people, and this requires a lot of interactions: meetings, informing others with presentations, and sharing the workload. You will have to negotiate with people from different backgrounds, and to learn that you cannot afford an attitude of looking down on salespeople or lawyers. Believe us: you will often be grateful for having had one around. The worst thing, but also the most challenging, is that you will have to be learning all the time (Figure 2-7). In a project you can never get by with the knowledge that you had before starting.

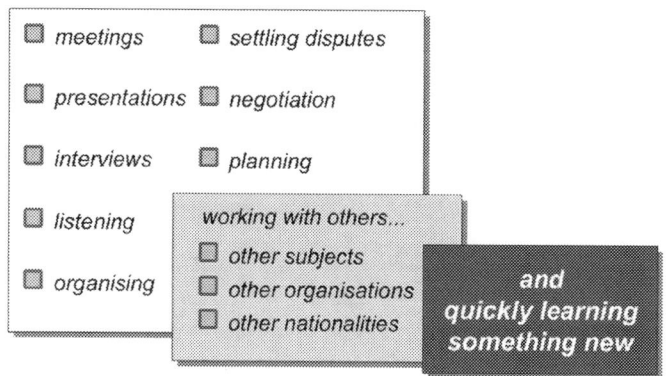

Figure 2-7 Some organization skills you will need

You will need to develop your science and engineering skills (Figure 2-8). There are many subjects that are both interesting and worthwhile to know as a developer. However, one can hardly become an expert in all of them. Nobody expects that.

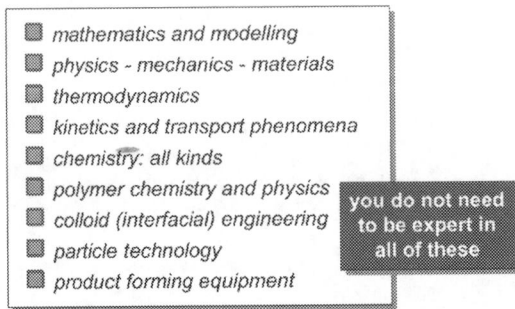

- mathematics and modelling
- physics - mechanics - materials
- thermodynamics
- kinetics and transport phenomena
- chemistry: all kinds
- polymer chemistry and physics
- colloid (interfacial) engineering
- particle technology
- product forming equipment

you do not need
to be expert in
all of these

Figure 2-8 Some technical skills you may need

Estimating Skills

As engineer in a team, you will have to answer 'how much' and 'how far' questions. 'If we reduce the enzyme concentration in our detergent by one third, *how much* longer will it take to remove fat stains? Can we compensate by increasing the temperature? By *how much* would the temperature need to be increased? Or could we do it by increasing the level of agitation? *How much* would we need to increase the agitator frequency? *How far* can we go?' It is not always possible to give exact answers to such questions, but even rough estimates are better than nothing. Such questions have to be answered in several stages of product development. There is every chance that you will be the one to work on them. Engineers and chemists are usually the ones who can best think quantitatively!

Should You?

Many people are attracted to product development, and we hope that will also be the case for some of you. Much of the appeal is in creating something new: a product that satisfies the needs of other people. Working closely together with people from other disciplines can also be very rewarding. On the other hand, product development has its difficult sides. In design one has to make trade-offs, to compromise on what one thinks would be technically or aesthetically better. Product markets can be extremely competitive, and plans can be ended early because the competition has come up with something better. You can get bogged down by the huge number of technical details that have to be worked out, and by the time pressure that exists in any development project. If you see these problems as challenges, you will feel at home in the world of product development!

Summary

Again we end with a summary.

1. Products are developed to please customers.
2. The people doing that are organized in firms: the organization can be by function, by project, or by some mix.
3. Functional organizations are stable and reliable, and allow development of expertise. However, they are too slow for product development.
4. Project organizations are flexible and renewing, but can lead to chaos.

5. Product development is done by project teams, even in functional organizations.
6. Team work is both frustrating and challenging. In a project team, there is often little time, and you have to develop skills yourself. (These are both scientific/engineering as well as communication/management skills.)
7. If you like challenges, you will like product development.

Further Reading

A good book on improving your team skills is Roger Fischer et al. *Getting It Done: How To Lead When You Are Not In Charge*, Harper Business 1999. You will need to do more than only reading.

The outcome of following large numbers of teams in management games: R. Meredith Belbin *Management Teams, Why They Succeed or Fail*, 2nd edition, Elsevier Butterworth Heinemann 2004. Some results are quite surprising.

Many practical problems with teams are analysed in Preston G. Smith and Donald G. Reinertsen *Developing Products in Half the Time*, 2nd edition, Wiley 1998, Chapters 7 and 8.

Lesson 3: Get a Method

You must do *many, many* things to develop a product: find or create customers with a need, make a design that pleases them, get the right personnel, learn the technology, find ways of making your product cheap enough; keep abreast of the competition, set up a marketing organization and so on. This can easily become chaotic. However, it does help if you have a *method*.

What a Method Is

Methods are summaries of ways that have been found to work well. They are not set in stone: most methods are continually being updated. Methods consist of steps to be followed. We give these as blocks. The arrows in method diagrams give the sequence of the steps in time.

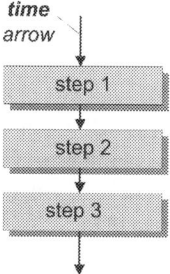

Methods are *not* strict rules, but guidelines. Use your common sense when applying them, and adjust them to your needs. For example, most of the method here has been developed for large projects, and some parts are overdone for a student project.

Development and Learning

Development *can* be seen as a series of steps; however, this is a bit limited. You can also see it as learning. You learn how to design a product that pleases your customer, how to make that product, how to bring it to the market, and how to sell it. You learn by experience. Learning is a series of cycles. These are like this:

(1) You look at something, and are not satisfied.
(2) You think about it, and come up with an idea.
(3) You try out the idea.
(1) You look at the result, and are not satisfied...

Design and Development of Biological, Chemical, Food and Pharmaceutical Products   J.A. Wesselingh, S. Kiil and M.E. Vigild
© 2007 John Wiley & Sons, Ltd

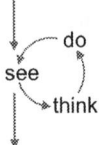

You never learn a complicated subject in one go: you need to keep looking, thinking, trying and looking again .... Learning is also looking back at what you have done, revising and improving, and thinking about how you might do things better next time. The line from top to bottom in the method diagrams is only the overall direction of development: in reality you often have to go back. There are little arrows pointing backwards on the steps to help you remember. Reality is not as linear as our method suggests.

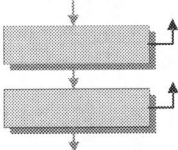

Phases in Projects

Development is usually done in several *phases*. Each phase can have any number of steps. In the course we run we assume four phases: a first one in which a firm orients itself and plans which products it will develop, a second one in which a core team forms concepts and plans the project, a third one in which the core team develops the selected concept to a product with its manufacturing and market, and a final phase in which the product is exploited (Figure 3-1). Each of these phases is a learning cycle for the firm, but there will be many sub-cycles in each. The subdivision into four phases is arbitrary: a complex project may need more phases. Regulations may force one to use more phases.

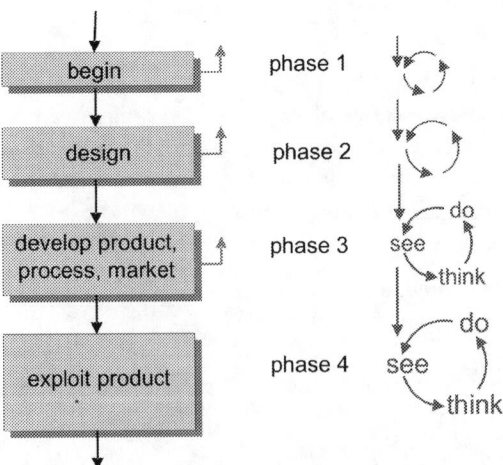

Figure 3-1 A subdivision in four phases

We use the four-phase method *in* the course on which this book is based. This is because it is typical, and gives a handy format for structuring the course. However, this is *not* the only (or always best) way of doing things. As an example, regard this course as a product. We are developing the course and trying to improve it all the time. However, each version of the course is 'marketed'. This is known as *evolutionary* development. It is more effective than development in phases, but is not applicable to products where each version requires a large capital investment, or when the reproducibility of the product is important. You will see that most development is to some extent evolutionary. Successful products are succeeded by improved versions – after another round of development.

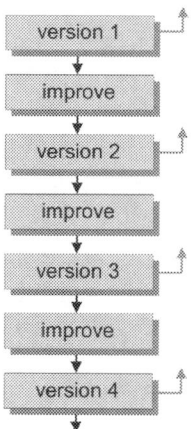

We go back to the phased method. As said, a team has to learn at least three important things – and often more. The three are learning to please the customer, to make the product, and to market and sell the product. One needs to look at all three, and at other important items, *in each phase again*. The team works on all aspects of design *in parallel*. This is also described as *concurrently*.[1]

The team develops in phases to allow management to monitor what is happening, and to keep a balance between risk and cost (Figure 3-2). In the first phase one does not know which of the many ideas will make it (if any). The risk that an idea will fail is large. That is why the team only spends small amounts of time and money on each idea. As you go to further stages, the product and development project must become more and more defined. The team has to focus, because the cost there increases greatly. If too much uncertainty remains management should stop the project.

In this diagram, and in several of the following ones, we have left out the 'exploit product' phase, as it is not really part of development.

---

[1] Formerly, development was often done sequentially. A design department would design a product. It would then be turned over to manufacturing to make the product. Only then would marketing and sales start advertising and promotion campaigns . . . Experience tells that this way of working is not successful. It leads to unbalanced designs and takes too long.

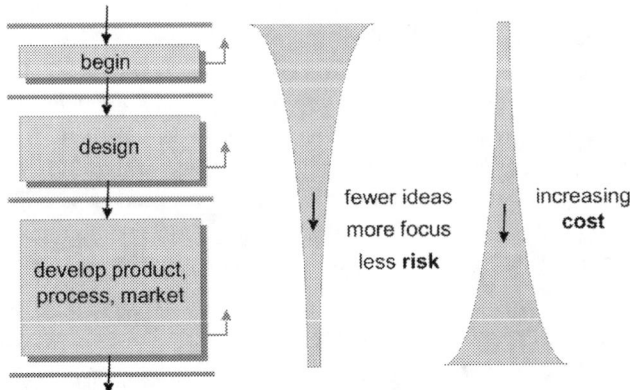

Figure 3-2 Decreasing risk and increasing cost

Diverging and Converging

At the end of the development, you want to have one single well-designed product (Figure 3-3). However, to get there the team has to consider many alternatives. In each phase, you will find that there are times where the team is looking for new ideas, and the list of possibilities increases. The team is *diverging*. To keep the work manageable, the list then has to be pruned: ideas that do not look good are removed. This is *converging*. Overall, focus should increase during a project, but not at each moment.

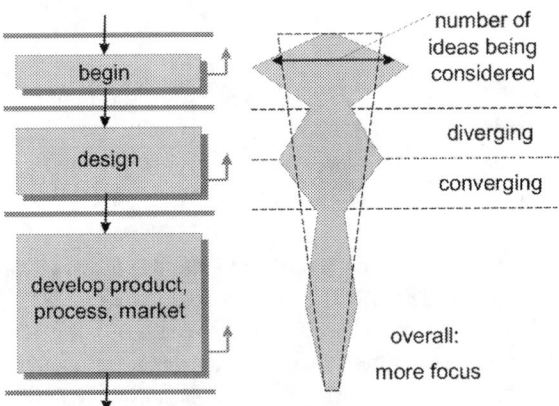

Figure 3-3 Diverging and converging sessions

As the team advances the development, its knowledge increases. The team learns more about customers, the competition, how to design the product, how to make it .... In the beginning, the team knows little and everything is uncertain. As you go on, you learn more and more – and the result becomes *overwhelming* (Figure 3-4). A team, and certainly a firm, has to find ways of managing this knowledge. Most of this has to be done by team members: computer database systems can help, but will not do the difficult part of bringing structure in the information. This can be a real problem towards the end of a project.

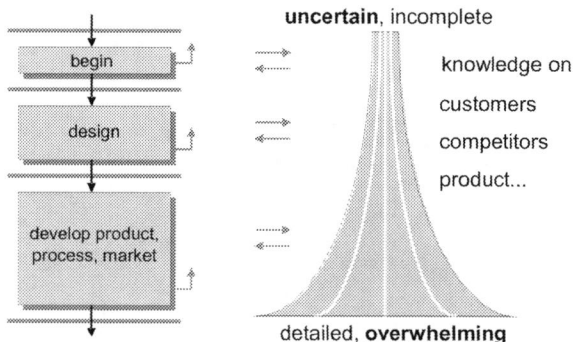

Figure 3-4 Knowledge explosion in a project

Gates (Milestones)

Back to our diagram. Between the phases is a point where decisions are taken whether to go on or not – or whether the team needs to change direction. Such points are called *gates* or *milestones* (Figure 3-5). A gate has to be opened to go on: at each gate, something must be finished. Before spending much time on analysing, the team needs a brief, but probably incomplete, description of the ideas. Before the concept formation phase is entered, the team needs a document describing the *scope* of the project: what the product is expected to be, how and in which amounts it might be made, the target markets and other things. After the concept formation there must be a *project plan* for timing and project resources. At the end of the development phase you expect to have developed the product, its manufacturing, and its marketing.

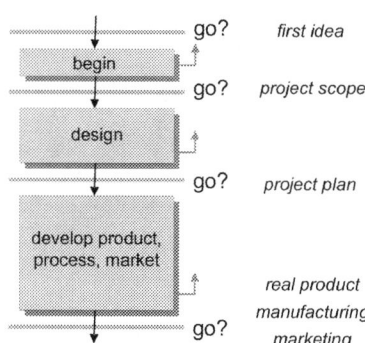

Figure 3-5 Gates (go/no go points) in a project

Our Phases

Now the phases of the method. In the initial phase – often called Product Planning – a small group of people collects ideas that might be worth developing. These people also check what can be done with the available resources, and make a first description of each product and the project needed to develop it. This *project scope* or *mission statement* is the starting point for a project team that is formed for phases 2 and 3. Phase 1 is a vague and uncertain phase. However, it is important for the long-term success of a firm.

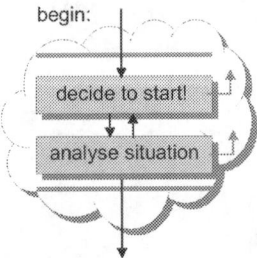

Before looking at the second phase, one remark. In your career you may expect to encounter two groups of products:

(1) *devices*, such as printers, batteries, spray dryers, distillation packings ...
(2) *matter*, such as peanut butter, paint, pharmaceuticals, adhesives ...

The development of these differs on several points. Devices are developed in a workshop, matter in a laboratory. Making of devices centres on *assembling*, making of matter on *processing*. A little bit of matter (say peanut butter) is still the whole product; a little bit of printer is not. With matter it is easier to do experiments on the whole product, and this shows in the ways of developing. In this course we focus on matter. However, we cannot neglect devices, as the design of a formulated product is often largely determined by the device with which it is applied.

Phase 2, called *designing*, is important. Much of the course is spent on this phase. We divide the second phase into the stages below:

(1) Find the needs of the customer.
(2) Set target specifications of the product.
(3) Explore (many) ideas that fulfil the specifications.
(4) Select the best idea and form a concept.
(5) Find ways to protect the concept.

This phase should end with a first plan of how the project is going to be run.

Phase 3 is the real *development*. Here the product is designed in detail, made and tested. There is usually a large amount of product testing, also with customers. Here the team starts developing the market. This is the most expensive phase, often by far.

In phase 3 the methods for devices and matter differ greatly. Production of devices (also chemical ones) is more a matter for mechanical engineers than for chemists and chemical engineers. As said, we will be focusing on matter in this course.

Phase 4 follows development. This book only considers the exploitation phase in as far as it influences development – not the daily operation of a company. The subjects that we will consider are how to organize the marketing of the product, forecasting costs and revenues (the money), a few aspects of selling, and finally how the innovation cycle is closed by planning of new products.

Development and Research

For a good design one often needs to do research – to make desk studies, try out things in the workshop, and – especially – experiment in the laboratory or in the field. This work can be applied and practical, but also very fundamental. However, the research part of product development differs from the largely curiosity-driven and exploratory research of many university departments in one important way: *it does not go further than needed for the development of the product*. Time is a real constraint in development!

This book is primarily about development, and not about research.[2] You will see research creeping in at many places in our examples, but we will not discuss it separately.

Plan of This Book

Now you know the method, we can show the plan of the book.

Phase 1 'Begin' has the lessons:

(1) Look Around
(2) Team Up
(3) Get a Method (this lesson)
(4) Analyse the Situation

Phase 2 'Design', has five lessons:

(5) Find Needs
(6) Specify the Product
(7) Create Concepts
(8) Select a Concept
(9) Protect the Concept

Phase 3 'Develop' also has five lessons:

(10) Formulate the Product
(11) Flowsheet the Process
(12) Estimate the Cost
(13) Equip the Process
(14) Scale Up

Phase 4 'Exploit' discusses the subjects:

(15) Organize the Market
(16) Forecast Money Flows

---

[2] Most of you will be learning to do research as part of your Master's thesis.

(17) Learn to Sell
(18) Plan Future Products

We end with a short review: 'Farewell'.

The subdivision may suggest that certain activities are only done in a certain phase, but this is not so. In each phase all aspects of the product are considered, although there are differences in emphasis.

Summary

1. In development you learn to please the customer with a good product design, learn to make the product, and learn to sell the product.
2. The method has four phases:
    (1) Begin
    (2) Design
    (3) Development
    (4) Exploitation
3. The phases are separated by gates: points where one decides whether a project should be continued. With phases and gates you reduce the risk of a project, but can also make it take longer.
4. Development proceeds from uncertainty – starting with many different ideas – to the focused certainty of the final product.
5. The risk of the project is high at first, but the expenses are low.
6. The risk has to be reduced as one goes from the first plans to the product launch, and expenses become much higher.
7. To do this the development team studies the needs of the customers, the products and marketing of competitors, and the properties of the own product.
8. In each phase all aspects are considered, albeit with differences in emphasis.

The plan of the course largely follows the steps in the method.

Further Reading

M. Myrup Andreasen and Lars Hein *Integrated Product Development*, Institute for Product Development, The Technical University of Denmark, 2000 (published earlier by Springer) tells why the different aspects of product development have to be done simultaneously. Very readable.

The set of methods used here is similar to that in Karl T. Ulrich and Steven D. Eppinger *Product Design and Development*, 3rd edition, McGraw-Hill 2003, Chapters 1 and 2. (That book is largely concerned with mechanical products.)

For an in-depth discussion of design methods and the difference between science and technology see N. F. M Roozenburg and J. Eekels *Product Design: Fundamentals and Methods*, Wiley 1995.

Lesson 4: Analyse the Situation

Using work of N. Bel for Unilever

Before beginning development, it is important to build up a basis to work from.[1] This means organizing the work of the team, but also collecting information and asking questions.

Suppose the team is to work on improving the detergent used for washing household textile. In the existing process, dirty textile goes into a washing machine together with water and detergent powder (Figure 4-1). If this is done well, the textile will be cleaned. Improving requires an understanding, not only of the product, but also of the surroundings. It requires the building up of an overview.

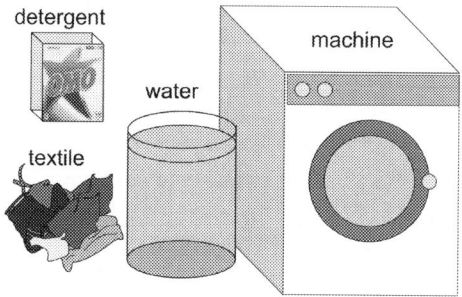

Figure 4-1 The washing system

Get Some Order

The start will probably be chaotic, but you might bring some order using the following steps:

(1) Set up a documentation system.
(2) Start collecting information.
(3) Consider where, by whom and how the product is to be used.
(4) Collect ideas on required performance.
(5) Analyse how existing products work and how they interact with the surroundings.

Except for the first one, these steps may have to be redone many times during analysis.

[1] In a real project the team has expertise from the beginning; you do not have that luxury in a student project.

Design and Development of Biological, Chemical, Food and Pharmaceutical Products   J.A. Wesselingh, S. Kiil and M.E. Vigild
© 2007 John Wiley & Sons, Ltd

Document the Project

Information will be in the form of documents (or it must be brought it into this form). The documentation system has to retain all information gained during development, by all people in the team – and later by others. Team members have to be able to find everything later. A method for a not too large a project is shown in Figure 4-2.[2] You will not have much idea of the structure of the information beforehand, so each document is marked with a unique number, a title, the author or authors, a date and perhaps five keywords to help find it again. Put these in a spreadsheet with a search capability.

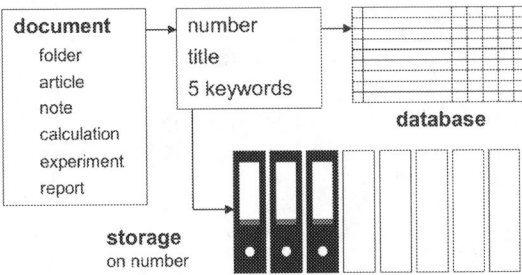

Figure 4-2 A simple documentation system

Store the documents in binders *by number*. Documents should never be removed, except for copying. They should be put back immediately. The archive is best organized by a single team member, but all have to participate in bringing in information and deciding what should be (or *not* be) archived and how the search system is organized.

Collect Information

The next step is to obtain information. You might talk with colleagues, with experts, or with (potential) customers. Or spend some time on the Internet, go to a conference or course, and read a bit.

Consider Product Usage

It is important not to focus only on the product, but also to find out who supplies it, who uses it, how it is used, in what kind of surroundings, and in which equipment.

In our example, it is fairly clear who the major customers are: people washing textile at home or in a laundry. There are other *stakeholders*: the company, retailers, water and sewage companies, and environmental authorities. You will also have to consider them. We come back to interactions with customers and stakeholders later, but the preparation begins here.

Collect Ideas on Performance

To find out what customers need, you may have to ask questions on which performance is required. It can help to think about this beforehand. In the example here, questions could be:

---

[2] For a small project, notes of the project meetings (with handouts and reports) may be good enough for documentation.

1. How well does the textile have to be cleaned?
2. Is textile degradation allowable?
3. Which kinds of dirt have to be considered?
4. Is the product easy to use?
5. Is the product safe?
6. What happens with the product and the dirt?

Start collecting such questions for later discussions.

How Existing Products Work

The engineer wants to know how things work – that is part of the fun of being an engineer. This is a point to start finding out. However, keep in mind that the goal is to get ideas for improving a product. This usually requires an overview of the whole system in which a product is used, and not only an understanding of some detail. To build up an overview one can try to look at a problem from different viewpoints: to *decompose* or *split* the problem. There are many ways of splitting: we introduce a few of them here.

In Which Systems?

Can you think of different systems in which the product is used? An obvious one here is the washing machine, but you could take the system as the household, or as the water and sewage system or .... For the rest of this lesson we consider only the machine as the system, but the other possibilities would probably give rise to other ideas.

In/Out Analysis

We have drawn the machine as a box, and shown

- what goes *in*: soiled textile and water with detergent
- what goes *out*: dirty water and clean textile.

The machine separates dirt from dirty textile, and delivers clean textile. For this purpose it needs water and detergent. This simple in/out analysis of the problem is good enough to explain to the lay-person how a washing machine works. It can also help to get further ideas on washing and detergents.

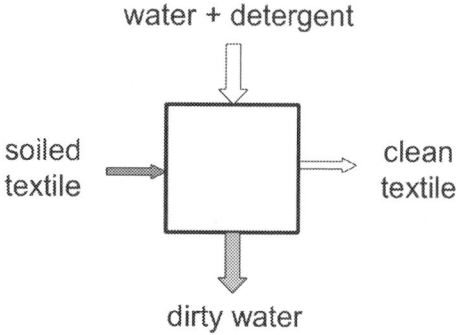

The taking-apart with amounts-in-and-out suggests ideas:[3]

1. One might expect the amount of water and detergent needed to go up with the amount of dirt in the textile. It might be an idea to provide the machine with a sensor for how much textile is loaded, or to input whether the laundry is very dirty or not.
2. If you reduce either the amount of water, or the amount of detergent, the textile may not be cleaned so well. Or perhaps one can do the same job, but in a longer time. There may be a trade-off if you want to minimize usage of water or detergent.

Our simple taking-apart is improved by considering the *amounts* involved. You can probably make a guess for this problem – and having a feel for amounts is often important in developing a product. The team will improve these figures as it goes on. This will lead to questions on *why* the amounts are such and such. Again these may give new ideas.

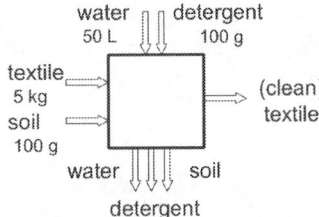

One step further is to consider not only amounts of matter, but also inputs and outputs of energy and information. Also these may lead to ideas. In our washing machine energy goes in as electricity, and comes out in the form of heat. You might be able to reduce the size of the machine (or increase its effectiveness) by adding more energy. Information might be on whether the textile is made from wool or from cotton. This allows the machine to 'know' whether a low temperature should be used (for wool) or a high temperature (for white cotton).

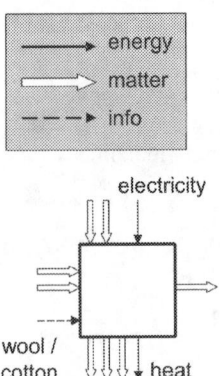

One can often get further understanding by dividing the system into sub-systems (Figure 4-3). In the older designs of washing machines, the washing drum and the centrifuge were actually

---

[3] Write down ideas when you get them: you may need them later. Do not start working them out at this stage. Can you see questions you would like to ask your customers?

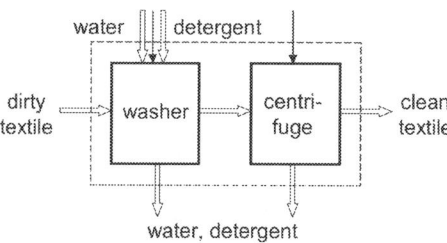

Figure 4-3 Splitting in two sub-systems

in different locations, and this was an obvious subdivision. This subdivision might lead to thinking about the working of the centrifuge. Subsystems do not have to be in different places: in modern machines centrifuging is done in the same drum as washing.

A different but related way of splitting is in terms of process steps (Figure 4-4). This gives some idea of how things happen in time or in which sequence they are done in a continuous operation. You might start wondering why things require a certain time, and whether to do something about that. Also here you can show the amounts going in and out, and the conditions in the different steps. Here these are the temperatures and the high acceleration in the centrifuge. A good question is often whether all these steps are necessary – or whether you might improve things by adding steps.

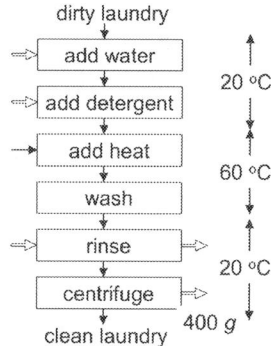

Figure 4-4 Splitting in process steps

Split the Product

Look at the product itself. The detergent considered here is matter. You may wish to look at the following properties:

(1) the chemistry of the product,
(2) the structure of the product,
(3) the application properties and
(4) how the product changes during application.

Looking at these may again give ideas on improving the product and on questions to take up with customers and stakeholders.

There are several sides to the chemistry of our product. We first consider compositions in our system. Dirt is poorly defined, but it can be divided into a limited group of similar types, such as the particles in mud and soot, the soluble salts and sugars, the calcium scum formed by washing, the fatty or oily types of dirt, stains such as those of wine or coffee, and blobs of polymers such as proteins or polysaccharides.

dirts
particles
soluble
calcium
fat / oil
stains (wine)
protein (egg)

These different types of dirt can be treated using different agents in the washing system: warm water for the particles and soluble components, a builder (ion exchanger) for the scum, emulsifying surfactants for the oily materials, a bleach system for the stains, and enzymes for the polymers. As always, you should dream up ideas and questions.

washing agents
water
'builder'
surfactant
bleach
enzyme

If the product uses chemical reactions, it is a good idea to try to get hold of the structural formulae of the chemicals, and the reaction equations (Figure 4-5). These may help to understand why certain components are used, and in which amounts. In our washing system there are at least three groups of chemical reactions:

(1) between calcium and the zeolite ion exchanger,
(2) the bleaching reactions to decolourize stains, and
(3) enzymatic reactions to degrade bio-polymers.

Trying to get data on reactions and reaction rates may trigger any number of ideas. In the early stages of development, you may only need a rough idea of how the reactions proceed.

The 'soapy' part of the washing powder is the surfactant. All surfactants consist of molecules with two parts:[4]

---

[4] Many of the subjects here are treated in the Notes on 'Colloids' at the end of the book.

- a non-polar, hydrophobic tail and
- a polar, hydrophilic, head.

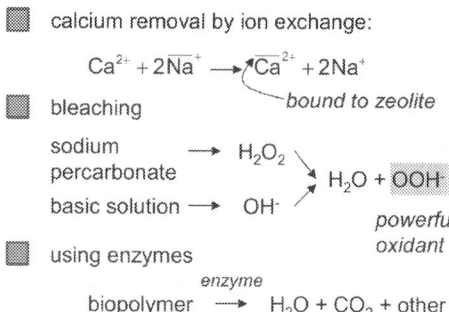

Figure 4-5 Chemical reactions in a washing machine

Surfactant molecules try to cover non-polar surfaces and displace oil and many other soiling components (Figure 4-6). An understanding of mechanisms may give ideas for product improvements. One might like to know the adsorption properties of the system to quantify its behaviour.

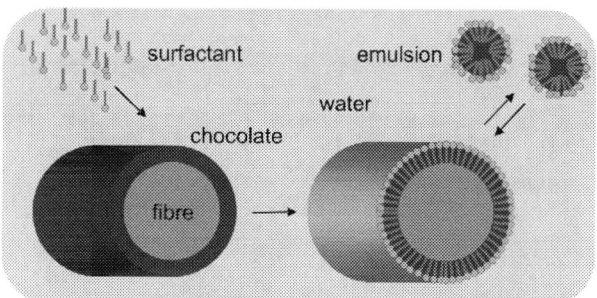

Figure 4-6 Adsorption and desorption in washing

Again another way of looking is at the *structure* of the product. Which phases does it contain? What are the volume ratios of the phases? What are the size and shape of the parts? Why is the structure as it is? How is it made?

An interesting structure in the washing system is textile (Figure 4-7). It is made of yarns of a few tenths of a millimetre. These in turn are spun from fibres, which might be only 10 μm in diameter. There are four kinds of space in the drum:

(1) space between the pieces of textile,
(2) voids between the yarns,
(3) voids between the fibres and
(4) the volume occupied by the fibres.

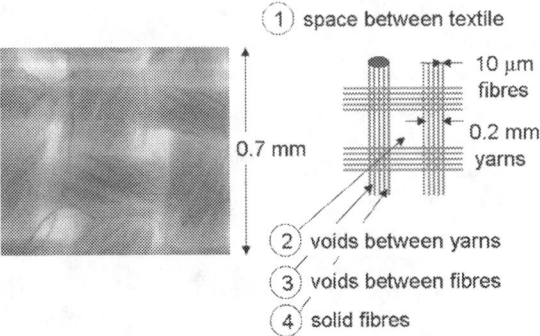

Figure 4-7 The structure of textile

Dirt tends to accumulate between the fibres; it has to be moved out into the liquid between the pieces of textile.

Product–System Interactions

At some point you will need to look at details of the interaction of the product with the system. In our washing machine, textile, water and detergent are contacted in a tumbling drum (Figure 4-8). The textile tumbles forward and backward. With a proper textile load, there is not much free water in the drum: the wet textile takes up water when stretched and releases it when bended. This allows detergent to move into the textile, and the dirt to move out.

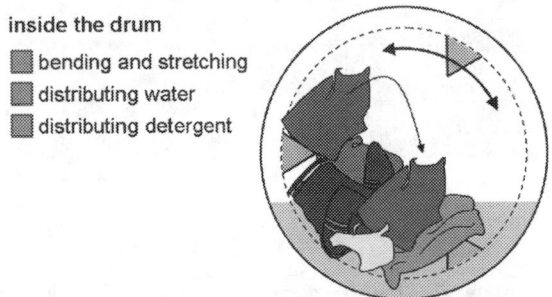

Figure 4-8 What happens in the drum

You can split this problem using the *model* shown in Figure 4-9.[5] This is a theoretical model that allows us to analyse how rapidly dirt can be moved out of the machine, and on which things that depends. You can even use it to understand what happens on the scale of textile fibres. Chemicals and dirt in region (3) mainly move by diffusion – a slow process. Transport in region (2) is mainly by liquid forced in and out of the textile by bending and stretching. This can be faster. Transport in region (1) is by flow (convection). Note that the four subsystems (regions) drawn are distributed over space. They are not located in any fixed position.

---

[5] You cannot calculate everything in this kind of product. However, a small sum can often improve your understanding, as you can see in Appendix 4-1 and at the end of this lesson.

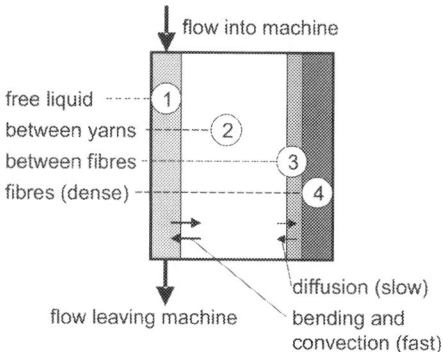

Figure 4-9 Four regions in the drum

In the early stages of product development, it is better not to use complex models. They require a large effort to develop and use – and that may well be wasted if one later chooses a different idea. Because the investment in time and effort is large, complex models tend to make it difficult to change ideas. Detailed models usually only yield ideas on details! These *can* be useful later in development.

Choosing Splits

Clearly there are many ways of splitting a problem. So what should you do? There is no definite answer: which splitting is 'best' depends on the problem. However, there are a few rules of thumb:

1. Use *very* simple splits early in the design process. Use these to decide what is important.
2. Try different splits; try as many as you can find, but keep them simple. Use them to get ideas.
3. Use more detailed splits (and models) as you get to know more about the product, and when you need more accuracy.
4. Beware of complex models except in the final stage of optimizing the product. Complex models tend to *deter* the formation of new ideas.

Remember that splitting and modelling is only an aid to develop understanding. If some way does not work, try something else. Finally, do not spend too much time on your first analysis. If the team has a week for a project, you might spend a few hours on it. If you have a year: perhaps a week. After that you will probably be better off getting on to the product development itself. You will have to keep on learning about your product anyhow. The analysis does not stop after the initial phase – it is a continuing process from which your knowledge and innovative potential will grow stronger and stronger.

Constructing an Overview

As you see, there are many sides to a product and a team can easily get lost. A simple technique that greatly helps to find the way is the construction of a *mind map* or tree diagram (Figure 4-10). Give the product a name such as 'Textile Washing Machine' and put this in the centre of the diagram. Then add a few legs – not more than five to seven – and jot down

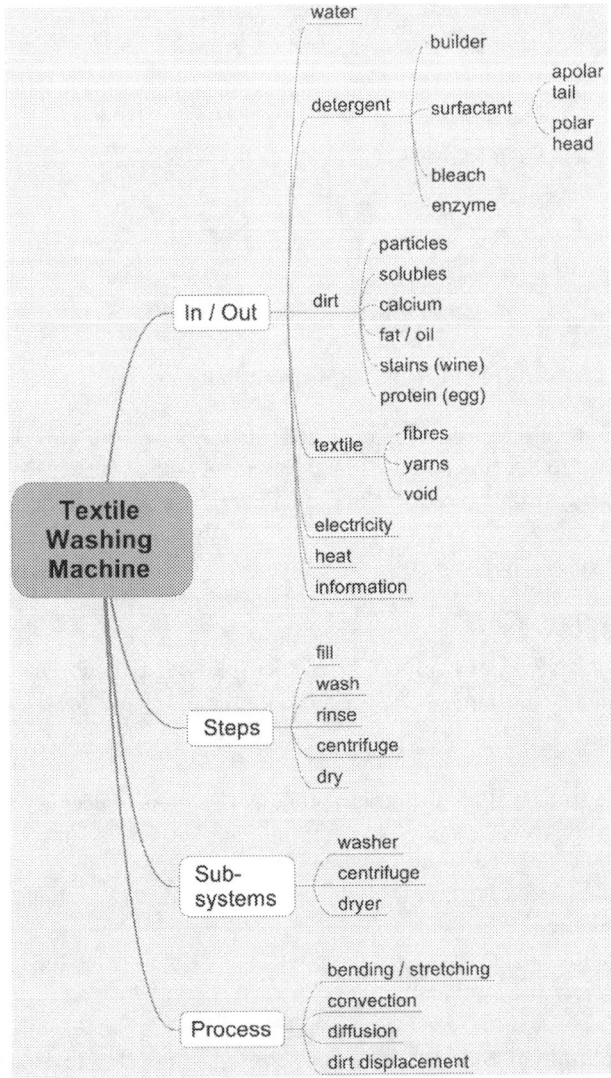

Figure 4-10 A mind map of the washing machine

the associations that you have on these legs. In our example these might start with 'In/Out'. For sub-associations you will need further legs. Soon the diagram will run full, and you will be trying to re-arrange the items. There is no fixed way of doing this: try to find something that you like and that looks sensible. The diagram will evolve as the understanding of the subject improves.

You will often find that tree diagrams lead to a hierarchy of subjects: an arrangement from *general* to *detailed*. This is clear on the 'In/Out' branch in the figure, but you can also see it in the others. Such a hierarchy can be useful for planning a development program.

The example in this lesson considers a development in a well-known product area. You will also encounter assignments where there are no good existing products to relate to. Such projects are different in several ways, but you will find that the techniques explained here are still useful.

Summary

We end again with a summary. When you start working on a new product, analyse the situation:

1. Set up a documentation system to order information.
2. Collect information by asking questions, using the Internet, reading, courses, conferences . . . .
3. Find where, by who and how the product is to be used.
4. See the product as part of a number of systems, and analyse these.
5. Analyse the parts of the product.
6. Analyse interactions between the product and its systems.
7. Analyse by splitting problems. Figure 4-11 shows some splits we have considered here.

devices	matter
customer needs	
in / out	chemical
matter	composition
energy	reactions
information	rates
process steps	equilibria
sub-systems	structure
looking inside	flow properties

Figure 4-11 Some splits for problem analysis

8. While you are doing this write down any ideas and questions that come up.
9. To keep an overview: construct a tree diagram of the subject.

Don't spend too much time on your first analysis.

The methods in the left side of Figure 4-11 are mostly related to devices; those in the right side to matter. However, this division is seldom straightforward: you will have realized that understanding detergent powder (matter) requires understanding of the washing machine (a device).

Further Reading

Analysis and splitting of the problem is well-developed in mechanical engineering design. A short and accessible text is Nigel Cross *Engineering Design Methods*, 2nd edition, Wiley 1994, Chapters 4 and 5.

The standard text on analysis in design is G. Pahl and W. Beitz *Engineering Design, A Systematic Approach*, 2nd edition, Springer 1999, Chapters 2–4.

On washing, detergents and washing machines: E. Smulders *Laundry Detergents*, Wiley VCH 2002.

Appendix 4-1
Detergent Requirements[6]

In this file we estimate the amount of detergent required for a single wash in a washing machine. Starting point is the structure of textile in Figure 4-7. The solid part '4' of the textile consists of fibres with a diameter of ten micrometres:

$$d_4 := 10 \cdot 10^{-6} \cdot m$$

The mass of textile for a full wash is:
$$m_4 := 5 \cdot kg$$

and the density of the fibres:
$$\rho_4 := 1400 \cdot kg \cdot m^{-3}$$

The fibres have a volume
$$V_4 := \frac{m_4}{\rho_4}$$

If we consider than to be cylinders, they have a surface area
$$A_4 := V_4 \cdot \frac{4}{d_4}$$

The diameter of the surfactant '5' is (Figure 1-5 in 'Colloids').
$$d_5 := 0.4 \cdot 10^{-9} \cdot m$$

The molar mass is (roughly)
$$M_5 := 180 \cdot 10^{-3} \cdot kg \cdot mol^{-1}$$

The surface occupied by one molecule of surfactant is
$$a_5 := \frac{\pi}{4} \cdot d_5^2$$

So the number of molecules required to cover the surface is
$$n_5 := \frac{A_4}{a_5}$$

With the Avogadro number
$$N_A := 6.02 \cdot 10^{23} \cdot mol^{-1}$$

the amount (number of moles) becomes
$$N_5 := \frac{n_5}{N_A}$$

and the mass required is
$$m_5 := N_5 \cdot M_5$$
$$m_5 = 3.4 \times 10^{-3} \ kg$$

You need a measurable amount, if only to cover all fibres. In reality you would need substantially more to get a rapid penetration and to displace dirst: perhaps ten times as much.

---

[6] This is a file written in Mathcad, a program for reporting engineering calculations.

Part 2   Design

You now have a rough idea of your interests and possible customers; of existing solutions and products; and some ideas on how to improve.

The coming five lessons consider steps you will need to design a better product. These steps are only roughly sequential: much has to be done more or less simultaneously.

Lesson 5: Find Needs

You *must* get customers for a new product, and this will have to satisfy some need. Finding (or creating) customers and customer needs is one of the first jobs of any development team. It should go on through the whole of development.

Finding Customers

There are two situations when looking for customers for a new product (Figure 5-1).[1] If the new product is a variant of existing products (but *better*), you can start with existing users. This *sustaining* (market-pulled) development is the most common. If the product is really *new* – such that it requires the customer to learn new working methods – then it requires a different approach. You will usually need to find *new* customers and may even need to develop the product in a new firm, as we discuss further on. Such *disruptive* (technology-push) changes are less common – but they are important.[2]

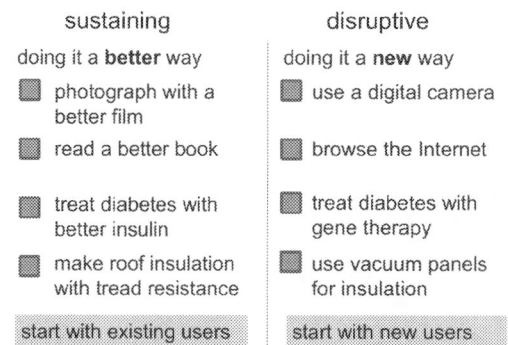

Figure 5-1 Sustaining and disruptive development

Sustaining Changes

We first look at a product that has to be sustained. Your firm produces the Attica™ windows used in sloping roofs of attics and penthouses (Figure 5-2). They have been in production for a long time, and their design needs to be improved. There are several problems with Attica™ windows. The most important one appears to be fogging due to condensation of water vapour between the two glass layers. This only appears after years of use, but even that is a problem.

[1] There are intermediate situations too.

[2] Sometimes a society has such urgent problems that developers do not have to worry about customers. The development of the atomic bomb in the Second World War comes to mind.

Design and Development of Biological, Chemical, Food and Pharmaceutical Products   J.A. Wesselingh, S. Kiil and M.E. Vigild
© 2007 John Wiley & Sons, Ltd

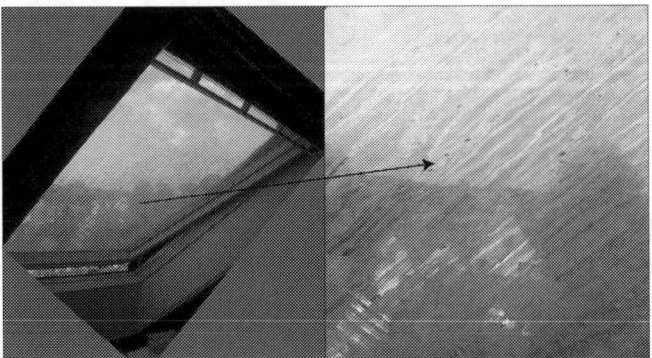

Figure 5-2 A twenty-year old Attica window

However, you may expect other comments from your customers, and must try to take these into account.

The window consists of two layers of glass, separated by a layer of stagnant argon (Figure 5-3). The glass layers are separated by an aluminium strip and glued to this strip by a polymer sealant. To improve the product, you will have to know your customers and what they need. When you have found the needs, they have to be translated into the product, via *product specifications*. This only works well if all design team members understand the needs of the customer, and are focused on them. Assessing customer needs is not at all simple. A firm has to learn to do it, and it should document the results.

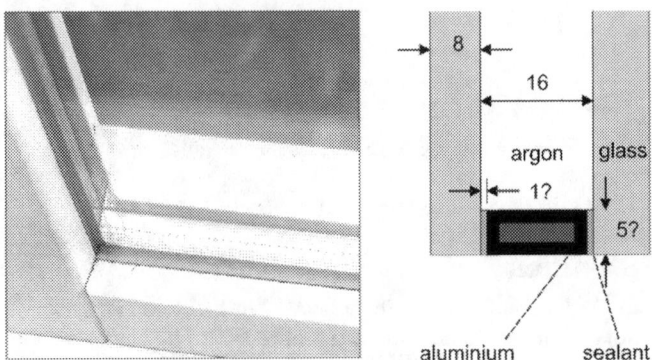

Figure 5-3 Construction of Attica windows

Figure 5-4 shows where we stand in our method. You must already learn a bit about your customers during the begin phase, but we start considering customers seriously in this design phase of our plan. At this point a design team has been formed: you are the team! The design team has been given a project scope. After analysing the situation, the first thing the design team does is to assess customer needs.

As said, the design team gets a project scope that has been put together during the begin phase (Figure 5-5). This gives the team some idea of what is expected. The project scope contains:

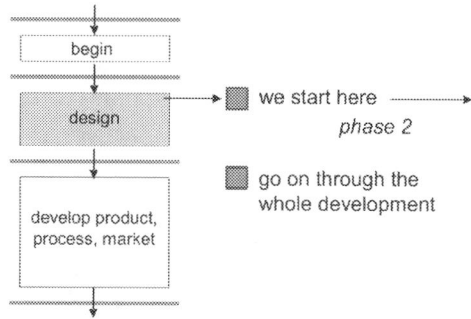

Figure 5-4 Where we are in our method

■ product: insulating window without
                   condensation problems

■ timing: available September 2005

■ markets: home, public buildings

                   current 10^6 m² per year ⎱
                                               ⎰ to be kept
                   turnover 10^8 € per year

■ constraints: on existing product line
                   (minor modifications)   cost as existing

■ stakeholders: building corporations, end-users,
                   house owners (private and
                   corporation), core team, management,
                   manufacturing...

Figure 5-5 Project scope for the Attica improvement

- a one-sentence description of what the product should do,
- desired timing; market and financial results,
- the markets for the product,
- constraints[3] on the development and
- a list of the stakeholders.[4]

When development starts, every team member must have this scope in his or her head.

We now turn over to assessing the customer needs. The method for this has the following steps:

(1) get customer data (mainly via interviews),
(2) interpret the data in terms of customer needs,
(3) tidy up the data,
(4) group and rank the needs,
(5) look back and reconsider the results.

---

[3] A typical constraint is that the product uses experience available in the firm.
[4] Stakeholders: people having an interest in the product.

At the beginning of this method, the team only has the project scope. At the end it has a ranked list of customer needs.

Customer Data

To get data from customers, you will need to know who they are (or are going to be). It is always a good idea to regard end-users as customers. However, others may be just as important – it may be a financial director who determines whether a product is bought, or a retailer. You will have to interview people from each group that you have identified, and preferably a number of them. Say a minimum of five. This easily adds up to tens of interviews. Some people will say that you need more, but this depends on the situation. Try to identify *lead customers*: those who are ahead in the use of the type of product that you are developing.

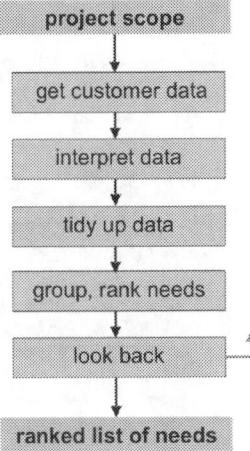

How do you get hold of customers for interviewing? For existing products such as Attica™ windows, the marketing department can help. Interviews nearly always start with a telephone call, or a personal request at some gathering. Asking for an interview by e-mail alone is seldom effective. To get data from customers, learn to be receptive to their ideas: to ask, to watch and to listen. Find things that are of interest to the customer. Engineers and scientists can be poor in this respect! The simplest – and often best – technique is the personal interview, which will typically take an hour per person. Sometimes groups of customers (focus groups) are invited for a discussion. However, these groups take longer, are more expensive, and may lead to group conduct that is either uncritical or over-critical.

All team members should take part in the customer interviewing. This is for three reasons: you can share the workload, distinguish more clearly between opinions, and you all get a feeling for the real customer.

Interviewing and Interpreting

One can set up a whole course on interviewing alone – indeed, there are many books on the subject. The thing to say here is that you should not interview unprepared. Get the name and position of the interviewed person, have a limited number of questions ready on your products and those from others, have some material ready to stimulate comment.[5]

Interviews have to be reported, so you will need to take notes. Using tape or a computer takes too much time and interferes with the interviewing: paper and pencil are best. Having a second person take the notes has advantages, but an interviewed person may feel a bit threatened by the 'two against one', unless this is carefully done. Working out of interview notes must be done immediately, not two months later.

The results from interviews will be a hodgepodge of positive and negative experiences with your products, totally irrelevant products, hobby-horses, good ideas, irrelevant ideas and what not. There may be tens of remarks from each customer, and tens of customers. So you have to bring some order out of the chaos. Below we will give a few ideas, but feel free to experiment. The trick is to rewrite each statement such that it tells *what the product should do*. Try to avoid losing information in rewriting: make the new statement as specific as the original. If necessary split a statement into several needs. Tell what the product *should* do, not what it should not. Express each need as an attribute of the product. Avoid the words *must* and *should*, as these imply which needs are important and you wish to take decisions on that later.

It is handy to put all questions, the original customer statements and the rewritten (interpreted) need in a spreadsheet. This will allow sorting and ranking later on. Keep in mind that the whole exercise is to help *you* get a good product design. If other ways of doing things look handier: do as you think best. A few examples of customer remarks and good rewrites are given in Figure 5-6. All this interpretation should be done as soon as possible after the interview.

question/prompt	customer statement	interpreted need
How do you use...?	It is difficult to clean the window on the outside.	The window is easy to clean on the outside.
What do you dislike...?	Seagulls leave droppings that are difficult to remove.	The window withstands bird droppings.
Suggested improvements	Couldn't you make the window so that it keeps sun out.	The window can keep sun out.

Figure 5-6 Customer statement list (shortened)

Tidying Up and Grouping

After rewriting all needs in a common form, write them out on Post-It notes. You can do the following in your spreadsheet, but it is better to do it with the whole design team. Decide together which needs can be combined into a single need. Then group similar (but not

---

[5] See Note 4 'Interview Your Customer'

identical) needs as customers would see them. It would be even better to let the customers group the needs.

Now choose a label (name) for each group (Figure 5-7). If there are many groups combine some into super-groups of a few needs each. You should preferably have not more than seven groups or super groups at this point: it is difficult to keep larger numbers in your mind. Here the team comes up with the grouping shown.

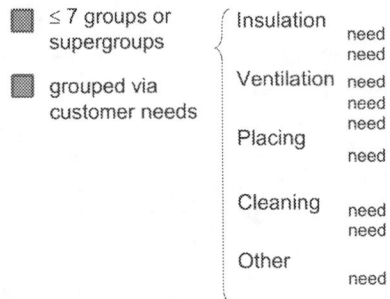

Figure 5-7 Grouping of the needs (shortened)

Ranking Needs

Now give each need a mark:

1. undesirable
2. not important
3. nice to have
4. highly desirable
5. essential

Usually the team will do this, although it would again be better, but cost more time and expense, to have it done by customers. The step ends with the grouped and ranked list of needs (Figure 5-8). Shown is part of the much larger list that is given separately in Appendix

need number	need description	rank
	Insulation	
1	the window gives good insulation, long term.	5
13	the window prevents rain blowing in	5
20	the window keeps sun out	4
	Ventilation	
18	the window can be easily closed / opened	5
19	the window closes automatically in storm	3
23	the window spreads air to prevent draught	4

Figure 5-8 Grouped list of needs (shortened)

5-1 at the end of this lesson. You may also find it handy to list the needs in order of rank: this is quickly done in a spreadsheet.

Finally look back and ask yourself a few things. Which of the customers should you keep in touch with during development? You might check whether these customers agree with your summary and ranking of needs, or whether they still bring up new ideas. At the very last decide what to do to improve things next time and write that up. This ends our first example, where we looked at the sustaining development of an existing product.

Disruptive Changes

Now we take an example of a disruptive change. Instead of the argon-filled double-glazed windows that are now the dominant design for insulating windows, one can also think of using double-glazed vacuum windows (Figure 5-9). The advantages – but also the disadvantages – are considerable.

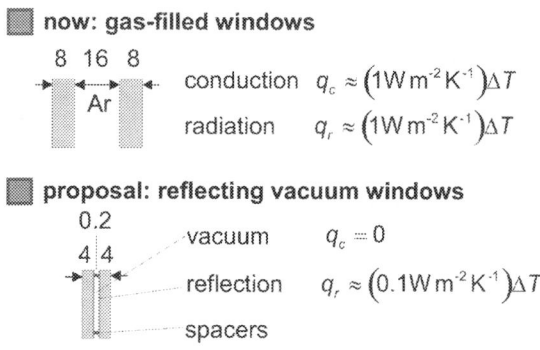

Figure 5-9 A disruptive proposal: vacuum windows

In gas-filled windows there are three heat transfer mechanisms: conduction and convection through the gas layer and radiation between the surroundings and the glass surfaces. The heat flow by conduction is minimized by using a fairly thick gas layer with a low conductivity. With even thicker layers, the effect of convection becomes important. Conduction and radiation cause similar heat fluxes, with heat transfer coefficients of a few watts per square metre per kelvin.

In the vacuum windows there is *no* conduction except through the spacers between the panes. There is also no reason to use a thick vacuum layer: the panes need to be only so far apart that they never touch due to bending. The transport due to radiation is the same as for gas-filled windows. However, it can be decreased by infrared-reflecting layers on the window. This can reduce heat transfer by an order of magnitude – at least in principle. Because the panes are connected via the spacers, they can be chosen thinner, leading to a lighter window construction.

The problems will also be clear. The manufacturer has to develop a new technology: one that will not be optimal initially. This requires anti-reflection layers, spacers and a vacuum. It will be more expensive than the existing system, certainly in the beginning. At the same time the windows may look less attractive than the existing ones: the spacers and the anti-reflection layers will make the windows less transparent (and probably cause some colouring), and the window will not be completely flat. The customers are fairly satisfied with the existing windows, so how do you think they will react if you come along with something more expensive and less attractive? In addition, the project will require a large part of the development capacity of the firm, jeopardizing improvements on the existing line of products. The new product will be cannibalizing their sales. You will be seen as pinching facilities. It is difficult to get support for a new development . . .

These are the problems of any inventor (Figure 5-10). First of all: others are not interested in *your* bright ideas. Secondly: customers do not like to change their working habits. As you have seen, firms do not like to change successful products, and there is always the excuse that the new product is not as good as the old one in some respects. New products usually start small, and initially they are not interesting for a big firm. Finally their development can take a long time: disruptive developments often have a slow start. So how do you ever get a disruptive development going?

- no interest in ideas from others
- customers won't change work habits
- firms won't change succesful products
- new products have disadvantages too
- new products start small
- their development can take long

Figure 5-10 Problems of any inventor

There are no general solutions – every case is different. However, here are a few suggestions (Figure 5-11):

(1) Find applications where the advantages are important and the disadvantages less so. Here one might think of insulation panels in refrigerators. These need to be good insulators but thin, and the optical properties are not important.

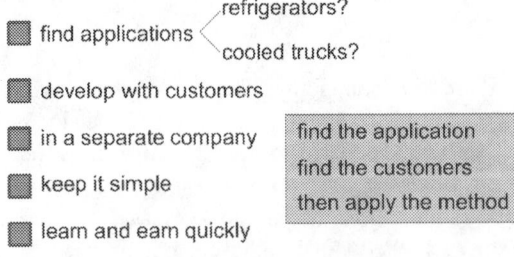

Figure 5-11 Suggestions with disruptive ideas

(2) Find people having such problems and try developing the new product together with them. The customers should think that the idea is also theirs. In this way both companies can learn and help each other.

(3) Get room for manoeuvring by the developers: disruptive products are best developed in a separate organization, perhaps even in a new firm. This will not have much money initially, so the team must learn to earn some money quickly.

(4) Once going, you may be able to develop the product for other applications. Here you might improve the optical properties to conquer the window market. But reckon on needing patience.

Once you have found customers and defined the new product, you can apply similar methods to refine the needs, as we have seen earlier.

Summary

The main points (Figure 5-12) in this lesson are:

1. learn to find customers and their needs,
2. do this by interviewing (potential) customers,
3. then interpret the result to specify the product, and
4. stay in contact with customers.

If you are considering a disruptive development, find suitable applications with new customers. Start the development *with* the customers, if possible in a separate organization. Reckon on needing patience and staying poor for some time.

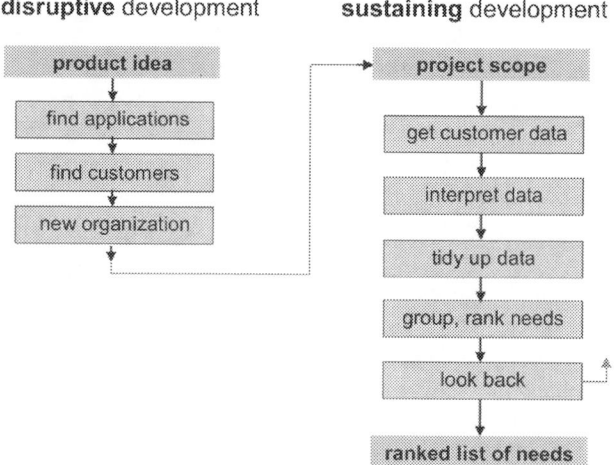

Figure 5-12 Summary of the method

Further Reading

For more on the method used here:

Karl T. Ulrich and Steven D. Eppinger *Product Design and Development*, 3rd edition, McGraw-Hill 2003, Chapter 4.

E. L. Cussler and G. D. Moggridge *Chemical Product Design*, Cambridge University Press 2001, Chapter 2.

For funny results of not considering customers: Donald A. Norman *The Design of Everyday Things*, Basic Books 2002.

Existing customers do not appreciate new developments: Clayton M. Christensen *The Innovator's Dilemma*, Harvard Business School Press 1997.

Appendix 5-1

This is the complete exercise described in the text.

Customer Data

There are two groups of customers:

> institutional owners of housing and
> single-home owners.

We consider their remarks separately.

Institutional Owners

(1) We doubt whether the windows are still in accord with the insulation requirements set by government. Insulation seems to get worse in time.
(2) In our experience, windows only last for 10–15 years. Then water vapour leaks in, and the windows become opaque due to condensation.
(3) There seem to be three kinds of leakage. Sometimes there is no damage to be seen, but even so condensate has formed. (continued)
(4) Sometimes the pane and the seal have parted, leaving a narrow slit where water can enter. (continued)
(5) Sometimes the window has cracked, with the same result.
(6) The windows jam because the outer frame has warped.
(7) Replacing the windows is expensive, because also the outer frame has to be removed.
(8) We sometimes have problems fitting a new window into an old roof. The size of the window and that of the rafter of the roof-tiles do not fit.
(9) We sometimes have problems fitting a new window into an old roof because the size of the window and the rafter of the roof beams do not fit.
(10) Water can get into the corners of the wooden frames, causing them to rot.

Individual House Owners

(11) It is difficult to clean the window on the outside.
(12) Sea gulls leave goo that is difficult to remove.
(13) In stormy weather, rain often blows into the window, even when it is almost closed.

(14) Water on the oiled wooden frame causes stains that are unsightly.
(15) My windows are no longer clear. There is water on the inside.
(16) My windows are no longer clear: they seem to be getting opaque on the outside. This may be due to salt or sand (I live near the sea).
(17) My attic can get much too hot in sunny weather with that large window in the roof.
(18) I cannot reach the top of the window easily to open or close it.
(19) It would be handy if the window would close automatically in stormy weather.
(20) Couldn't you make windows such that they keep too much sun out?
(21) It can be cold underneath the window, even when it is closed.
(22) My roof does not slope very much, and water accumulates at the bottom end.
(23) With the window open, I often get a draught in my neck.

Customer Needs

When translated into needs, these might read:

(1) The window gives a good insulation, also after a long time.
(2) The window shows no condensation between the panes.
(3) The window shows no condensation due to diffusion of water through the sealant.
(4) The window remains sealed, also after a long time.
(5) The window does not crack.
(6) The window retains its form and size, also under stress.
(7) The window can be easily replaced.
(8) The window is available in sizes for all roof-tile rafters.
(9) The window is available in sizes for all roof-beam rafters.
(10) The window frame is rot-proof.
(11) The window is easily cleaned on the outside.
(12) The window glass withstands bird droppings.
(13) The closed window prevents rain blowing in.
(14) The window frame is not stained by water.
(15) The window shows no condensation of water between the panes.
(16) The window glass withstands salt and sand.
(17) The window prevents entry of (too much) heat from the sun.
(18) The window can be easily closed when it is high up. (And opened!)
(19) The window closes automatically in stormy weather.
(20) The window keeps (too much) sun out.
(21) The window gives good insulation.
(22) The window prevents water accumulating at the outside bottom.
(23) The window spreads air entering (to avoid a draught).

Customer Needs, Tidied Up

Several of the needs are duplicates (or almost so): 1 and 21; 2 and 15 are covered by 3; 4 and 5; 17 and 20;

(1) The window gives a good insulation, also after a long time.

(3) The window shows no condensation by water going through the sealant.
(4) The window remains sealed, also after a long time.
(5) The window does not crack.
(6) The window retains its form and size, also under stress.
(7) The window can be easily replaced.
(8) The window is available in sizes for all roof-tile rafters.
(9) The window is available in sizes for all roof-beam rafters.
(10) The window frame is rot-proof.
(11) The window is easily cleaned on the outside.
(12) The window glass withstands bird droppings.
(13) The closed window prevents rain blowing in.
(14) The window frame is not stained by water.
(16) The window glass withstands salt and sand.
(18) The window can be easily closed and opened, also when it is high up.
(19) The window closes automatically in stormy weather.
(20) The window keeps (too much) sun out.
(22) The window prevents water accumulating at the outside bottom.
(23) The window spreads air entering (to avoid draught).

Needs, Grouped

A. Insulation

(1) The window gives a good insulation, also after a long time.
(13) The closed window prevents rain blowing in.
(20) The window keeps (too much) sun out.

B. Ventilation

(18) The window can be easily opened and closed, also when it is high up.
(19) The window closes automatically in stormy weather.
(23) The window spreads air entering (to avoid draught).

C. Placing

(7) The window can be easily replaced.
(8) The window is available in sizes for all roof-tile rafters.
(9) The window is available in sizes for all roof-beam rafters.

D. Cleaning

(11) The window is easily cleaned on the outside.
(12) The window glass withstands bird droppings.
(16) The window glass withstands salt and sand.

E. Problems

(3) The window shows no condensation by water going through the sealant.
(4) The window remains sealed, also after a long time.
(5) The window does not crack.
(6) The window retains its form and size, also under stress.
(10) The window frame is rot-proof.

(14) The window frame is not stained by water.
(22) The window prevents water accumulating at the outside bottom.

Needs, Ranked

The needs are ranked according to:

1 feature is undesirable
2 feature is not important
3 feature would be nice to have
4 feature is highly desirable
5 feature is essential

A. Insulation

(1) The window gives good insulation, also after a long time. 5
(13) The closed window prevents rain blowing in. 5
(20) The window keeps (too much) sun out. 3

B. Ventilation

(18) The window can be easily opened and closed, also when it is high up. 5
(19) The window closes automatically in stormy weather. 3
(23) The window spreads air entering (to avoid draught). 4

C. Placing

(7) The window can be easily replaced. 4
(8) The window is available in sizes for all roof-tile rafters. 4
(9) The window is available in sizes for all roof-beam rafters. 4

D. Cleaning

(11) The window is easily cleaned on the outside. 5
(12) The window glass withstands bird droppings. 4
(16) The window glass withstands salt and sand. 4

E. Problems

(3) The window shows no condensation by water going through the sealant. 5
(4) The window remains sealed, also after a long time. 5
(5) The window does not crack. 5
(6) The window retains its form and size, also under stress. 5
(10) The window frame is rot-proof. 3
(14) The window frame is not stained by water. 3
(22) The window prevents water accumulating at the outside bottom. 3

Needs, Ordered by Rank

Essential

(1) The window gives good insulation, also after a long time. 5
(13) The closed window prevents rain blowing in. 5

(18) The window can be easily opened and closed, also when it is high up. 5
(11) The window is easily cleaned on the outside. 5
 (3) The window shows no condensation by water going through the sealant. 5
 (4) The window remains sealed, also after a long time. 5
 (5) The window does not crack. 5
 (6) The window retains its form and size, also under stress. 5

Highly Desirable

(23) The window spreads air entering (to avoid draught). 4
 (7) The window can be easily replaced. 4
 (8) The window is available in sizes for all roof-tile rafters. 4
 (9) The window is available in sizes for all roof-beam rafters. 4
(12) The window glass withstands bird droppings. 4
(16) The window glass withstands salt and sand. 4

Desirable

(20) The window keeps (too much) sun out. 3
(19) The window closes automatically in stormy weather. 3
(10) The window frame is rot-proof. 3
(14) The window frame is not stained by water. 3
(22) The window prevents water accumulating at the outside bottom. 3

Lesson 6: Specify the Product

You now have a list of customer needs, but most of these are qualitative. They are too vague to guide design. What are needed are *product specifications*: these describe what a product should do in measurable terms.[1] At this stage of designing you do *not* specify how a certain result could or should be obtained. Experience tells that *what* and *how* are better dealt with after each other. As an example, you will set up specifications of a toothpaste. Before doing this, you will have to know the method of application – here with an ordinary toothbrush (Figure 6-1).

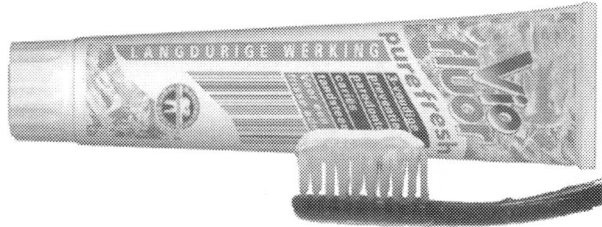

Figure 6-1 Toothbrush with toothpaste

Setting up specifications is a large job – one might wonder why they are needed. We have already noted that the main reason is to translate subjective customer needs into precise targets. These allow comparing the plans of a team with the competition. This helps in predicting whether the design will be a success in the market or not. In any design there will be conflicting requirements, both between technical aspects and between quality and cost. Having thought about the specifications greatly helps in the trading-off (compromising) on such points. The team will need this later in designing.

List of Needs

Start with the ranked list of needs such as those obtained after the previous lesson (Figure 6-2; see also Appendix 6-1). We have given this as a mind map to keep it short. Note that all the *regulations* have a rank 5 (essential): you *must* obey these.[2] Some needs in the map are a bit cryptic because we had to keep them short. 'Tartar' is a calcified deposit on your teeth; 'caries' is the dental name for holes or cavities. 'Simulates water' is short for 'brushing with paste simulates drinking water with a suitable fluoride content'.

---

[1] What has to be attained; not how!

[2] You cannot change regulations **yourself**.

Design and Development of Biological, Chemical, Food and Pharmaceutical Products   J.A. Wesselingh, S. Kiil and M.E. Vigild
© 2007 John Wiley & Sons, Ltd

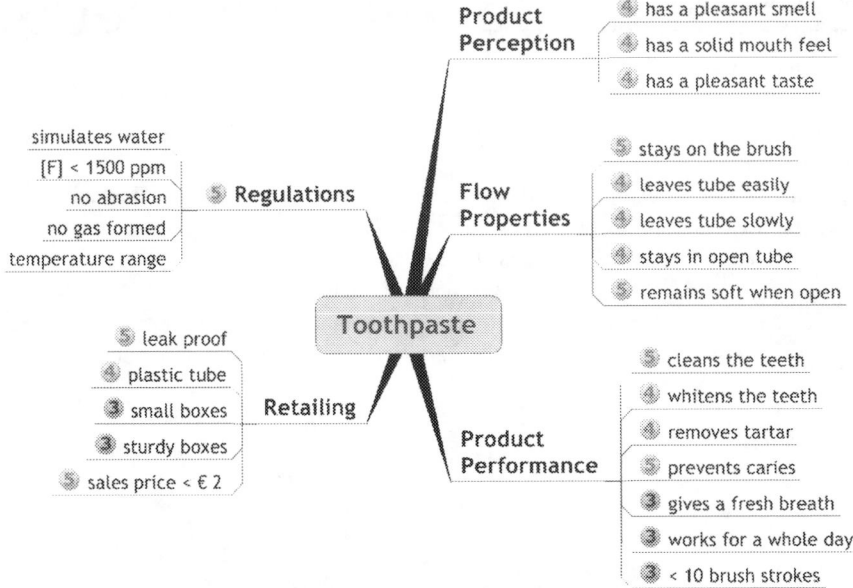

Figure 6-2 List of needs with ranks

The Method

Figure 6-3 shows a method for setting specifications. The list of needs gives a first list of specifications. Quantify the specifications with metrics; more about these in a moment. Then benchmark: compare your ideas with the competition. Finally discuss what the ideal values would be for the metrics, and which would be just acceptable: use these values to set the list of specifications.

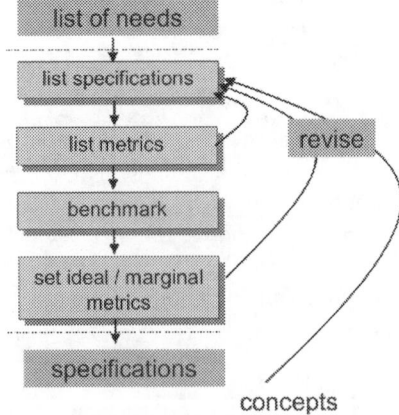

Figure 6-3 How to set specifications

Ideally, you would set the specifications at the beginning of a project, and then design the product such that it meets your specifications. However, most products are too complicated to allow a team to do this. Usually there have to be at least two rounds: one at this point and one later on when the team has decided which concept is going to be used for the product. In the first try, set *target specifications*. These are hardly more than guesses of the team: they will need improving.

List of Metrics

Each specification consists of a *metric* – a quantifiable property of the product – and a *value*. For example, customers require toothpaste to be stiff so that it does not flow off the brush. Here the metric could be the yield stress, of which the value would be given in the *unit* Pa (pascal). Not all needs can be quantified well as you will see in a moment.

A good way to get a first list of metrics is to consider each customer need in turn. The team then thinks of ways in which these can be quantified and measured: these will become the metrics. Ideally, there will be one metric per need, and this will be a measure that the designer can influence. This ideal is seldom possible: you often need several metrics to describe a need, and a given metric may be important in describing several needs. Two additional points: your metrics should be easily measured and not too expensive. They *must* cover the requirements of the market – requirements of retailers and authorities.

The first list of metrics will look like that in Figure 6-4.[3] Each metric has a number and a name. It will be associated with one or more needs. In this first list, need and specification numbers coincide, but later you may add or delete metrics. Note that some metrics have a straightforward unit. However, others may be given in terms of a list, or a binary (yes/no; pass/fail). One of the units is given as subj or *subjective*: this one is measured by a panel of users. You will want to avoid these, because it takes a long time to measure them. Some metrics have the 'unit' RDA: these use the Radioactive Dental Abrasion test, a standard test used in the toothpaste world. When such tests exist, you should use them. This makes comparison with measurements from others easier. Also it is often a large job to develop a test. The rank of a metric is determined by the rank of the need it describes – this may require some discussion in the team.

It is important to check whether all needs are well described by the list of metrics. A *matrix of needs and metrics* as shown in Figure 6-5 can help. This would hardly be necessary for the very short list in the figure, but in real projects the matrix can be much larger. You can see at a glance whether specifications are missing or superfluous.

The Competition

Unless you are the only firm in a market, you must try to find out what your competitors are up to! When developing a new product, you should collect products from competitors, try them out, analyse them, and get to understand them. You must find out how well competing

---

[3] Figure 6-4 is a selection from Appendix 6-1: the metrics numbers are not sequential.

metric number	need(s)	specification(s)	metric unit	rank
1	pleasant smell	aroma	subj	5
4	stays on brush	yield stress	Pa	5
6	leaves tube slowly	viscosity	Pa·s	4
11	removes tartar	tartar rem	RDA	4
16	sales price	price	€	5
21	storage temperature	store temp	ºC	5
22	no gas evolution	no gas	y/n	5
23	no abrasion	abrasion	RDA	5

Figure 6-4 A part of the first list of metrics

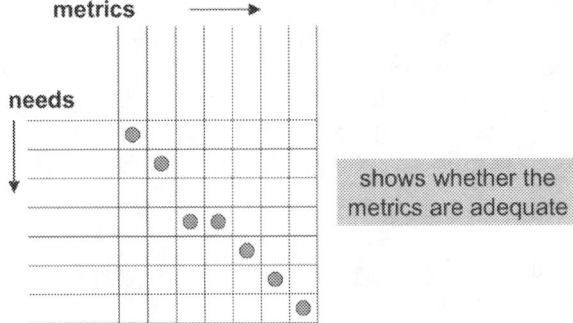

Figure 6-5 A matrix of needs and metrics

products satisfy the needs of your customers (according to your list). Customer tests are lengthy and expensive. So you may have to rely on the (biased?) judgement of the team. It is difficult to compete if you do not assemble this information properly. Also measure the metrics of competing products using your own list of specifications.[4] This can be quite a job, but is similar to the testing of the own product. Sometimes you can already get part of the data from competitor's catalogues and product descriptions, but these data are not always reliable.

With toothpaste it is not difficult to get samples from competitors. Just walk into a few shops and buy them (Figure 6-6). It is not always that easy, especially when you want to get the first of the latest products. You may wonder why there are so many toothpastes. This is because the different manufacturers have tried to *position* themselves. They try to cover a certain segment of the market where they will have less competition.

Some data on toothpaste composition are printed on the back side of the tubes. These are instructive. You will find abrasives (such as silica) which remove plaque, humectants (such

---

[4] This is often too much work for a student project.

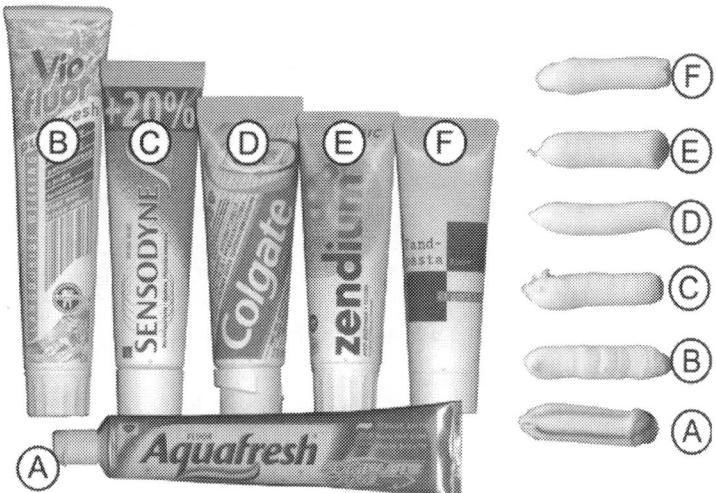

Figure 6-6 Some competing toothpastes

as sorbitol) which retard drying out, water (here called aqua), binders such as cellulose gum to make the paste solid, a detergent (soap) such as sodium lauryl sulphate and a number of other additives including therapeutic ones such as fluorides. Try to identify them.

Now construct a needs chart (Figure 6-7), which is just an extension of your former chart. Leave a column to fill in the results for your own product later. Give scores in the way seen in consumer magazines. The same applies to your second chart for metrics, but here most metrics can be given a value (Figure 6-8).

need number	need description	rank	scores own	competitors
1	pleasant smell	5	●●	●
4	stays on brush	5	●●●	●
6	leaves tube slowly	4	●●	●●●
11	removes tartar	4	●	●●●
16	sales price	5	●●	●
23	no abrasion	5	●	●●

Figure 6-7 Parts of the needs chart

You now know how needs are satisfied by competing products, and what their metrics are. More important: you have gained experience and technical knowledge, and have a frame of reference for dealing with toothpaste. The team should now be able to set up two values for each metric:

– an ideal value: the best you could hope for, and
– a marginal value just acceptable for your customers.

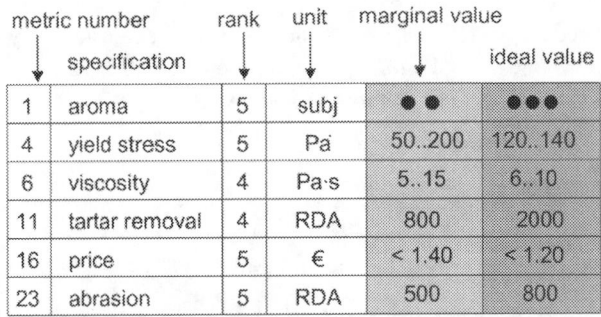

metric number	specification	rank	unit	metrics — own	metrics — competitors
1	aroma	5	subj	●●	●
4	yield stress	5	Pa	118	77
6	viscosity	4	Pa·s	9.1	6.7
11	tartar removal	4	RDA	1900	600
16	price	5	€	1.98	1.20
23	abrasion	5	RDA	1900	600

Figure 6-8 Parts of the metrics chart

You will need trade-offs: not all metrics will get their ideal value. All this gives a first idea of your design space; this will have to be sharpened as you go further into the design process.

List of Specifications

The last chart, the list of specifications, is nothing but the list of metrics of your firm's own product, with the ranges of metrics values added (Figure 6-9). This is what you will use to guide our design. As said, the list is still only dreams and hopes. There is a lot of hard work ahead.

metric number	specification	rank	unit	marginal value	ideal value
1	aroma	5	subj	●●	●●●
4	yield stress	5	Pa	50..200	120..140
6	viscosity	4	Pa·s	5..15	6..10
11	tartar removal	4	RDA	800	2000
16	price	5	€	< 1.40	< 1.20
23	abrasion	5	RDA	500	800

Figure 6-9 List of specifications (incomplete)

Using Models

Specifications nearly always have to be revised once – and often many times. A good point is two steps further in our scheme, where you have selected one concept or a few for further working out and have started testing them. However, already at this point you may start developing models of the behaviour and cost of our product. These can be a great help in improving specifications.

There are two groups of technical models (Figure 6-10):

- numerical ones (also called analytical models) and
- physical models made of real materials.

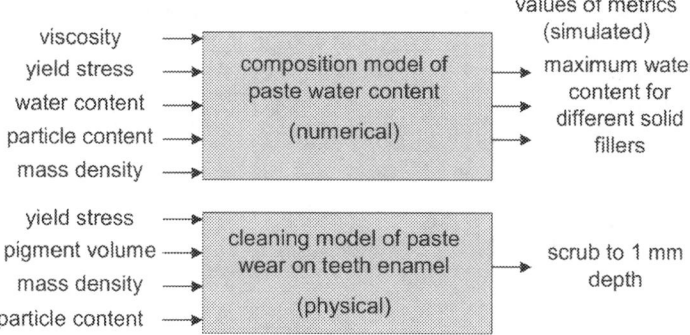

Figure 6-10 Two models of toothpaste

The numerical models are usually implemented on a computer while the physical models can be test versions of the actual product. Both types of models help in estimating part of the product properties without making a complete product. One can seldom model *all* properties of a product in one go. An example of such a model is that for flow properties of the toothpaste given in Appendix 6-2. We used it for the first guesses of the yield stress and viscosity.

In these 'front-end' stages of design you need models to help understand product behaviour and to improve your ideas. So here the models should be *simple* and you often construct them yourself. Further on in the design models are used to accurately predict product properties: these are often 'black boxes' for the users and less useful for concept development.

Parallel with the technical models, you will be constructing a cost model of the product. We discuss this in lesson 12. At this stage it will contain a list of components, estimates of their material and processing costs, and of the cost required for packaging. It should include investment and overhead costs, even though you will not know them accurately at this point. For a not-too-large project the whole can be done in a spreadsheet. The cost model allows the

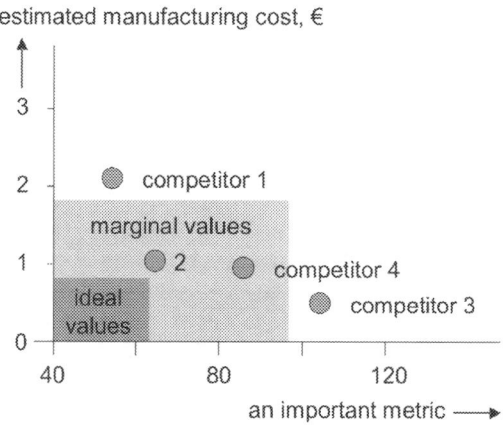

Figure 6-11 Comparing different designs

team to estimate the effects of design and manufacturing methods on cost. It is a powerful tool to help make decisions on what a team should or should not do. The cost model will be continually refined and updated during development. With the cost model and data on competitors, you will be able to construct charts like that in Figure 6-11. These will give a further idea of where you stand with your product design in comparison with the competition.

Looking Back

As always, you should look back on the results. At the point that product specifications have been set, consider the following questions.

1. Is your product really a winner? If it is not, and you cannot improve it, this is the time to stop!
2. Is the market that you have in mind the best for your product? If your design looks very good, you might aim for a more profitable section of the market.
3. You should not only look back, but also ahead. For example, this is a good point to ask whether the company should not be setting aside resources for developing or acquiring better models. These may be useful later in the project, but their full use will come in further projects.

Summary

In this lesson we have discussed how to specify what a product is to do.

1. Begin with the list of needs.
2. For each need try to find a metric – something that is measurable and that describes the need quantitatively.
3. Look around for competing products and determine how well they fulfil the needs; also measure the values of their metrics.
4. Your new product will have to be better than existing products – this gives you an idea for your first specification.
5. This will guide you in the next steps: making and selecting product concepts.
6. You will probably have to refine your specifications several times during development.

Further Reading

For methods similar to those used here:

Karl T. Ulrich and Steven D. Eppinger *Product Design and Development*, 3rd edition, McGraw-Hill 2003, Chapter 5.

E. L. Cussler and G. D. Moggridge *Chemical Product Design*, Cambridge University Press 2001, Chapter 2.

We are still looking for a good reference on toothpaste!

Appendix 6-1

Below is a first (very incomplete) attempt to construct metrics for toothpaste.

metric #	need description	metric name	unit	rank	value
(1)	pleasant smell	fragrance	subj.	4	
(2)	solid mouth feel	mouthfeel	subj.	4	
(3)	pleasant taste	taste	subj.	4	
(4)	stays on brush	yield stress	Pa	5	>300
(5)	leaves tube easily	viscosity	Pa·s	4	<30
(6)	leaves tube slowly	yield stress	Pa	4	>20
(7)	stays in open tube	yield stress	Pa	5	>1
(8)	cleans the teeth	cleanpower	subj.	5	
(9)	whitens the teeth	whitepower	subj.	4	
(10)	removes tartar	abrasiveness	mg	4	>15
(11)	prevents caries	cariesprevent	ppm F	5	>1000
(12)	gives fresh breath	fresh breath	subj.	3	
(13)	works for a whole day	longevity	subj.	3	
(14)	requires <10 brushstrokes	cleanpower	subj.	3	
(15)	leakproof tube	leakage	per million	5	<0.1
(16)	plastic tube	tubetype	y/n	4	y
(17)	small boxes	boxtype	y/n	4	y
(18)	sturdy boxes	falltest	y/n	4	y
(19)	sales price	salesprice	€	4	<2
(20)	simulates fluorided water	fluormax	ppm F	5	$500 < F < 1500$
(21)	maximum fluoride	fluormax	ppm F	5	<1500
(22)	no abrasion	abrasiveness	mg	5	<30
(23)	no fermentables	gas-evolution	y/n	5	n
(24)	storage temperature range	temprange	°C	5	$-10 < T < 45$

Appendix 6-2

Flow Properties of Toothpaste[5]

Toothpaste is a material that has to be solid at rest and liquid when sheared.[6] We will assume that it behaves as a Bingham fluid, and is described by two parameters:

a yield stress $\qquad \tau_Y$

a differential viscosity $\qquad \eta_D$

The relation between shear stress τ and shear rate γ is

$$\tau = \tau_Y + \eta_D \cdot \gamma$$

We would like to have an idea of the required values of these parameters, so as to set specifications. We begin with the yield stress. This will be highest when the brush is held vertically:

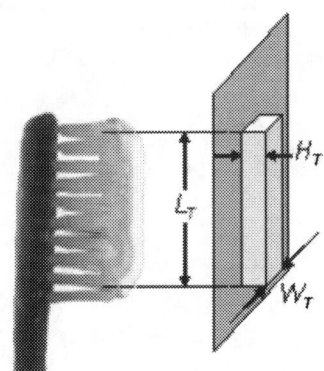

We might regard the brush as a flat plate, and the toothpaste as a little box of solid with dimensions:

$$L_T := 40 \cdot 10^{-3} \cdot m \quad W_T := 6 \cdot 10^{-3} \cdot m \quad H_T := 6 \cdot 10^{-3} \cdot m$$

and a density $\rho_T := 1200 \cdot kg \cdot m^{-3}$

The mass of the toothpaste is then

$$m_T := \rho_T \cdot L_T \cdot W_T \cdot H_T \quad m_T = 1.73 \times 10^{-3} kg$$

---

[5] This is another Mathcad file.
[6] Flow properties (rheology) are introduced in the Notes on 'Colloids' at the end of this book.

If we hold the brush vertically, the stress at the brush is:

$$\tau_0 := \frac{m_T \cdot g}{L_T \cdot W_T} \qquad \tau_0 = 71 \text{Pa}$$

If the yield stress is lower than this, the toothpaste will flow off the brush. In reality, we might need a higher yield stress to allow for acceleration forces when one moves the brush. Assume that the brush is at the end of the arm with length

$$L_A := 0.5 \cdot m$$

and that it is moved with a velocity: $v_A := 1 \cdot m \cdot s^{-1}$

The centrifugal acceleration is $\qquad a := \frac{v_A^2}{L_A} \qquad a = 2 \frac{m}{s^2}$

This does not greatly increase acceleration above that of gravity alone. So we conclude that the minimum yield stress of toothpaste should be around 100 Pa.

Now the differential viscosity. In the following we assume that the shear rate is high, so that the effect of the yield stress is unimportant. When you squeeze a tube of toothpaste, you increase the pressure inside. We have estimated the force exerted by clenching a personal weighing scale:

$$F_T := 40 \cdot N$$

the area squeezed is

$$A_T := 40 \cdot 10^{-4} \cdot m^2$$

giving a pressure difference $\Delta p := \dfrac{F_T}{A_T} \qquad \Delta P = 1 \times 10^4 \text{ Pa}$

The toothpaste should flow onto the brush in about $\qquad t_T := 1 \cdot s$

so with a velocity $\qquad v_T := \dfrac{L_T}{t_T}$

The flow rate of a viscous liquid through a tube is given by the Poiseuille equation: $\qquad v = \dfrac{1}{32} \cdot \dfrac{D^2 \cdot \Delta p}{L \cdot \eta}$

Here D is the diameter of the tube, L the length and η the viscosity. A circular opening behaves like a tube with a length of six times the diameter:

$$v = \frac{1}{32} \cdot \frac{D^2 \Delta p}{\eta \cdot 6 \cdot D}$$

In our case the diameter of the opening and the velocity are equal to that of toothpaste:

$$D := W_T \qquad v := v_T$$

So

$$\eta := \frac{1}{32} \cdot \frac{D^2 \cdot \Delta p}{v \cdot 6 \cdot D} \qquad \eta = 7.8 \text{ Pa} \cdot \text{s}$$

So we require a differential viscosity of the order of 10 Pa s (ten thousand times that of water).

Lesson 7: Create Concepts

With C.E. Weinell from Hempel A/S

Using the list of specifications, we look for ways to make a good product. We create *concepts*: brief descriptions of the working principle or form of the product. These are usually in the form of a sketch, of a written description, or of a model.

Bio-fouling of Ships

As an example we look at bio-fouling of ships. A ship has to load and unload, and in these periods it is lying still, often in tropical waters. Then all kinds of organisms start growing on the ship, and it will be no surprise that this greatly increases the roughness (Figure 7-1). This is bad for fuel consumption – how bad we will see in a moment.

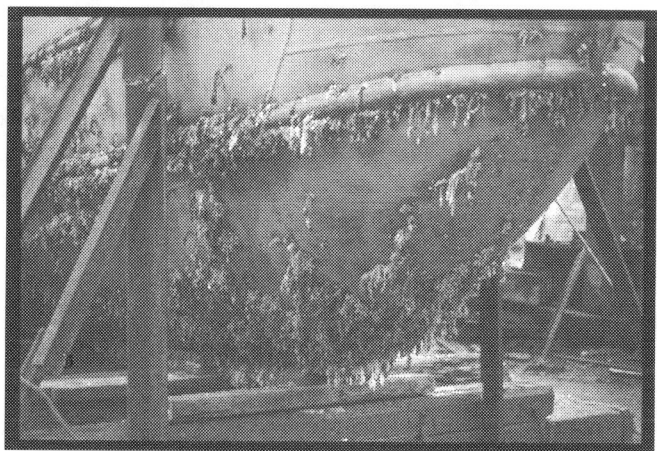

Figure 7-1 Biofouling on a ship. Reproduced with permission from Hempel A/S

There is a solution to this problem. The ship can be coated with a layer of a tributyltin copolymer, in which a fine copper oxide pigment is embedded. The layer gradually erodes, giving small concentrations of dissolved copper and tin outside the skin (Figure 7-2). These kill organisms adhering to the skin. Also erosion helps remove any fouling. Unfortunately, the tin and copper not only kill the organisms that we want to prevent: they have consequences for much of sea life.[1] As a result this method was banned world-wide in 2003. This created a problem, but also an opportunity, for manufacturers of paint for ships.

[1] This came up around the year 2000.

Design and Development of Biological, Chemical, Food and Pharmaceutical Products   J.A. Wesselingh, S. Kiil and M.E. Vigild
© 2007 John Wiley & Sons, Ltd

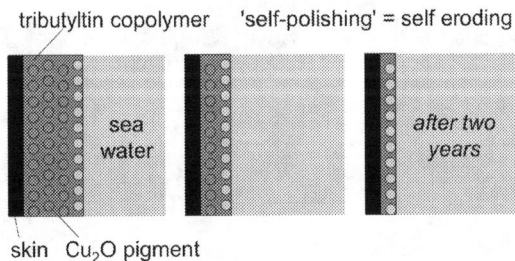

Figure 7-2 A self-polishing[2] antifouling layer

To get an idea of the size of the problem we will look at the transport of oil. The amount of oil used worldwide is enormous: of the order of 100 tons per second! The greater part of this is found in the Middle East and has to be transported to the industrial centres of our world, to the United States, Europe and Eastern Asia. The oil has to be transported over distances of around 10 000 km, so a typical round trip is 20 000 km.

The oil is transported in tankers, which have dimensions like those shown in Figure 7-3. To give some idea of the size: a walk around the deck is almost a kilometre. It is not surprising that bicycles are used on such ships. Even though these are huge installations, they are run by a small crew of perhaps 25 people. The tanker can be seen as a large double-walled box, with a small propulsion system. The weight is largely that of the contents. About a thousand super tankers are required to cover world transport.

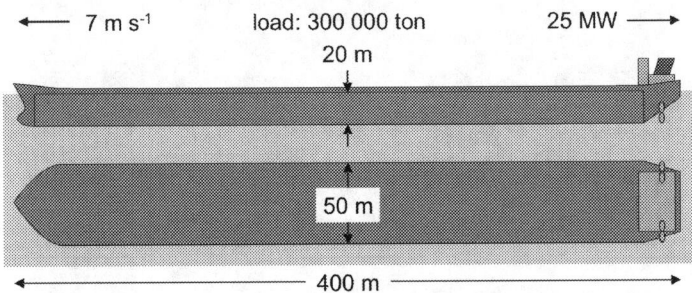

Figure 7-3 Dimensions of an oil tanker

A tanker uses about 1% of its content as fuel on a round trip. This is a major part of the cost. The propulsion system has an efficiency of perhaps 40%. The propulsion has to overcome the drag forces on the ship.

There are two major drag forces:

1. form drag, due to water being accelerated and decelerated in front and behind the ship;
2. skin drag, caused by the flow past the sides of the ship.

---

[2] The layer is very thin: about 500 μm initially.

Form drag is proportional to the wetted cross-section of the ship; skin drag to the wetted area. For a tanker, skin drag is fairly important. Skin drag also depends on the *roughness* of the skin. For a tanker, a roughness of 0.1 mm already has an appreciable effect. For small, fast ships there is third drag mechanism: wave drag. However this is not important for tankers. The effects are worked out in Appendix 7-1.

The consequences for cost and operation are large. There is an optimum speed for running a tanker (Figure 7-4). Low speeds do not utilize the transport capacity well; at high speeds the fuel consumption is excessive. The optimal speed goes down as the tanker gets rougher. This means that more roughness not only increases fuel costs, but also forces one to use more tankers. The effect of doubling of the roughness (say from 0.1 mm to 0.2 mm) is about 260 000 euros per tanker per year. As the roughness can easily increase by a factor of 10, we see that we are talking about a million euros per year for a single tanker.

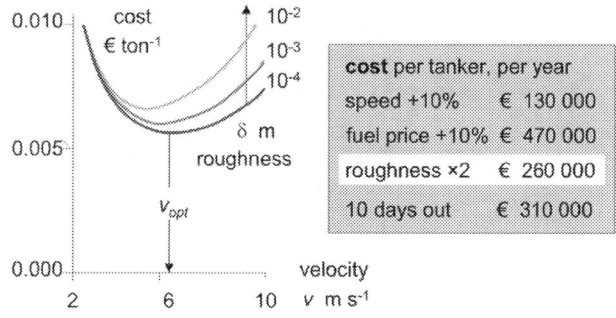

Figure 7-4 The minimal transport cost

Your Project

Suppose you are working for a firm making marine paints. Changes in international laws governing the use of copper/tin anti-fouling paints have been announced. The firm has decided to take up the challenge, and you are part of the development team. Figure 7-5 gives an abbreviated form of the project scope. This scope has been created using the model of the tanker operation in Appendix 7-1.

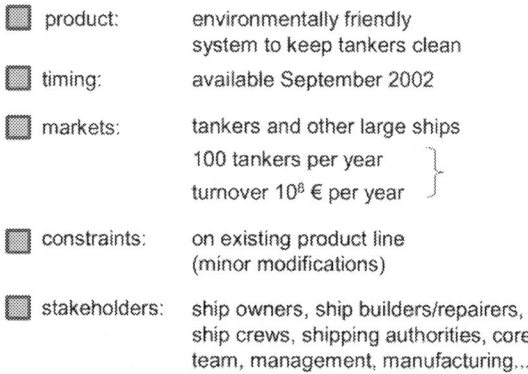

Figure 7-5 The scope of the project (simplified)

After analysing the situation and searching for customer needs you have formed a first idea of the specifications of the product (Figure 7-6). The main points are summarized below. You will have a fairly good idea of the problem, and a list of ideas and questions that have come up during orientation, and will be using these to start forming concepts.

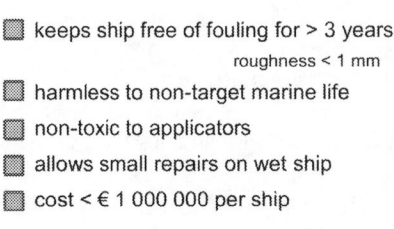

Figure 7-6 First set of specifications

Creating Concepts

A team must create many concepts.[3] How many? It depends, but start thinking in terms of tens – not one or two. There are good reasons why a team should create many concepts. You can only expect to get a good product starting with a good concept, and the chances of finding one are larger with more alternatives. You will not get *stuck* so easily when there are many concepts to fall back on. Considering many concepts can also help in understanding the competition – essential if your product is to be a success in the market. Finally, there is little reason *not* to consider many concepts; a team can do this quickly and cheaply.

Here are types of behaviour to avoid in this stage. The first is to consider only one or two concepts (usually from the most assertive member of the team) and to start working these out. This causes the team to miss opportunities and is bad for team commitment. A second is to neglect concepts from others (especially the competition). This we-know-better or not-invented-here has led to the end of many a firm. Most good products are the result of *combining* concepts: you should consider combining when creating concepts. A third counter-productive kind of behaviour is to be critical and to kill ideas when they are first proposed by others. Finally, at this stage try not to forget categories of solutions. We will give a few tricks to help you do this.

We will consider creating concepts using five steps (Figure 7-7):

(1) splitting into smaller problems (decomposing),
(2) searching for existing ideas[4] or concepts,
(3) searching for new ideas or concepts,
(4) exploring combinations of these concepts, and
(5) looking back.

Actually this looking back happens during the whole process: creating concepts is an iterative process. It can be a lot messier than the diagram suggests. The team ends with a large list of concepts.

---

[3] Later you will choose a small part of these to work out seriously.
[4] We use the word idea for a precursor of a concept: something vague and not worked out.

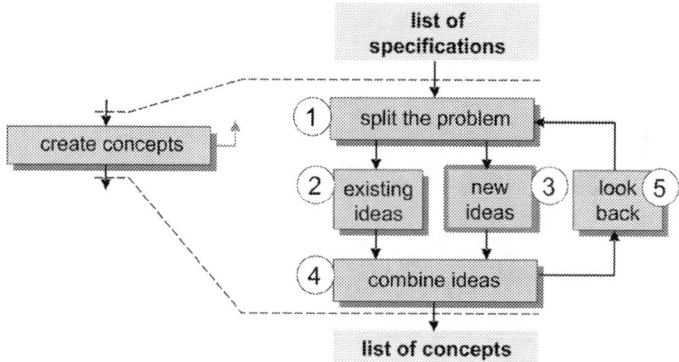

Figure 7-7 The method for creating concepts

Splitting (Decomposing)

The first step is to split the problem into sub-problems and to analyse sub-functions. Focus on sub-problems that appear to be critical to the product. We have already discussed splitting (or decomposing) in Lesson 3. Here we look at only a few splits of our problem. You should try more of them. A way of splitting that is often surprisingly effective is to give the problem a long name, and to start looking at the different parts of the name (Figure 7-8). This is not science, but it can work.

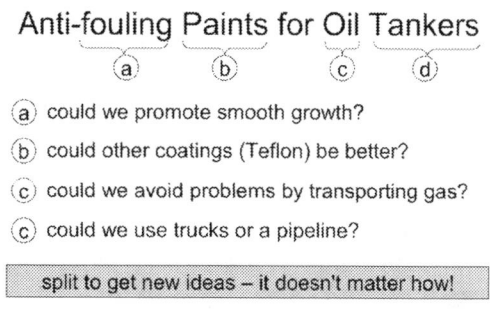

Figure 7-8 Splitting a problem by splitting its name

A second split is to consider what happens on a non-protected ship (Figure 7-9). This starts with a clean skin. Growth probably starts with micro-organisms adhering to the skin, and forming an environment in which larger organisms can grow. These are followed by even larger ones.... From shipping experience you get the impression that growth is serious when a ship is lying still – this suggests that organisms are easily sheared off initially. The impression is that the problem is especially serious in warm waters. How could you influence adhesion? How growth rates? How shearing? Your paint company might have a job for a biologist! However, she would have to be oriented towards problem-solving, not problem-description. This might be difficult for a research biologist.

A third split looks at the current method of protection (Figure 7-10). We have again jotted down questions that come up. Any of these can lead to ideas for solutions. 'Which substances

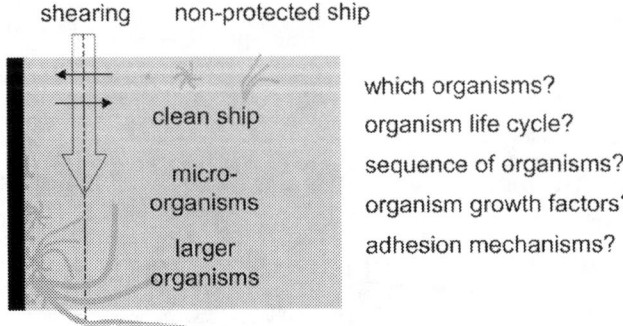

Figure 7-9 What happens on a non-protected ship?

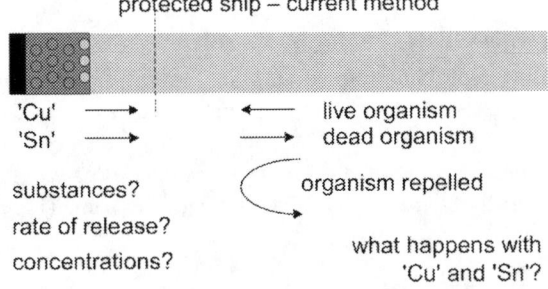

Figure 7-10 Getting ideas from the current method

are we releasing' leads to whether there might be other, less detrimental ones, perhaps biodegradable. 'What are the concentrations' suggests you might find ways of maintaining a high concentration near the skin but with a lower release rate. 'What happens with the poisons' might lead to the idea of recovering them from the sea with selective ion exchange. Or of considering why they are so bad for the environment (because they accumulate somewhere?). Anyhow, try to look at the problem from as many viewpoints as you can, noting questions and ideas as they come up.

You have already been looking at existing ideas while analysing and splitting and may find it worthwhile to do this systematically. Good sources of existing ideas are *lead users* – customers who are ahead of others in exploiting the limits of your products. Obvious external sources are experts (consultants or university people), patent literature, open literature, meetings such as trade fairs or symposia[5], and the products and product descriptions from the competition. The search for external information actually goes on throughout the whole project, and not only while forming concepts. When the right knowledge can be found elsewhere, it is usually much cheaper than developing it yourself.

---

[5] There is even a large annual gathering of shipping companies, marine authorities, ship builders, paint manufacturers, environmental people . . . You only need to search the Internet and find money to go there.

Forming New Concepts

The third step is for the team members to create *new* concepts. Again, you have already been doing that, and should have a list by now. You can form ideas individually (which is quite effective), but some group work is desirable if only to exchange ideas and to keep every team member involved. These *new* concepts are the ones that may give the firm a competitive edge.

A few guidelines for forming concepts: suspend judgement on ideas in this stage – do not criticize – welcome daft ideas as these often lead to other ideas – use graphical and physical media such as blackboards and flipovers in group sessions. The trick in forming ideas is to *avoid vertical thinking* (Figure 7-11). Vertical thinking is the logical way of thinking, in which one proceeds step-by-step through a problem. It is the way of thinking required to solve examination problems, or when doing a mathematical analysis. Engineers and scientists are trained, trained and trained to do this. So much so that they often have lost abilities to use our other mode of thinking: *lateral thinking*. In lateral thinking logic is of no importance. The important thing is to generate new ideas. Whether these are any good you will see later, perhaps via vertical thinking. *Suspend judgement*. Each time step aside or think laterally to come up with something different. Artists, writers, architects, industrial designers and other groups of people not considered by engineers and scientists are often very good at this. But even engineers can learn the tricks! We have listed a few tricks at the bottom of Figure 7-11. We will be using mind mapping and brainstorming.

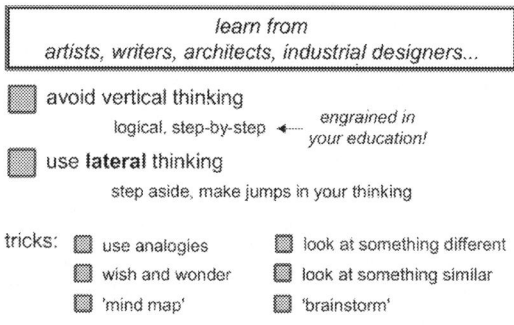

Figure 7-11 Using lateral thinking

Using Concept Trees

For a *concept tree* or *mind map* note the problem somewhere on a large piece of paper or a blackboard.[6] Then draw branches (say five or seven) radiating from the problem, and start noting any associations that come up on the branches. If these give new associations, add new branches, and so on. It is important to keep thinking laterally, and to avoid evaluating when first setting up a mind map. *Suspend judgement*. A concept tree is no magic, but you will find that it works much more naturally than just making lists.

The concept tree helps finding new ideas in several ways:

---

[6] You can also do this in a program such as Mindmanager.

(1) It identifies independent approaches.
(2) It leads to further splitting of the problem.

In a further stage use the concept tree to tidy up ideas:

(1) to prune branches of which you have no expectations,
(2) to bring some order in the ideas,
(3) to consider a lack of knowledge of any branch.

Figure 7-12 shows a concept tree of ideas that are already in use to avoid the problems of tanker fouling. Note that just drawing this provokes associations. Think of a series of release mechanisms of chemicals, and of whole groups of chemicals that might be used, or of any combination of these.

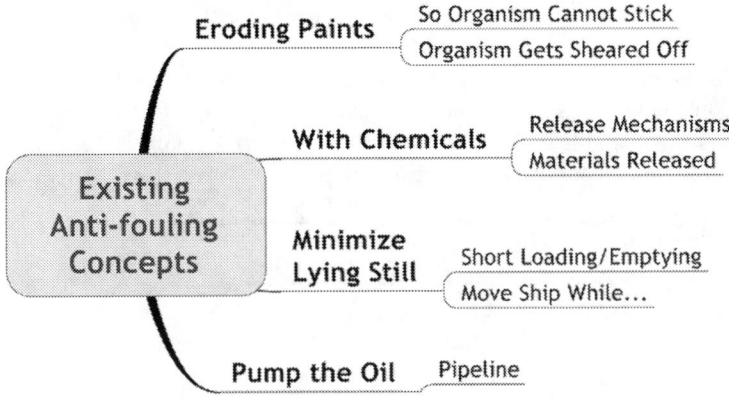

Figure 7-12 Concept tree of existing anti-fouling concepts

At this point you may be tempted to think: 'I am a paint manufacturer, so minimizing the amount of time that a tanker is lying still is none of my business.' However, it may be that this is a better solution than the one you have in mind – and then you can better get out of the business quickly! It may also turn out that combining this with some new paint (which is less effective, but also less harmful) leads to an acceptable solution. So be careful with discarding ideas too quickly.

Brainstorming

Brainstorming is a group technique: one to use in a team. The group should neither be too small nor too large, say six to ten people. The group can include people from outside the team. Get together in a place where you will not be disturbed, and have some method of showing text that everybody can read (such as a blackboard).

One person – not necessarily the team leader – leads the discussion. She first explains that, from this moment on, criticism is not allowed. Every idea that is brought forward (including nonsense) is to be accepted for the moment. The group is to suspend judgement: everybody is allowed to 'make mistakes'. The leader puts up a brief description of the problem on the blackboard, so that everybody can read it. Then each person is asked in turn to bring up some idea on the problem. This is added to a list. The leader encourages associations: ideas that follow from earlier ideas. The mind map form is good for brainstorming as it allows associations to be added as new branches. After some time – say half an hour – the forming of ideas begins to dry up. The leader stops the session. The group goes out to get coffee, and one or two people try to bring some order in the ideas. After coffee the new list of ideas is discussed to see whether the original ideas have come across.

Figure 7-13 shows a set of new ideas that has come up in a brainstorming session. For some of them we only have a vague idea of whether they might work. Others are probably nonsense.

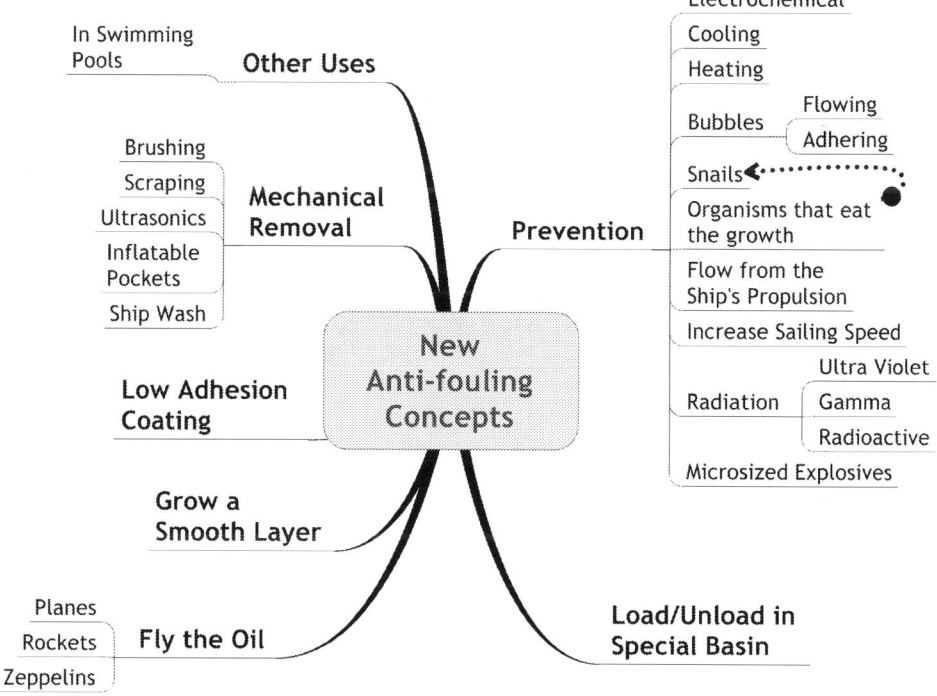

Figure 7-13 Ideas from a brainstorming session

The combination of Figures 7-12 and 7-13 gives the list of ideas to begin with. In the next lesson we investigate how to choose from this disparate and disorganized lot. In a first round we will scrap all nonsense and 'no-go' solutions and rearrange the remaining items such that you can see who might work on them. The result for this lesson might look like Figure 7-14.

While forming concepts, but certainly at the end of this phase, you should look back on what you have learned. Have you explored the concept space fully (well, far enough)? Have all ideas brought up been considered at least briefly, or have they fallen by the wayside? Could you find better ways of splitting the problem? If you get a similar job in the future, what will you do differently?

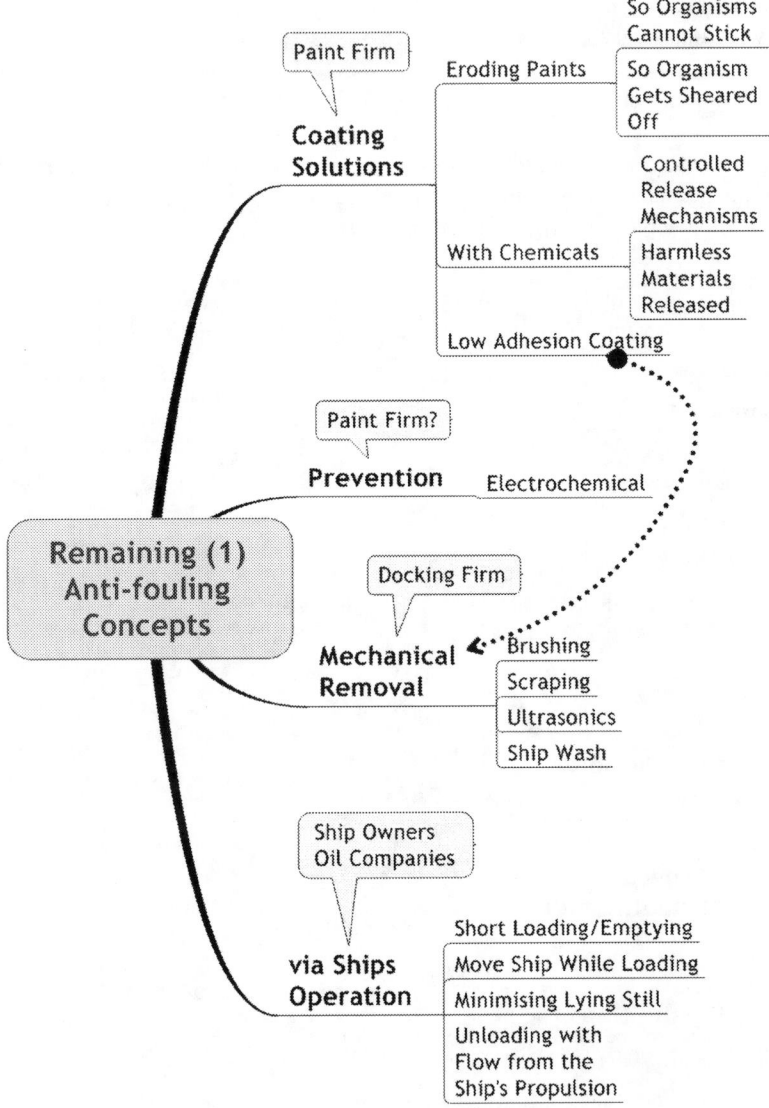

Figure 7-14 Concepts remaining after a first selection

Summary

Creating concepts begins with the list of customer needs and the first target specifications. The team generates a great number of ideas, from which 2–8 will be considered somewhat seriously. The method used here has six steps:

1. Clarify the problem: split it into simpler sub-problems.
2. Find existing ideas: contact lead users, experts, patents, other products . . . .
3. Find new ideas with both individual and group methods.
4. Explore ideas with concept trees.

5. Look back before trying a new iteration.
6. Finish with a list of concepts.

Creating concepts is seldom a linear process – it usually requires several iterations.

Further Reading
The method used here is largely from:

Karl T. Ulrich and Steven D. Eppinger *Product Design and Development*, 3rd edition, McGraw-Hill 2003, Chapter 6.

The standard book on creativity is Edward de Bono *Lateral Thinking*, Penguin Books 1990 (Other books by de Bono such as *The Five Days Course in Thinking* are at least as creative, but they are out of print.) A lively and humoristic one is Roger von Oech *A Whack on the Side of the Head*, Warner Books, 3rd edition 1998.

On the many applications of mind maps:

Tony Buzan *How to MindMap®*, Thorsons (Harper Collins) 2002. A bit simple, but short and stimulating.

On roughness of ships: R. L Townsin et al., Speed, Power and Roughness: The Economics of Outer Bottom Maintenance, *Trans Royal Institute of Naval Architects* 1980, pp 459–483.

Appendix 7-1
Running an Oil Tanker
This is a Mathcad model of the running of an oil tanker. It contains technical and cost sub-models and helps to find requirements for an anti-fouling system. The parameters are guessed!

Technical Model
The ship has dimensions:

depth	length	width	speed
$D_S := 20 \cdot m$	$L_S := 400 \cdot m$	$W_S := 44 \cdot m$	$v := 7 \cdot m \cdot s^{-1}$

The sea water and oil have densities:

$$\rho_W := 1000 \cdot kg \cdot m^{-3} \qquad \rho_O := 850 \cdot kg \cdot m^{-3}$$

The mass of oil transported by the ship is:

$$m_O := \rho_O \cdot D_S \cdot L_S \cdot W_S \qquad m_O = 3 \times 10^8 \ kg \qquad 300\,000 \text{ tons}$$

There are two drag forces working on the ship:

1. form drag, which is proportional to the cross sectional area:

$$F_{form} := 0.1 \cdot \frac{\rho_W \cdot v^2}{2} \cdot W_S \cdot D_S \qquad F_{form} = 2.2\times10^6 \text{ N}$$

2. skin drag, which is proportional to the longitudinal wetted area, and also depends on the skin roughness:

skin roughness $\qquad\qquad\qquad\qquad \delta_S := 10^{-3} \cdot \text{m}$

skin friction coefficient $\qquad\quad C_S := 0.03 \cdot \left(\dfrac{\delta_S}{W_{S+2 \cdot D_S}}\right)^{0.25}$

$$F_{skin} := C_S \cdot \frac{\rho W^{\cdot v^2}}{2} \cdot L_S \cdot (2 \cdot D_S + W_S) \quad F_{skin} = 1.5\times10^6 \text{N}$$

The form and skin friction coefficients are explained in books on Fluid Flow or Transport Phenomena (for example W. J. Beek et al. *Transport Phenomena*, Wiley 1999). We derived that for skin friction using data for rough tubes.

The fuel power required by the ship is then

propulsion efficiency $\qquad\qquad\qquad\qquad \eta := 0.4$

$$P_S := \frac{1}{\eta} \cdot (F_{form} + F_{skin}) \cdot v \qquad P_S = 63\times10^6 \text{ W} \qquad 63 \text{ MW}$$

Each roundtrip of the ship has a length.

$$L_T := 20 \cdot 10^3 \cdot \text{km}$$

So a trip requires

$$t_T := \frac{L_T}{v} \qquad t_T = 33\times10^0 \text{ day} \qquad 33 \text{ days, loading and unloading excluded}$$

Cost Model

The model considers fixed costs and variable costs (Lesson 12).

Fixed cost items are:

(1) capital cost (for borrowing money)
(2) depreciation cost (for replacing worn out ships)
(3) maintenance cost

(4) registration taxes
(5) personnel cost

We first define the cost unit: $\quad$ Euro $:= 1 \cdot C$

The price of the ship is $\quad c_S := 50 \cdot 10^6 \cdot$ Euro

For the first four costs we set aside a certain fraction of this:

$f_{cap} := 0.05$ $\qquad$ $f_{dep} := 0.05$ $\qquad$ $f_{maint} := 0.05$ $\qquad$ $f_{reg} := 0.02$

For the cost per person and the number of people required we take

$c_p := 50.10^3 \cdot$ Euro $\qquad$ $n_p := 40$ $\qquad$ not only the crew!

This yields a fixed cost:

$c_{fixed} := (f_{cap} + f_{maint} + f_{reg}) \cdot c_S + n_p \cdot c_p$
$c_{fixed} = 10.5 \times 10^6$ Euro $\qquad$ per year

The variable cost is that for fuel, with a price:

$p_{fuel} := 5.10^{-9} \cdot$ Euro $\cdot J^{-1}$

The ship runs 85% of the time, so the fuel energy required per year is:

$E_F := 0.85 \cdot (1 \cdot \text{yr}) \cdot P_S$ $\qquad$ $E_F = 1.693 \times 10^{15} J$

This yields a variable cost:

$c_{variable} := E_F \cdot p_{fuel}$ $\qquad$ $c_{variable} = 8.5 \times 10^6$ Euro

The total cost is then

$c_{total} := c_{fixed} + c_{variable}$ $\qquad$ $c_{total} = 19 \times 10^6$ Euro $\qquad$ per year

Cost per Mass of Oil

The number of trips made per year is:

$n_T := 0.85 \cdot \dfrac{1 \cdot \text{yr}}{t_T}$ $\qquad$ $n_T = 9 \times 10^0$

So the amount of oil transported is:

$$m_{OT} := n_T \cdot m_O \qquad m_{OT} = 2.8 \times 10^9 \text{ kg}$$

The cost per kg of oil is then:

$$c_O := \frac{c_{total}}{m_{OT}} \qquad c_O = 6.8 \times 10^{-3} \text{ Euro} \cdot \text{kg}^{-1}$$

The curves in Figure 7-4 were obtained by varying the parameters in this model.

Lesson 8: Select a Concept

With A. Bressendorff (Novo Nordisk A/S)

You have now created a large number of concepts for the new product and 'just' have to select the best one ... If only it were so simple; this is the point where many developments run into problems. Deciding what to develop – and what not – is far from easy. It can disrupt a team.

The first difficulty is that decisions have to be taken before you *have* the products. At this point you do not know enough to make a proper decision! A second difficulty is that one often has to compare ideas that are incomparable: ideas of a very different level. A third difficulty occurs when team members invest time in a certain concept, and become attached to it. If 'their baby' is killed this can lead to bad feelings. A fourth problem is not getting lost in the almost infinite number of ideas, variants and combinations that one might consider.

Trying to select from a number of concepts nearly always gives rise to new ideas – and often not the worst ones. It would be foolish not to consider these, but it does disrupt the selection process. All these things can lead to indecision in the team, bad feelings and political compromises – usually with poor results. In this lesson we discuss methods that can help. However, do not expect miracles. Decision making remains difficult, even with a good method.

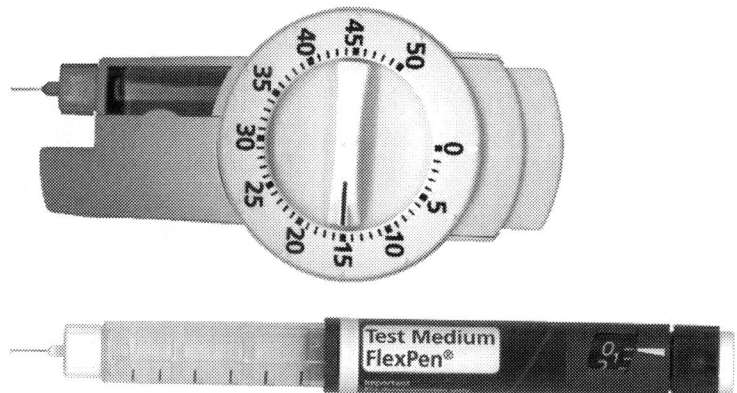

Figure 8-1 Dial and pen injectors for insulin (on the same scale)

Design and Development of Biological, Chemical, Food and Pharmaceutical Products J.A. Wesselingh, S. Kiil and M.E. Vigild

Treating Diabetes

The example we will use in this lesson is the selection of alternatives for treating the illness known as diabetes. This will lead to the most common method of this moment, where the patient treats himself with insulin injections. Figure 8-1 shows two current injector designs: 'dial' and 'pen'.

Insulin is a hormone (protein) that plays an important role in the regulation of the glucose level in our blood. More insulin causes this level to fall; less causes it to rise. It is important that the glucose level stays within certain limits, and so the insulin level has to be regulated. Insulin is formed in the pancreas, and is both excreted by and destroyed in the body. The body needs a certain base level, but during and after meals (when glucose is being taken up) the level needs a temporary increase. In the healthy body this all happens automatically. Not so in bodies of people with diabetes. For these people it is often essential that they have injections of insulin – a wrong level can be deadly.

Insulin was first extracted from the pancreas of cows and pigs in the 1920s. This first material was very impure, causing side effects. So manufacturers began a long campaign to produce purer insulin. They also managed to make the insulin long-lasting, so that patients could do with a single injection per day. Finally, they managed to get micro-organisms to produce human insulin – one of the first big successes of modern biotechnology. All these developments had occurred before 1980 and the marketing director of Novo, then a small Danish manufacturer, realized that there was little scope of improving the product further along these lines. However, the situation was far from perfect for diabetes patients. They needed injections once a day, which were painful. These long-lasting injections provided a constant insulin level in the blood, but this meant that normal eating habits were impossible. This made it difficult for patients to lead anything like a normal life.

Now suppose you are in the position of the marketing director. You have been gathering ideas from customers, co-workers and outsiders. Perhaps the team has also brainstormed. The ideas are summarized in the mind map of Figure 8-2.[1] In reality the list would probably be longer. This is quite a mess, so what to do?

---

[1] We have limited ourselves to this set of ideas: it is not difficult to generate more of them.

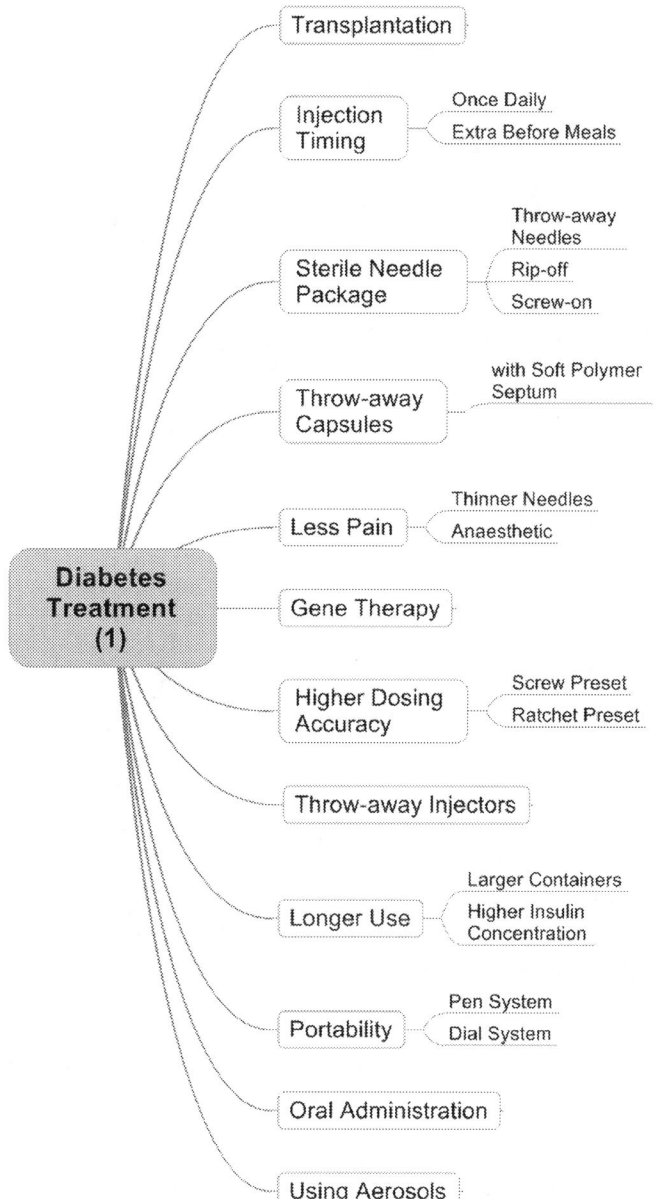

Figure 8-2 Ideas collected for diabetes treatment (further explanation in the text)

Explanation of Figure 8-2

Transplantation A possible way of dealing with diabetes would be to transplant cells or the complete organ that produces insulin in the body.

Multi-injection Treatment You have heard about experiments by a doctor in Scotland. The doctor has tried giving patients supplementary injections before meals: this allows more natural eating habits (Figure 8-3).

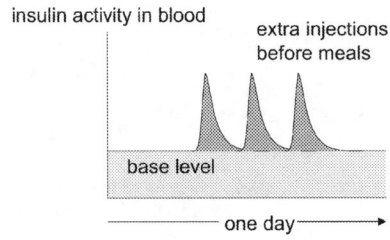

Figure 8-3 Using extra injections before meals

Improved Injection There are several suggestions for this:

(1) You might use throw-away insulin capsules with a septum: that would avoid filling of the injector.
(2) You could do the same with a throw-away injector.
(3) You might use throw-away needles: that would avoid cleaning of the needle. The needles would have to be in a sterile package, such that they could be attached to the injector without risk of contamination.
(4) You could make the injection less painful in several ways. One is to use very thin needles, a second to add an anaesthetic to the insulin. It might also help if you could reduce the force required for injection.
(5) You might improve the dosing accuracy with a good scale and by presetting the dose.

Injection by the Patient If you want the patient to do the injections, the injector should preferably be portable and have an easy and accurate setting of the insulin dose.

Oral Administration This means applying the insulin via the mouth (perhaps as a tablet).

Gene Therapy Insufficient production of insulin in the body is often caused by deficiencies in the genes of the patient. If these genes could be replaced, the sickness could be cured. The technique is being tried out in the lab, but so far with little success.

Aerosol Administration You have heard of a small start-up firm that is developing techniques to apply drugs via the lungs. The drug is sprayed to form a fine aerosol that is then inhaled.

The Top-Down Method

A method that often works for arranging the ideas in the selection process is called *top-down*. First decide which ideas to consider as the most *general* (Figure 8-4). Don't worry about the other ones (the *details*) – they come later.

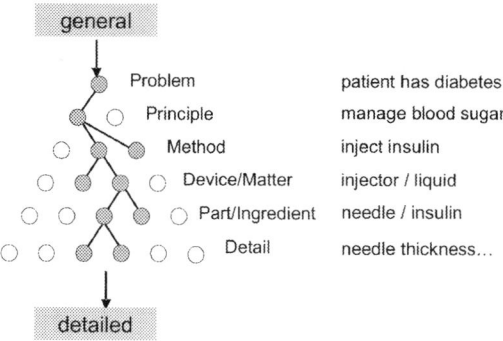

Figure 8-4 Arranging ideas from general to detailed

Then follow Figure 8-5. Scrap nonsense ideas, or ideas which will not work anyhow and tidy up the remaining list. Consider the remaining ideas separately as little projects and divide these among team members. Try to keep this number low (say less than seven). Investigate details of those solutions briefly. Then choose the most promising route or routes together.

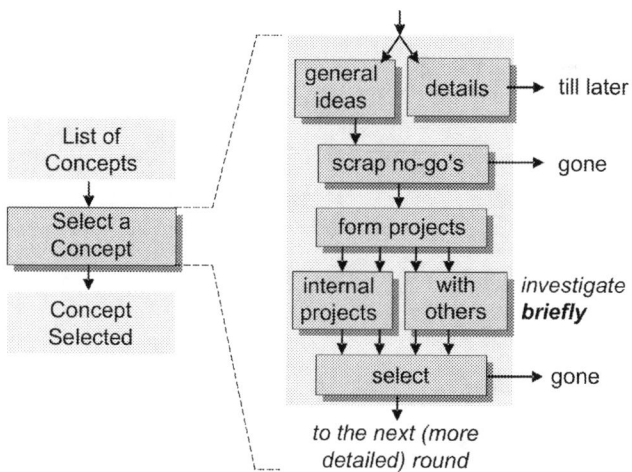

Figure 8-5 The top-down method of selecting

Now go further with your choice or choices, forming and investigating ideas on a more detailed level. Keep on scrapping the less attractive ideas. You may have to do this several times, but after a few rounds you will hopefully have a well chosen product.

The Diabetes Problem

Let us see how this works out for our diabetes problem. The only concept on the 'principle' level in Figure 8-4 is to manage sugar in the blood. There are several groups on the 'method' level: those that use insulin and those that do not (Figure 8-6). Those with insulin can be divided again into three, with insulin provided by injection, via the mouth and via the lungs. The other ideas are on the device, part or detail level.

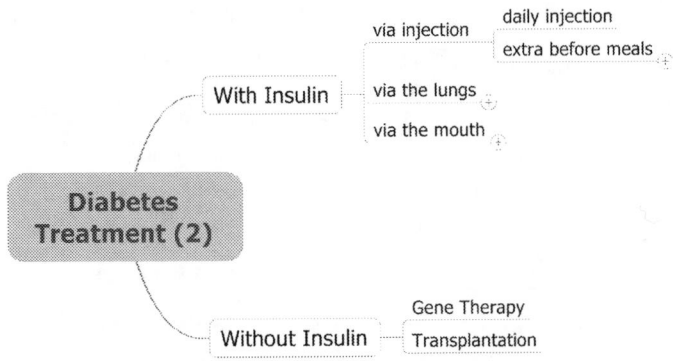

Figure 8-6 Ideas on the 'methods' level

We now try to scrap nonsense and 'no-go' ideas on the 'principle' level (Figure 8-7). In this scrapping you will need to use any information that you can get:

(1) your common sense and that of your fellow team members;
(2) an idea of the competences and interests of your firm;
(3) information from the project scope, list of needs and list of specifications;

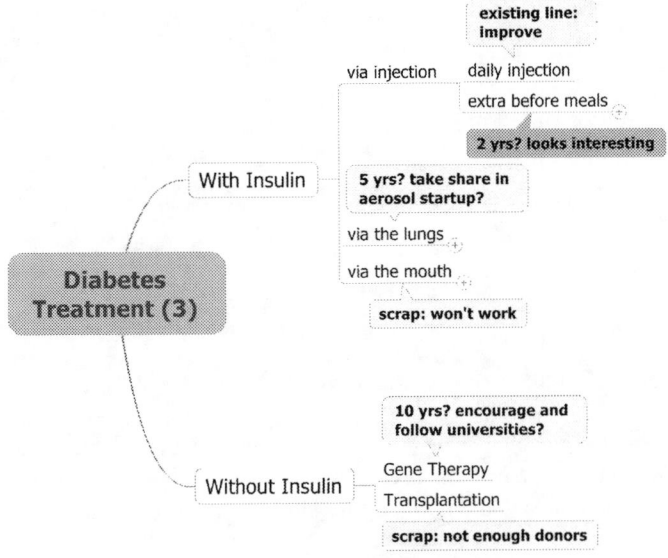

Figure 8-7 Scrapping of no-go ideas

(4) information from the Internet, journals, books and interviews;
(5) information from experience, calculations and experiments;
(6) and so on.

You quickly find that with the number of diabetes patients around, it is not probable that there will be enough donor organs – unless organs can be grown separately, but that seems a long way off. Scrap this possibility. A talk with people at university confirms that gene therapy will not be a solution within 10 years – also scrap this concept. A biochemist in the firm says that insulin will not permeate the stomach or intestine walls in an active form; you also have to scrap this idea. Information from the aerosol start-up tells that the idea looks promising. However, there is a lot to be worked out. You keep this idea on hold, but it does not look attractive on a medium term. The idea that looks as if it has most chance within a timescale of, say, 2 years is that of improving the injection method. It is a technology that you already know a lot about. This is the concept chosen to continue working on.

In this example it looks as if the method has worked well – you have narrowed the search to a single concept with relatively little work. Also the search is helping to form an idea of what the research and development program might look like. Things do not always work that well; it may be that you end with too many ideas or with none at all. Also the broad brush way of scrapping may cause one to overlook some important possibility.

Extra Injections Before Meals

You have now chosen the concept for diabetes treatment and need to work it out. The real advance will be when patients can look after themselves, and keep correct insulin levels in their blood also during and after meals. You look on the Internet, read anything you get hold of, talk with doctors, nurses and patients, and even try out a few injectors on yourself. You follow the experience of a few patients who are willing to try out the new method. You discuss what will be needed, and find out that the main requirements are:

(1) new rapid-working insulin,
(2) blood glucose monitoring by the user,
(3) insulin injections by the user and
(4) education and responsibility of the user.[2]

All these items will have to be in order if the concept is to succeed. You will need to get projects running on all four, but resources are limited, so you may not be able to do everything at the same time.

Already you are trying to get customers by listening to patients and trying to help. You are collecting data on the market to convince your bosses to go on.

Working Out Some Details

We now start looking at devices and matter in our concept, starting with the new injector. The existing injectors are simple instruments as in Figure 8-8. The patient sucks up the required amount of insulin solution from a bottle (vial) and injects it at a suitable point and a suitable

---

[2] It is important that the user gets good information, also on the dynamics of using 'fast and slow' insulins.

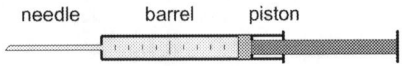

Figure 8-8 The existing injector

depth. Then the injector is cleaned to be used another time. The needles are coarse, and the injections painful.

You have interviewed patients, nurses and doctors to get hold of their needs, and realize that the new system will require something different. It will be hygienic – also when used by a patient who is not too handy. It should not be too painful because more injections are required. It will deliver a small amount, accurately dosed, also when applied by the not-too-handy patient. Finally it will be carried around by the patient, with a store of insulin sufficient for some time, say a few days or a week. These items are summarized in the short list of specifications in Figure 8-9.

metric	unit	marginal	ideal
hygiene	yes/no	yes	yes
pain	subjective	low	none
dosing	insulin units	2..30 ± 1	1..60 ± 0.1
long use	days	2	7
readability	letter size pt	14	20
cost	€	<10	<1

Figure 8-9 A first list of specifications

Figure 8-10 shows ideas that have been collected. There are two ideas to increase dosing accuracy: a screw preset to fix the amount injected and a ratchet preset, where the piston is pulled out a certain distance beforehand. The force for pushing the fluid through the needle should not be too large even when very thin needles are used. There are two proposals for this: using a screw and gears.

Again the list of ideas is a mess, but a little thought allows you to separate the three general ideas (Figure 8-11) into sub-projects

(1) the insulin solution,
(2) the injector itself, and
(3) the injection needle.

All other ideas can be seen as details of these sub-projects. The sub-projects can be largely tackled independently, although there are interfaces. For example, the size of the insulin container will depend on the insulin concentration of the solution, and the needle does have to fit on the injector.

Here you will again consider what can best be done internally and what externally. Designing the insulin solution clearly is the strong point of Novo, so that will be an internal project. You

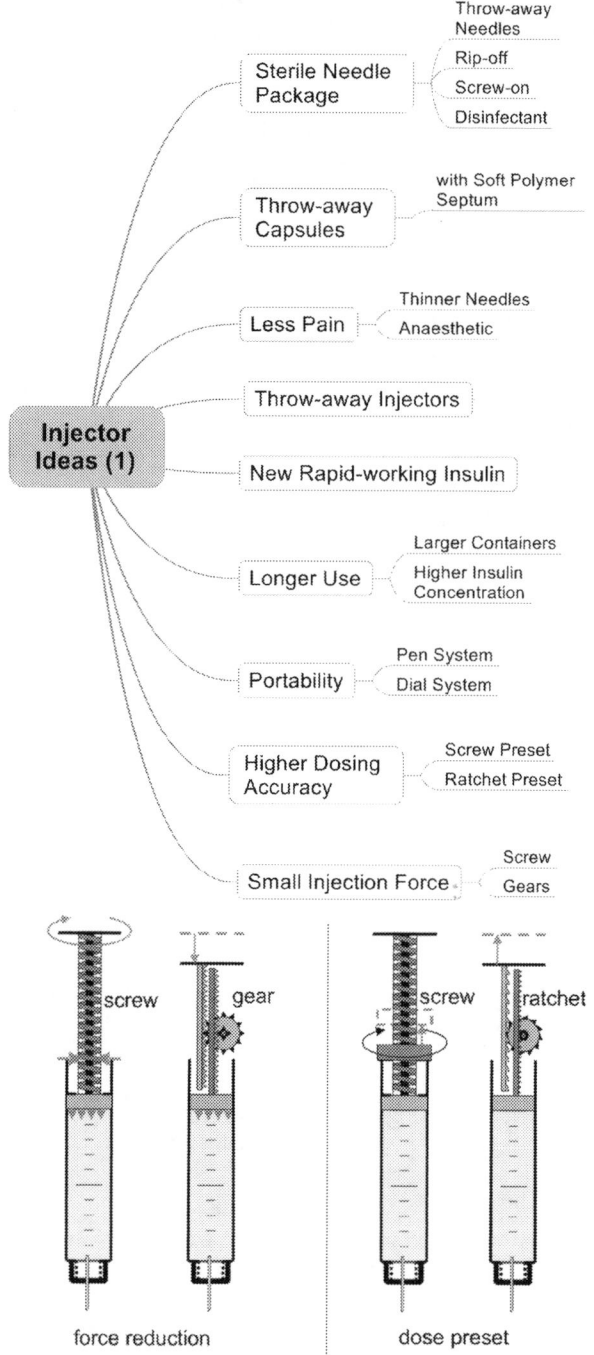

Figure 8-10 Ideas collected for improving injectors

would like to outsource the other projects because they are not 'core business'. However, it turns out to be difficult to get other firms interested, and most of this development will have to be done internally.

In the sub-projects (and perhaps sub-sub-projects) the problems become more and more detailed. Here we look at two techniques that are often used there:

(1) using engineering estimates and
(2) using concepts–criteria matrices.

Using Engineering Estimates

In much of design work, but certainly in the detailing stage, simple estimates can greatly help when taking decisions. As an example we look at the development of the needles. Experiments indicate that thin needles are less painful than thick ones. Indeed, the 'needle' of a mosquito is thought to be ideal. How thin could you make the needles? You get a good idea with the two sets of calculations in Appendix 8-1. These tell us that a needle that is too long and thin may buckle, and may require a force or time of injection that is too long. The calculations indicate that the needle cannot be made much thinner than about 0.3 mm. You prefer to find somebody who can make these needles: you do not want to do that as a pharmaceutical firm.

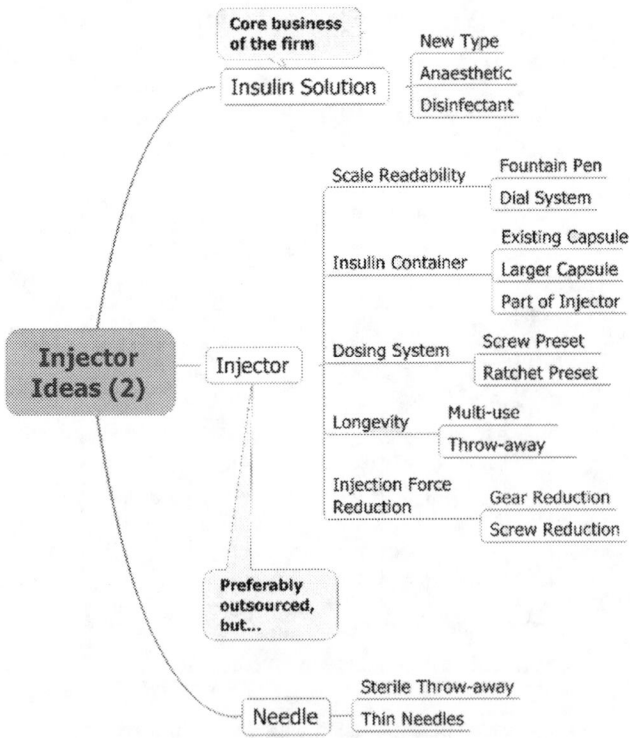

Figure 8-11 Ideas for the injector after rearranging

pen		
screw preset	gear reduction	A
	lever reduction	B
ratchet preset	gear reduction	C
	lever reduction	D
dial		
screw preset	gear reduction	E
	lever reduction	F
ratchet preset	gear reduction	G
	lever reduction	H

Figure 8-12 The remaining concepts[3]

Choosing with a Concepts–Criteria Matrix

For the injector there still is quite a list of ideas, and many of these can be combined. The question is which combination to choose. The trick again is to first scrap the no-goes: choices that you do not really have. For example, an important choice will be between throw-away injectors and those with replaceable cartridges. However, the first injectors will probably be rather expensive, so throw-away is not a good first choice. You may develop that later if the concept turns out to be a success. This means that you will need a capsule. You think (hope) you will be able to use the existing capsule, as there are a lot of other things to do . . . Somebody will have to check this; if not . . . Sterile single-use throw-away needles are going to be a must, so there is no choice there either. The remaining choices are those in Figure 8-12. There are eight possible combinations, which is a number that you can reasonably consider. You will do this using a 'concepts–criteria matrix'.

In reality you will now make more detailed sketches or models of the injectors so that everybody will know what is being discussed. However, we do not need these to explain the method.

Begin by defining *criteria*. Criteria include the most important customer needs, but can also include needs of the firm – such as ease of making (which is hardly relevant for customers). A need of the firm that is often included at this point is cost of manufacture, and there may be others. Choosing criteria is important: with more than five to seven criteria, discussions become difficult, so look at only those things that are really important. This will require some discussion in the team. Here you have chosen those in Figure 8-13.

Construct a matrix with the concepts along the horizontal axis and the criteria along the vertical axis (Figure 8-14). You can do this and the subsequent calculations in Excel. There

---

[3] The pen and dial systems are those from Figure 8-1. We have pitted these against each other to demonstrate the use of CC-matrices. Actually the dial was developed for patients with poor sight, which is often caused by diabetes.

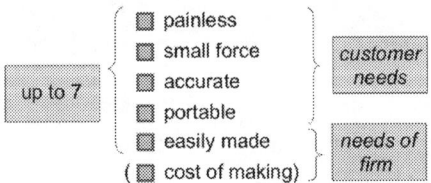

Figure 8-13 Criteria chosen for the injector

are two columns for each concept. Leave a column to the right for weights and a row at the bottom for adding up totals. Make a copy for all team members.

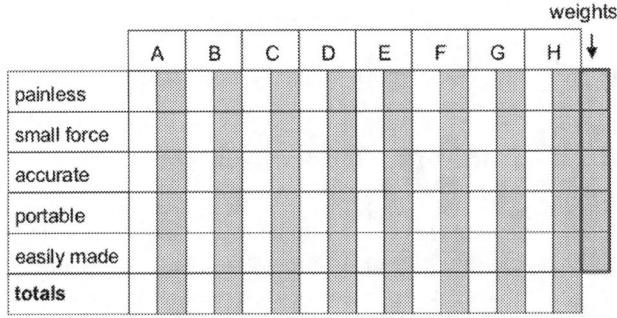

Figure 8-14 The concepts–criteria matrix

Before going on you must decide on:

(1) how to mark the concepts, and
(2) how to weight the criteria.

It is important to decide these things before going further.

Marking is best done on a scale with numbers and better-is-larger. It is important to standardize on this: the alternative first-is-best can lead to great confusion. Every team member will give a mark to each cell of each concept–criterion combination. There are three common ways (Figure 8-15):

(1) give a mark using some scale decided on beforehand,
(2) compare each concept with a reference concept, or
(3) distribute a given number of points for each criterion.

The first method is the simplest. If there is a concept that every team member knows, for example an existing design, it may be more accurate to use this as a reference for comparing. In our example the existing injector is not a good reference as it is poor on nearly all criteria. If you want to sift through large numbers of concepts without too much thinking and discussion beforehand the third method has its uses. Here each team member is allowed to distribute a

with a pre-decided scale		for comparing with a reference		for large lists
excellent	5	much better	2	distribute a number of points...
good	4	better	1	
adequate	3	the same	0	
poor	2	worse	-1	
terrible	1	much worse	-2	

Figure 8-15 Three ways for marking

fixed number of points (say ten) over each criterion (row). Often some constraint is put on this, for example that no criterion should get more than half of the points.

A criterion can be more or less important: this is reflected in the weight given to it. The more important the criterion, the higher the weight. Also here the choice of the scale is arbitrary; you might use

(3) very important,
(2) important,
(1) not very important.

Weights are often chosen such that they sum to 100%, but there is little reason for doing that.[4]

Each team member completes his matrix: one example is in Figure 8-16. He uses the second columns to multiply the results along the rows by the weights. Then the second columns are added: the columns with the highest markings are the ones preferred by the team member (Figure 8-16). This is a good point for a sensitivity check: seeing whether the figures have much meaning by varying the weights.

weights

	A		B		C		D		E		F		G		H		↓
painless	3	9	1	3	3	9	1	3	3	9	1	3	3	9	1	3	3
small force						all the same											
accurate	3	3	3	3	3	3	3	3	4	4	4	4	4	4	4	4	1
portable	4	8	4	8	4	8	4	8	3	6	3	6	3	6	3	6	2
easily made	5	5	3	3	5	5	3	3	4	4	3	3	4	4	3	3	1
totals		25		17		25		17		23		20		24		16	

Figure 8-16 A completed matrix

---

[4] You can dream up other variants. The details are not important, as long as everybody uses the same method. The main reason for the exercise is to force the team to compare alternatives and to discuss.

The team then compares the different outcomes, and uses these to discuss which concept or concepts to develop further. The discussion *is* important, as the decision that you take has large consequences for the development phase of the project. Development is usually by far the most work, so a wrong decision here is serious. Is everybody happy with the result? If not, what are the reasons why? If one person knows more about a certain problem than the others there may be good reasons to listen carefully and change the choice. You may also find that you do not really know enough about some concepts. Then you will either

(1) have to take a risk or
(2) spend more time and redo the whole procedure.

You will also have to go back if better ideas or combinations come up during the discussion. Good teams learn to do these things quickly.

There is one other reason why the discussion is important: it always leads to turning down of proposals. It is easier for a team member to accept this if she understands why. It is important that the whole team accepts the decision.

At the end of this exercise you will have made a decision which product you are going to develop. (Even now, there is no guarantee that you will not come up later with a new, marvellous idea.)

Summary

To select the final concept from your list, use the following steps:

(1) Select the general ideas (put the detailed ones aside).
(2) Scrap the nonsense and no-go ideas.
(3) Arrange the remaining ideas in what might become projects. Consider who might be involved in these.
(4) Get more information and briefly work out project plans.
(5) Select using the limited information that you have.
(6) Go into the next (more detailed) round of designing using the same method, and so on until you have a good choice and a rough development plan.
(7) Techniques useful in making choices are engineering estimation and concepts–criteria matrices.

Further Reading

Karl T. Ulrich and Steven D. Eppinger *Product Design and Development*, 3rd edition, McGraw-Hill 2003, Chapter 7.

E. L. Cussler and G. D. Moggridge *Chemical Product Design*, Cambridge University Press 2001, Chapter 4.

N. F. M. Roozenburg and J. Eekels *Product Design: Fundamentals and Methods*, Wiley 1995, Chapter 9. Discusses different evaluation and decision methods.

Jørn Rex *The NovoPen® Story*, Novo Nordisk A/S 2003.
(*Hvordan finder man på at lave en NovoPen®?*)

Historical Remark

We would like to end with one experience from the real Novo story. As you remember it started with a marketing director having the idea of patients looking after their own injections before meals. It was not all that simple to get it running.

Research and Development in Novo was dominated by medical and biological scientists, and they were not enthusiastic. Medication by a patient was against medical traditions, and why would you want to develop a rapid-working insulin after you had spent 40 years developing a long-lasting one? The marketing director could not get R&D to work on this project, and for lack of better he went to the manufacturing department. This was a large department with hundreds of people running fermenters, purification and packaging equipment. These people did get the idea and started developing it, without a budget and more-or-less unauthorized. It was not easy, but they soon realized that they were on to something important. We will not describe their struggles, but they succeeded in getting their ideas accepted in the firm. Already the first of their products – the NovoPen – was a great success.

Appendix 8-1

The example below shows two engineering calculations that can be very useful for setting specifications, to help choose design parameters, and in helping reduce the amount of experimental work in development.

Injection Needle

One of the secrets to the success of the NovoPen has been the use of very thin needles (Figure 8-17). It is interesting to check how close they are to their limit. The needles must extend 6 to 8 millimetres to inject insulin at a proper depth. Then there are two probable limitations:

1. if the needle is thin it will buckle too easily,
2. if the channel is thin, the force on the piston will be large.

Let us have a look how close the current design is to these limits.

Buckling

We can predict the force at which buckling will occur using a formula from Euler:

$$F = 2 \cdot \pi \cdot \frac{E \cdot I}{L^2}$$

This is for a thin column with one fixed and one free support (a cantilever). Here E is the modulus of elasticity or stiffness, I is the second moment of area and L is the length of the

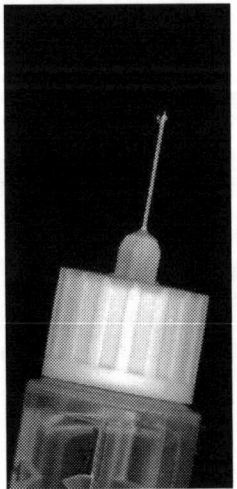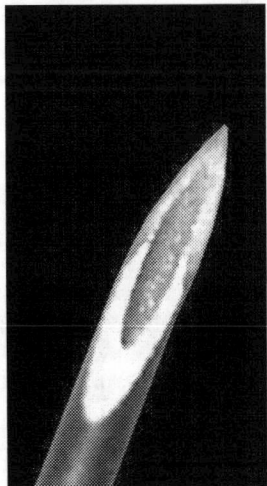

Figure 8-17 The NovoPen needle

profile. We have it from J.E. Gordon *Structures, or why things don't fall down*, Penguin 1978, still the most readable introduction into structural engineering.

For a tube with radius r and thickness w:

$$I = \frac{\pi}{4} \cdot [r^4 - (r-w)^4]$$

A few figures:

$$E := 2 \cdot 10^{11} \cdot N \cdot m^{-2} \quad \text{for steel}$$

$$r := 0.15 \cdot 10^{-3} \cdot m \quad w := 0.08 \cdot 10^{-3} \cdot m \quad L := 8 \cdot 10^{-3} \cdot m$$

This yields a buckling force:

$$I := \frac{\pi}{4} \cdot [r^4 - (r-w)^4] \quad F := 2 \cdot \pi \cdot \frac{E \cdot I}{L^2} \quad F = 7.4 \, N$$

This is a magnitude that one would expect if the pen were pressed by accident on a hard surface, so we are indeed close to this limit.

Force Needed for Injection

The syringe is to deliver a maximum dose of 0.60 mL in a fairly short time–say two seconds. We will calculate the force required on the piston.

The pressure difference along the needle is given by the Poiseuille equation:

$$\Delta p = 8 \cdot \frac{\eta \cdot L' \cdot v}{(r-w)^2}$$

Here Δp is the pressure difference along the capillary, η the viscosity of the liquid, r and w are as before, and L$'$ is the flow length in the capillary. The volume transferred in time t is:

$$V = \pi \cdot (r - w)^2 \cdot v \cdot t \quad \text{so} \quad v = \frac{V}{\pi \cdot (r - w)^2 \cdot t}$$

The piston has a diameter D and the force on it will be:

$$F = \frac{\pi}{4} \cdot D^2 \cdot \Delta p = 2 \cdot \frac{\eta \cdot V \cdot L' \cdot D^2}{(r - w)^4 \cdot t}$$

The viscosity will be at least as high as that of water (probably higher):

$$\eta := 10^{-3} \cdot \text{Pa} \cdot \text{s}$$

Part of the capillary is inside the needle holder, so the flow length is longer that that of the protrustion of the needle:

$$L' := 12 \cdot 10^{-3} \cdot \text{m}$$

and the other values are:

$$V := 0.6 \cdot 10^{-6} \cdot \text{m}^3 \quad t := 2 \cdot \text{s} \quad D := 9.4 \cdot 10^{-3} \cdot \text{m}$$

This gives

$$F := 2 \cdot \frac{\eta \cdot V \cdot L' \cdot D^2}{(r - w)^4 \cdot t} \quad F = 26 \text{ N}$$

Even this lower limit is substantial: the weight of two and a half kilograms. The force rises rapidly if we try thinner channels; we cannot make them much thinner.

Lesson 9: Protect the Concept

With G. Kontogeorgis and G.A. Pogany

As soon as you seriously start to think about developing a concept, begin to protect your work. Ensure that you can benefit from what you develop, and try to make it difficult for others to do so. Nearly all countries have a legal system to make this possible, but the ways are not easy or straightforward.

There are several ways in which a firm can protect itself. These make use of three kinds of intellectual properties:

(1) trade secrets
(2) patents and
(3) publications.

In addition the firm can register trade names and trademarks. SHELL is a name; the shell emblem is a mark. Aspirin is a name; the BAYER cross is a mark (Figure 9-1). You may also use copyright, which restricts the copying of written, printed or artistic material. Intellectual property rights can be to your advantage, or disadvantage (especially when others own them). To avoid getting into trouble, you must find out what your position is.

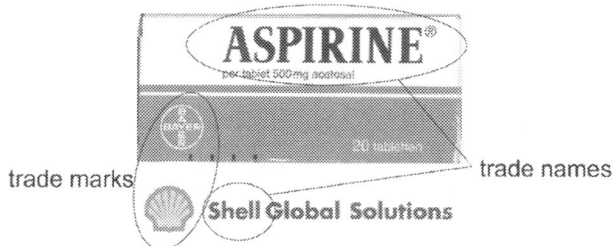

Figure 9-1 Trade marks and trade names

Trade Secrets

Trade secrets (or know-how) are what the name says: secrets. Anything used to make or sell your product that is not disclosed to outsiders is a trade secret. This even includes things like a list of customers. You can try to keep things secret by only informing small numbers of

Design and Development of Biological, Chemical, Food and Pharmaceutical Products   J.A. Wesselingh, S. Kiil and M.E. Vigild
© 2007 John Wiley & Sons, Ltd

people, and having them under contract not to tell others.[1] However, if they do, you can only sue them personally, and that may hardly be worth the trouble. Another problem with trade secrets emerges when they are patentable. Anyone who finds out can patent your secret and make it difficult for *you* to use it! Even so, most protection relies for a large part on trade secrets: on the competition not knowing how you do things. With modern analysis methods one can find composition, but even then it is often impossible to find out how things have been made.

Patents

If parts of your product or process are 'useful, novel and non-obvious', you may be able to patent them. Patents are the most complicated of the intellectual rights. A patent is a contract between government and inventor. The inventor discloses to the public how to do certain novel things; in response the government gives a right to the inventor to stop others from using his invention, typically for a period of 20 years. Patents can cover most of the things we consider when developing a product: the process, the machines, the product, its composition . . .

Before we go into details, one important remark about patents. One can only patent things that are not public knowledge at the moment of the patent application (Figure 9-2). This means that you must keep your own doings secret until you apply for the patent. Any *prior* public knowledge can invalidate the application even after a patent has been granted. So a product that you wish to patent should not be sold before the patent application. This is also the reason why companies often appear so paranoid about publications and conferences. Meetings between people who are under a *signed* secrecy agreement are not considered to be public; to avoid problems reports have to be *handled* as confidential. It is not sufficient to mark them as such.

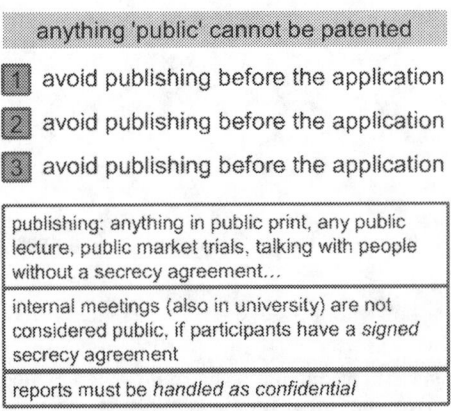

Figure 9-2 Avoid disclosure before applying!

Showing that an invention could be useful is usually not a problem. If it is not useful, don't patent! However, showing that an invention is novel and non-obvious to people in the field of

---

[1] This is a good reason why firms want loyal personnel.

the invention is a different matter. The inventor has to show that the invention is not described in an existing patent or other public literature. He also has to show that the invention is not obvious to a person knowledgeable in the field. Experimental proof that the invention works will be required. The preparation (Figure 9-3) may require several years. This all has to be shown to the officials who decide whether a patent will be granted. The officials will look critically at the proposal, and often want changes. Everything has to be reported in well-defined legal forms. The final application might take another year.

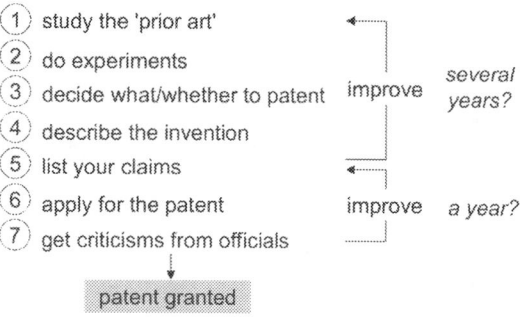

Figure 9-3 How to prepare a patent

A good patent will claim a lot of things (Figure 9-4). It may claim a new product, a new process and a new application. There might be 25 claims or more, listed from wide to narrow. The inventor tries to make the first claims as wide as possible. However, a claim must work: if the wider claim does not, it can be abandoned in favour of the narrower ones.

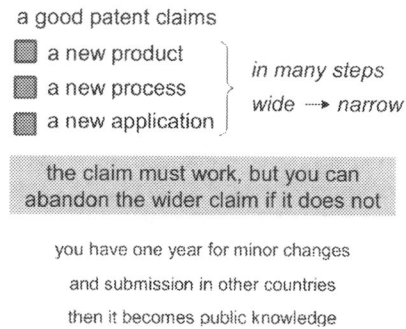

Figure 9-4 The many claims in a patent

Once the patent is granted,[2] the inventor has several rights. He decides who *cannot* use the patent. He can licence it to others, typically for a fee of a few per cent of the turnover generated. The inventor can cede or sell the rights to others. Finally, he is allowed to enforce his rights. But he must do that himself: find out whether others infringe his patent, inform the infringer, pay lawyers, negotiate, set up a lawsuit . . . The police will not do this for him!

---

[2] 'Patent pending' on a product may mean very little.

A patent also has its disadvantages. The owner has to maintain it – usually by annual payments, which often increase in time. When the patent is maintained in many countries this can become expensive: up to €100 000 over the life of the patent. If others challenge the patent, it may have to be defended in court. There is always a chance that competitors will be able to show that the patent was granted on poor grounds and that it is declared invalid. A patent application often gives away more information than is realized by the applicant. Finally: competitors will be looking for loopholes in the patent; for ways to work around it. And you will be doing that with their patents. If you are not too certain about a patent, you can avoid a lot of trouble by licensing it to your competitors!

You will have realized that there is another downside to patents. Also others have them, and not only your competitors. If you infringe their patents, they can sue *you*. This can even happen when you do not realize that you are infringing. So find out what the rights of others are.

A few final words on legal aspects of patents. Infringing a patent is not a criminal act, although the lawyers of patent owners will do their best to let you feel bad if they find out. Patent infringement is part of civil law: any legal processes have to be started by the patent owner as we have already noted.

Infringement can be *very* expensive for the infringer. This is especially so if the infringement can be shown to be wilful. The infringer must reckon on having to recall product, to pay licensing costs, and to pay the cost of the legal process. Legal processes are risky for both parties, and expensive. So they are often settled out of court.

Publications

The third way to protect intellectual property is by publication. A publication is any knowledge that is made available to the public – not only articles in academic journals! You might wonder how you could use publication to protect yourself. The answer is that publication prevents anybody – also competitors – from patenting. There are many cases where you do not need more. Information *in* a patent, which is not part of the claims, is a publication just like anything else. Also this will prevent anybody from patenting the knowledge.

Which methods of protection should you use? That depends (Figure 9-5). If you want to prevent others from using your knowledge, either keep it secret or patent it. If you want to prevent others from patenting, either patent the knowledge or publish it. Do remember: patents are expensive, and there is no guarantee that you will get them.

To protect yourself you need a combination of these methods. The ideal is that:

(1) you can do what is needed, using public information, own patents, licences, knowledge, know-how . . .

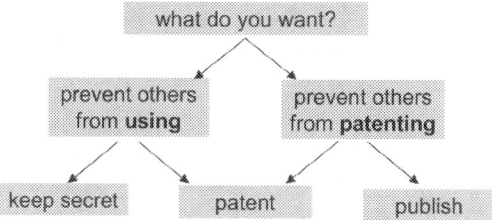

Figure 9-5 Which methods?

(2) you can make it difficult for competitors by having patents in a few key areas and keeping secrets in other areas;

(3) you can do this with a minimum of fuss and cost.

'Secrecy' has to be balanced, as you must keep your surroundings informed of what you are doing!

A patent typically gives 20 years of protection. This may seem a lot. However, look at the, rather extreme, example of the pharmaceutical industry (Figure 9-6). Say that preparing the application takes 2 years; it may take another year before the patent is granted. Approval of the product – with many tests on patients – may take 10 years. You then have 10 years of protection left, for an investment that has taken 13 years to develop. There is a lot of pressure to apply late, to extend the protected time. However, this does have its risks, as competitors may sneak in and patent your ideas. It is up to you to decide.

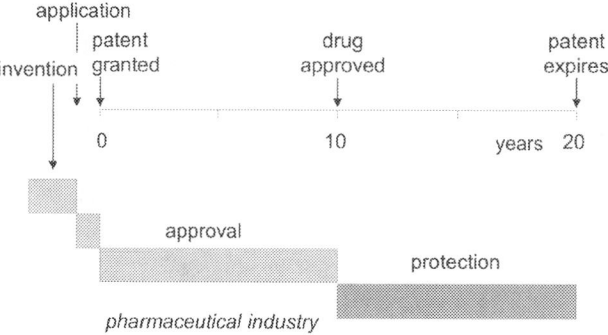

Figure 9-6 Protection of a pharmaceutical product

A Warning

This lesson has introduced protecting: don't assume that you now know the subject. For one thing patent rules differ in different countries: what is described here is roughly the European situation. That of the United States differs on several points.

Realize that patent laws are *rules*: there is some rationality behind them, but also a lot of politics and history. You have to learn to understand these rules. Do not expect them to have much in common with your 'feeling of justice'. Another problem is that they are stated in the language of Legalese. This can look like everyday language, but it uses terms that are more strictly defined. Its meanings are subject to interpretation by courts (jurisprudence). Don't try to find your own way. Protection is a minefield for engineers – do it together with lawyers.

A final word on the value of patents. A patent can greatly increase the value of a business. So when starting a business there are good reasons to try to patent the essential parts. However, a patent on its own – without a business – is seldom worth much. Most patents *cost* money. Most firms need patents to keep on working. They may use them to have a position in negotiations. They may licence (part of) their patents. Only a few firms, mainly development ones, regard patents as core business.

Summary

1. When you develop a concept protect the work, so that you can exploit it and (preferably) competitors cannot.
2. There are three main ways of protecting yourself:
    (a) by keeping the work secret (know-how);
    (b) by patenting the work;
    (c) by publishing the work.
3. The disadvantage of trade secrets is that others may find out (and may even patent your work). However, many things are not patentable, but can be kept secret . . .
4. You can patent a product or process that is useful, novel and non-obvious. This gives you the right to deter the use of the patent by others for a period of (usually) 20 years.
5. Patents are expensive: you have to maintain and defend them.
6. By publishing your work you make it impossible for others to patent that work at a later date.
7. Protection is a minefield for people who are not at home in patent law.

Further Reading

A fairly good introduction:

K. T. Ulrich and S. D. Eppinger *Product Design and Development*, 3rd edition, McGraw-Hill 2003, Chapter 14.

You will probably have access to the major US and European patent databases in your university library. Have a look.

Part 3 **Develop**

You have a concept and the approval to develop it. This part discusses important things to be done – formulating the product and setting up the process with its equipment. You will have started this earlier – here it has to be worked out.

Lesson 10:
Formulate the Product

With M.A. Wesselingh (formerly with UCB)

Your first real product will usually be made in the laboratory. That is the place to develop the recipe for full scale production. Experimenting in the lab takes much less time and is much cheaper than on a full scale. The laboratory techniques used in product development are no different from those used in chemical research and education. However, there are differences in the way you need to organize experiments. In research and education, you can choose freely which variables you want to investigate. This is not so in product development. In product development you must try to get a feeling for the effect of all important variables. If you miss any, there is a large chance that competitors will find your weak spot. However, you must be clever if you want to 'investigate everything' with limited means and a limited amount of time.

Powder Coatings

As an example we look at the development of a powder coating for a refrigerator (Figure 10-1). You can often see whether you are dealing with such a coating by looking *along* the surface. You will see that it is not quite smooth, but has little bumps left from the melting of the powder particles. The photograph does not catch this 'orange peel' very well; you can better have a look yourself. The bumps are not simply those of the individual particles: the bumps are larger.

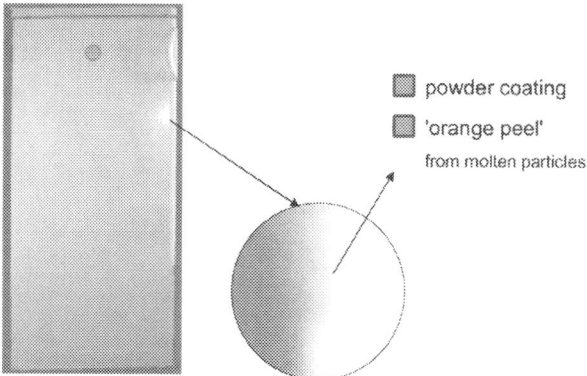

Figure 10-1 Door of a refrigerator

Design and Development of Biological, Chemical, Food and Pharmaceutical Products J.A. Wesselingh, S. Kiil and M.E. Vigild
© 2007 John Wiley & Sons, Ltd

The big advantage of powder coatings over paints is that they use no solvents; coating material that is not used, can be recycled.[1] This yields a low price and is better for the environment. In addition, powder coatings allow a fairly thick layer to be applied in one go. A big problem in the development of powder coatings was the conflicting requirements for flow (melting) and reaction. To solve these required a good concept and a large experimental program.

Three main components for the final polymer layer are shown in Figure 10-2. They are a di-ol (here neo-pentyl-glycol, NPG) and two di-acids (terephthalic acid, TPA and isophthalic acid, IPA). Together they are to form a linear polyester (that will later be cross-linked).

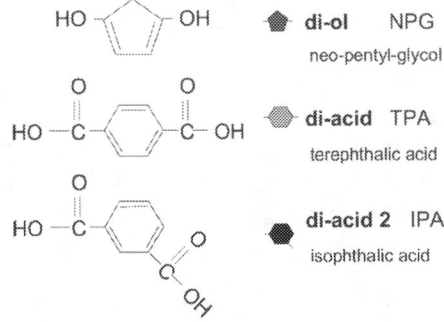

Figure 10-2 Three monomers for the polyester

The polyester is formed in two steps. In the first (Figure 10-3) NPG and TPA react to form a polyester. This happens at 240 °C where both the polymer and the monomers are liquids. The water formed is removed by vaporization through a refluxer. The average length of the polymer chain depends on the ratio of the amounts of reactants. With the numbers shown, we get an average chain length of 19 groups with hydroxyl groups at the end (check that you understand). The first step has to use an excess of di-ol, otherwise the reactants do not mix well. The polymer has a distribution of chain lengths, but we do not consider that further.

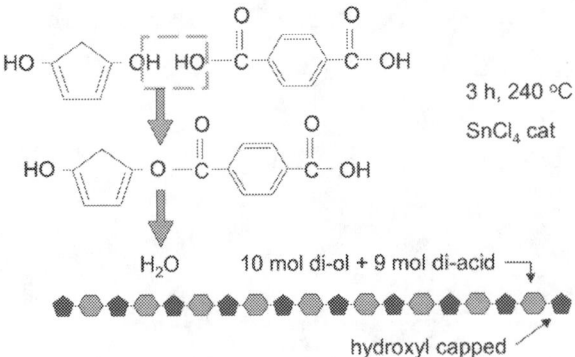

Figure 10-3 The first step in the polymerization

---

[1] However, you cannot use powder to coat a tanker, as you would have to place the whole ship in an oven.

In the second step (Figure 10-4) we add just enough IPA to cause the polymers to become acid-capped. We use IPA and not TPA; IPA makes the chain less regular, so that it will not crystallize (crystalline polymers are difficult to process). The melt is then cooled and milled to a powder.

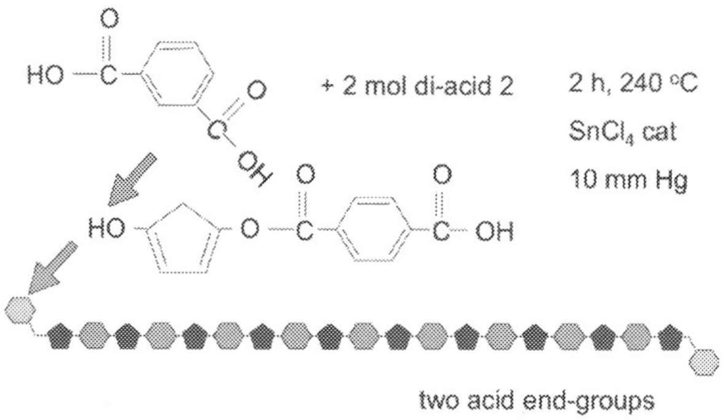

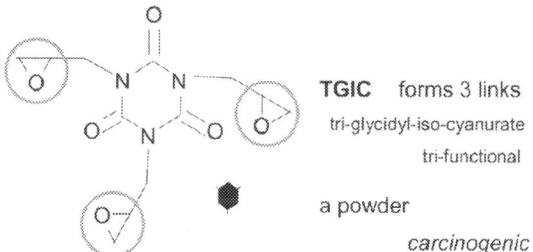

Figure 10-4 The second step in the polymerization

Thermoplastic films from linear polyesters do not have good mechanical and chemical properties. These are obtained by cross-linking. The cross-linker used in our example is tri-glycidyl-iso-cyanurate or TGIC (Figure 10-5). It is a solid at room temperature, and made in the form of a powder. It has to be handled carefully because it is carcinogenic. The final polymer product is not!

Figure 10-5 The cross-linker for the final polymer

TGIC and polyester powders are mixed intimately in an extruder at about 120 °C. At this point other components such as pigments can be added, but we do not consider that further. The result is milled to get the powder that is used for the coating. Figure 10-6 shows a schematic picture of the particles we get. The extruder is operated below the melting temperature of all components. As a result, the particles of polyester and TGIC stick together, but do not mix on a molecular scale. *This is essential to avoid cross-linking before the powder is applied.* We can distinguish four parameters in the design of the powder particle: the diameter of the powder particle, the diameter of the polyester particles, the diameter of the TGIC particles and the volume fraction occupied by TGIC.

The cross-linking reaction (Figure 10-7) only starts above the melting temperature of the powder, but then it is rapid. It takes only 100 s at 220 °C. So there is only a short time for the molten particles to spread out and form a closed flat layer of polymer.

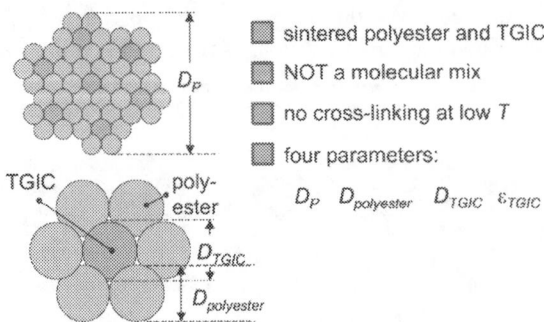

Figure 10-6 Particles before application

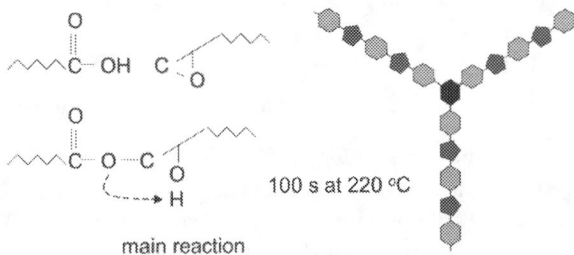

Figure 10-7 The cross-linking reaction

Your Job

That was the introduction. Now you are to find conditions for getting a good film; these are to become the full scale production recipe.

Before beginning your experimental program seriously, it is usually a good idea to spend a bit of time on orienting yourself – *by experiment*. You may already have done this in an earlier stage of development, for example when selecting a concept. If not, now is the time. We cannot give many guidelines on how to do this. You may use your own experience or that of others around you. Sometimes literature can give a starting point. Then you must get laboratory techniques to work – including analysis methods – and find conditions that make a product that is good enough to start improving. A few experiments with extreme conditions may help to find limits to the space to investigate. Otherwise, we can only wish you patience and good luck.

As an engineer, you have been taught to work systematically. So you may be tempted to investigate your design space systematically by doing experiments that cover the whole range of variables. However, this is not a good idea. Figure 10-8 shows important variables in the design of the powder. There are 12 of them, and the list is not complete. For example, we have omitted all variables of the extrusion process, the spraying process, the influence of pigment and additives, and of the preparation of the substrate. If you want five measurements per variable, you will need 5^{12} experiments. At one experiment per day that will take 700 000 years. Forget it. You need a different approach.

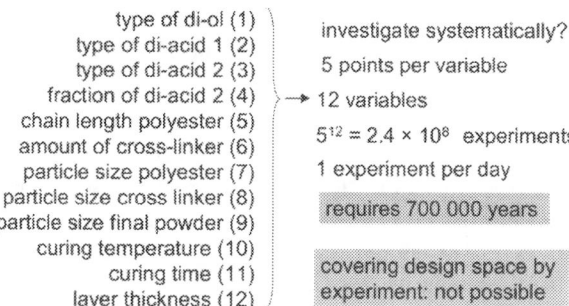

type of di-ol (1)
type of di-acid 1 (2)
type of di-acid 2 (3)
fraction of di-acid 2 (4)
chain length polyester (5)
amount of cross-linker (6)
particle size polyester (7)
particle size cross linker (8)
particle size final powder (9)
curing temperature (10)
curing time (11)
layer thickness (12)

investigate systematically?

5 points per variable

→ 12 variables

$5^{12} = 2.4 \times 10^8$ experiments

1 experiment per day

requires 700 000 years

covering design space by experiment: not possible

Figure 10-8 Handling twelve variables systematically

Limiting Experimental Work

There are several ways to reduce the amount of experimental work, and combining them can be very effective. First try to understand how the product is to work. We have already described that for our example. This helps to split off parts of the work that are independent – parts that can be studied on their own. Another way to reduce the number of experiments is to use models of the process or parts of it to find suitable starting values. Then we have seen that systematic coverage of the design space is not an efficient way of finding the best solution: there are better search methods. Finally, it is often possible to do many experiments simultaneously. Together these techniques can reduce the time needed enormously, and that is just as well.

Setting up an experimental program is usually iterative – you learn to understand your problem while working on it. You will find out later which experiments could have been avoided – don't have the illusion that you can plan this.

Figure 10-9 gives a repetition of our understanding of the process. The powder is sprayed on the cold substrate; it adheres because it has been charged electrically. The substrate with adhering powder goes into a curing oven, where it is heated above the softening temperature of the polyester. This causes two things:

(1) polyester flows and spreads over the substrate, and
(2) TGIC diffuses into the polymer and starts cross-linking.

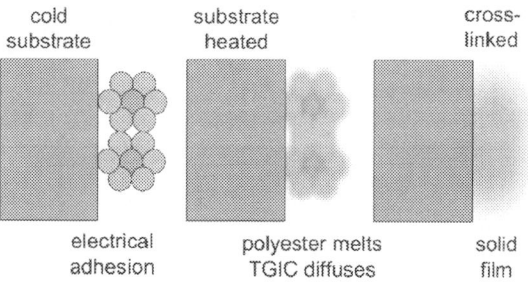

cold substrate · substrate heated · cross-linked

electrical adhesion · polyester melts TGIC diffuses · solid film

Figure 10-9 Forming of the final film

We end with a solid cross-linked film. (The powder particle is drawn as if it contains a single TGIC particle. It actually contains a large number of these.)

You can greatly reduce the number of variables to test by one simple observation (Figure 10-10). The film needs to have certain values for elasticity, impact strength and softening temperature. These are properties of the bulk polymer, and they also apply to the film. Look for polymers with the desired properties separately (for example in literature), and then choose one or two of them. This eliminates the first six variables from the coating program. In passing, note that the amount of cross-linker has to be just sufficient to link all of the polyester. So the volume fraction of TGIC in the powder is fixed by the choice of the chain length (it has a value of a few per cent).

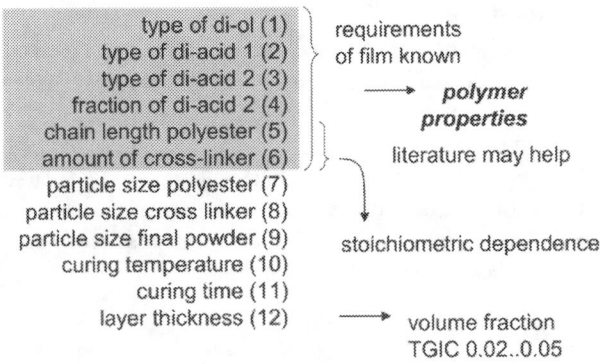

Figure 10-10 Removing the first six variables

We next look at the dimensions in our powder particle (Figure 10-11). As we have seen, there are three of them:

(1) the diameter of the particle,
(2) the diameter of the cross-linker sub-particle, and
(3) the diameter of the polyester sub-particle.

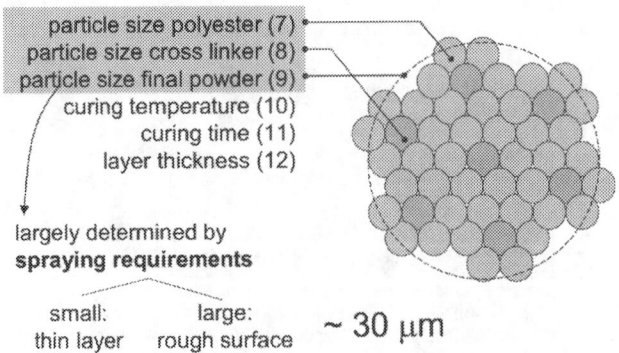

Figure 10-11 Dimensions in the particle

The first two are important; for the last one it is only important that the polyester is fine enough to allow a good distribution of the cross-linker throughout the particle. You take its diameter equal to that of the cross-linker sub-particle. To get an idea of the optimal particle size, you will need to analyse the spraying operation. We will not do that here; we only note that it requires particles of the order of 30 µm in diameter. The spraying analysis will also tell us that the maximum layer thickness is a few times the diameter of the particles.

When the powder particle melts, it wets the substrate (Figure 10-12). The liquid is pulled over the surface by a line tension σ. This depends on the interfacial tensions of liquid, solid and gas; it is lower than the surface tension. This tension is counteracted by forces due to the viscosity η. The flattening will also depend on the initial size R_0 of the drop. Finally you would expect the drop to become flatter with increasing time t.

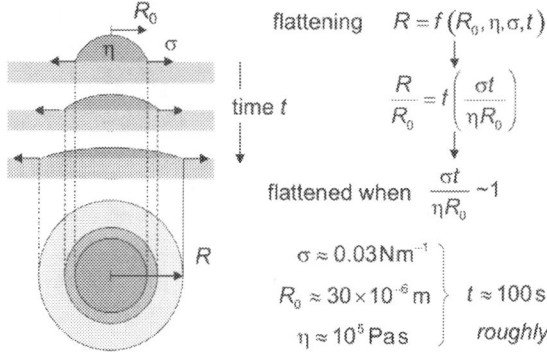

$$\text{flattening} \quad R = f(R_0, \eta, \sigma, t)$$

$$\frac{R}{R_0} = f\left(\frac{\sigma t}{\eta R_0}\right)$$

$$\text{flattened when} \quad \frac{\sigma t}{\eta R_0} \sim 1$$

$$\left.\begin{array}{l} \sigma \approx 0.03\,\text{Nm}^{-1} \\ R_0 \approx 30 \times 10^{-6}\,\text{m} \\ \eta \approx 10^{5}\,\text{Pas} \end{array}\right\} \begin{array}{l} t \approx 100\,\text{s} \\ \textit{roughly} \end{array}$$

Figure 10-12 Melting and flattening of a particle[2]

Dimensional Analysis

One can learn more by using *dimensional analysis*.[3] This assumes that the two sides of the first equation must have the same dimensions. If you make the left side (the flattening) dimensionless, as in the second equation, then the right side must also be so. This is only possible when the flattening is a function of the dimensionless group in the right side of the second equation. This shows the right kind of behaviour: flattening increases with time; it happens more rapidly when the wetting tension is larger, and more slowly with a higher viscosity, or with larger drops.

Experience also tells that interesting things often happen when dimensionless groups attain a value of about one.[4] Here flattening will be substantial when the right hand number has this value. For typical values of our parameters, we find a flattening time of the order of 100 s. This is a rough estimate, but much better than nothing.

---

[2] When working on a new subject you must learn to guess values such as those in Figure 10-12.
[3] For more on Dimensional Analysis see Further Reading section.
[4] There is a lot more behind this than we can cover here.

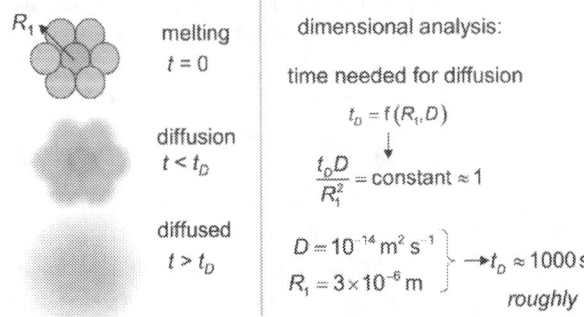

Figure 10-13 Time required for diffusion[5]

Flattening stops when the polymer gets cross-linked. This will not happen before TGIC has diffused into the polymer. You can again estimate how long that takes using dimensional analysis (Figure 10-13). First the polymer melts. Then the TGIC starts diffusing into the polymer. When enough has diffused over a distance R_1 (one half of the distance between the TGIC particles) diffusion will be complete. The time t_D required only depends on the distance and the diffusivity D. There is one way to get both sides of the equation dimensionless, as in the second equation. Diffusion is complete when the group of variables in this equation has a value of one. For a diffusion distance of 3 μm the cross-linking time is of the order of a 1000 s – larger than the flattening time.[6] A distance of 3 μm corresponds to a TGIC particle radius of about 1 μm. For larger TGIC particles the cross-linking time is predicted to increase rapidly.

Your Final Parameter Space

Where does this bring you? See Figure 10-14. You choose a few polymers using data on bulk properties. So items (1)–(6) form one variable. The diffusion argument tells that (7) is

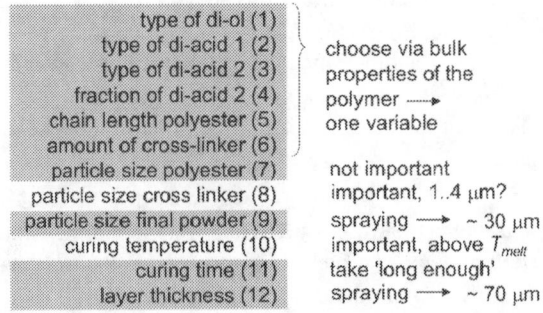

Figure 10-14 Final program with three variables

---

[5] Also the values in this figure are guesses
[6] If our guess of the diffusivity is more than ten times too low, the conclusion will be wrong.

not important. You have found limits on spraying operations which make it unnecessary to investigate (9) and (12). The particle size of the cross-linker seems to be important: it should be a few micrometres. The curing temperature has to be above the melting temperature of the polymer, but probably not much. Perhaps you can omit the curing time (11) in the program by taking it to be a multiple of the cross-linking time. There are now two variables left. Not only that, you have a fair idea in which band to vary them to get good results.

You can further reduce the amount of work required by using a good search method. One that is often used in practice is shown in Figure 10-15.[7] To keep things simple, we consider only the particle size of the cross-linker and the curing temperature. You might be measuring the smoothness of the film – with units from zero to ten, ten being completely smooth. Start with three conditions where you expect to be able to make a coating (not necessarily a good one), and measure the result. Suppose you get values of 5, 3 and 4. This indicates that you should be searching in the direction of the arrow in the first figure.

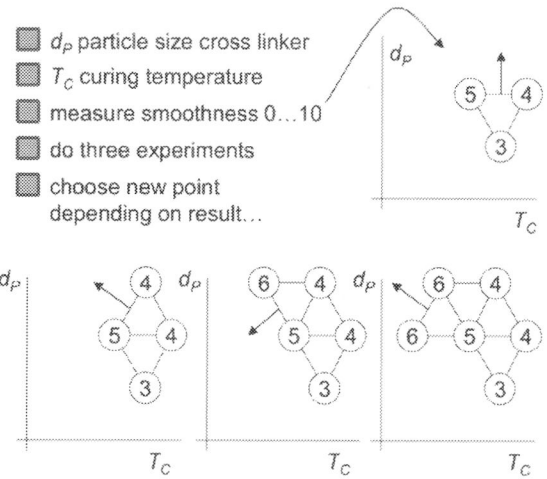

Figure 10-15 A simple search method

It is then just a matter of searching further, each time going in the direction of the greatest change. You may be varying more than two variables, and recording more than one result. However, the principle remains the same: you are trying to find a combination of variables that gives a good combination of properties. Note that there is no reason to change only one variable at a time – changing them simultaneously can be faster. The method does assume that there is a single optimum in the desired set of properties. You run a risk of ending on a local optimum.

It can help to do different experiments simultaneously. In some areas of technology (perhaps not in powder coatings) techniques are coming or are available to do large numbers of experiments at once, with automatic registration of the results.

---

[7] You will find more clever ways of doing this in literature under the name of 'Experimental Design'. However, these are not helpful in the early, exploratory part of development.

A final remark: the real development of the powder coating process was not as straightforward as in our story. It was the result of many smaller projects, with many dead ends. Even so, it did not take 700 000 years!

Summary

In this lesson we have looked at some of the aspects of developing a recipe in the laboratory. The techniques used there are the same as in research and education. However, you often must learn to understand the interaction between many variables. The key to this is to try to get an understanding of the process and its variables. Then to split off parts that can be done independently. In these parts we can often use models to understand the interactions (roughly) and to find where we should experiment. Search good conditions using experimental results as a guide. The experiments can often be speeded up by doing tests in parallel. All this is an iterative job: do not expect to only need one set of experiments!

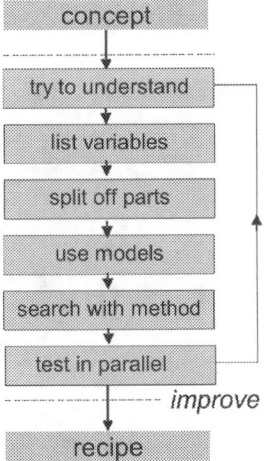

Further Reading

The example is based on T. A. Misev *Powder Coatings, Chemistry and Technology*, Wiley 1991.

A book on the design of experiments is Douglas C. Montgomery *Design and Analysis of Experiments*, 6th edition, Wiley 2005. However, realize that its statistical techniques only become useful after you have played quite a bit and begin to understand your system.

On dimensional analysis: our favourite is still Edward S. Taylor *Dimensional Analysis for Engineers*, Oxford University Press 1974. You will also find introductions in several chemical engineering texts such as W. J. Beek et al. *Transport Phenomena*, 2nd edition, Wiley 1999, Chapter 1.

Lesson 11:
Flowsheet the Process
Based on work by G.E.H Joosten and J. Schilder (formerly from Shell)

You have played in the lab and now have the product as you want it. You have a recipe: a list of ingredients, the lab-equipment required, and a description of the procedures to make the product. However, this is all on a scale of perhaps 100 g in a laboratory setting. We still have a lot to do before the product is in the market. Here we start thinking about making the product on a larger scale, say a thousand or a million times more than in the recipe. We first do this on paper.

This is the last point in the method used here where you can go back to the lab and improve the process without needing to redo expensive large scale experiments.

Start with the recipe; with this in hand, construct a process diagram showing the steps in the process, and how they are connected. At this point do not worry about equipment – that comes later. Then consider the ingredients and where they are added to the process. It is often instructive to look also at the amounts of energy that go in and out of the process. And to look at the waste produced.

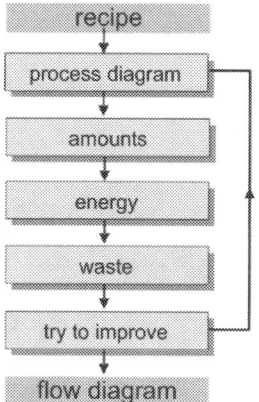

All too often you will find that the lab recipe is no good on a large scale. The ingredients cannot be obtained with the same quality, they are too expensive, or the source is too

Design and Development of Biological, Chemical, Food and Pharmaceutical Products   J.A. Wesselingh, S. Kiil and M.E. Vigild
© 2007 John Wiley & Sons, Ltd

uncertain. The waste streams are large and such that you cannot get rid of them. Processing times and volumes look too large to be practical. You then have to devise something better, make a new recipe, and go back to the lab to test it. You end with a flow diagram of the process.

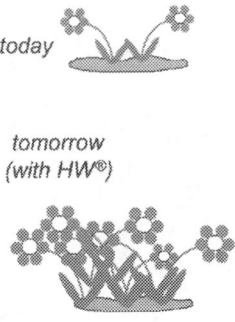

Killing Weeds

We illustrate this procedure with an example. This is an old one, from more than 30 years ago. It is a real story (though a little disguised). Some of the technique used is dated, but the lessons to be learned from this project are just as valid as they were then. The story is about a weed killer or herbicide. A product that lets your flowers grow, but not the weeds: the dream of many a gardener. Our company has been producing it for some time and selling it with an attractive margin. The future of the company looks bright, but then all of a sudden alarm bells start ringing . . . They are the bells of our marketing people, who are in panic. Our product has a release characteristic such as shown in Figure 11-1. Directly after application, the product is too active, but it gradually loses activity and after a week it is no longer effective. The competitor has released a better product. It shows a constant release rate; this is thought to be much better for the performance of the product. Roses like it, they say. Our customers are leaving in droves.

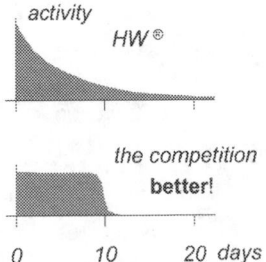

Figure 11-1 The competition is better

During a hastily set up brainstorming session, we come up with an idea to beat them (Figure 11-2). We are to develop a herbicide that only releases active material when it is required: during wet weather. This will be better for the roses, for the environment (the garden) and possibly for the gardener. We assume without further work that it will be better for our sales. The idea is to use a capsule made of a biopolymer such as gelatine. Such

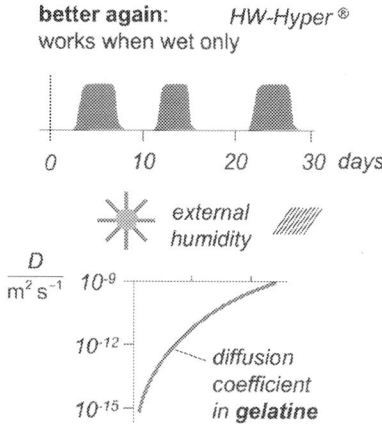

Figure 11-2 Humidity-controlled release using gelatine

polymers swell when they are wet and then become much more permeable than in their dry state. The graph shows the diffusivity of water in gelatine as a function of the water content. It varies by many orders of magnitude. It is this effect that we want to use. This technique should allow a low but adequate release rate over long periods.

Designing a Capsule

This does require us to develop capsules: a technique with which we are not familiar (Figure 11-3). The first question that comes up is which diameter d should they have? Closely behind that which wall thickness δ do they need? And what should the permeation and mechanical properties of the wall be like?

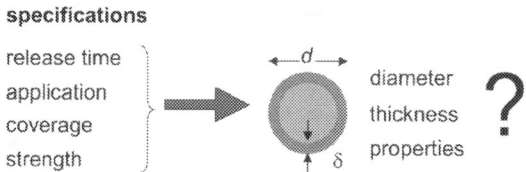

Figure 11-3 From specifications to capsule design

The release of the active ingredient from the capsule is governed by a number of steps. The active material will have a high concentration c_0 inside the capsule. It must first dissolve in the wall – as we shall see, the solubility K has to be low. It then diffuses through the polymer wall into the surroundings.

Figure 11-4 shows the laws governing the different steps in the transport process and how they are combined to obtain a flux relation. In the end we obtain an expression for the mass flow leaving the capsule. This is proportional to the surface area A of the capsule, to the diffusivity D in the wall, and to the solubility and concentration of active material in the capsule. It is inversely proportional to the wall thickness. From this it is easy to derive a relation for the release time.

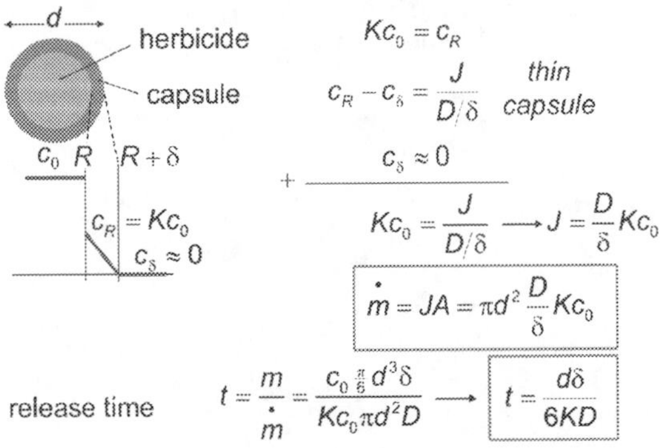

Figure 11-4 Release time of the capsule

release time depends on:

solubility	K	kind of polymer cross linking size of HW molecule	$t_r \propto K^{-1}$
diffusivity	D	kind of polymer cross linking size of HW molecule humidity	$t_r \propto D^{-1}$
thickness	δ	to be chosen	$t_r \propto \delta$
diameter	d	to be chosen	$t_r \propto d$

Figure 11-5 Parameters governing the release time

Figure 11-5 repeats the main parameters that determine the release time of the active component. A good chemist can vary the distribution coefficient and diffusivity of the active material by many orders of magnitude. This can be done by varying the kind of polymer chosen and its cross-linking. He can also vary these parameters by adding non-active chemical groups to the active material. The effects of changing the distribution coefficient and the diffusivity are in the same direction: a low distribution coefficient will usually lead to a low diffusivity. It is just as well that we can manipulate the first two variables, as we shall see the other two are more or less fixed by other requirements.

The method of delivery has important effects on the design of our capsule. If we use a spray can, the capsules have to pass through the opening of the sprayer. They must then be very fine, say with a diameter of 10 µm or less. On the other hand, if we use spraying by aeroplane, the capsules should not be too small. Otherwise they will be blown away and not land where we need them. Actually we are thinking of something in between, with the gardener dispersing dry capsules either by hand, or with some kind of disperser.

A requirement that is easily overlooked is that the capsules should give a reasonably homogeneous coverage. The active material is extremely active, so we only need very small amounts per unit area (in this example: 1 kg per hectare). With capsules of one millimetre diameter, we only get 200 capsules per square metre. This is not sufficient for a good coverage. For a given mass, the number of particles rises rapidly as the particle diameter goes down: with particles of a few tenths of a millimetre we get sufficient coverage.

Another requirement is that the capsule should have sufficient strength. Mechanics tells us that the strength is determined by the mechanical properties of the (dry) wall polymer and by the *ratio* of the wall thickness to capsule diameter. We settle on a wall thickness of 3% of the diameter. Because capsule diameter and wall thickness are coupled, the release time turns out to be proportional to the capsule diameter squared. This makes it difficult to use very small capsules. With our dispersing method we do not want very small capsules anyhow: the gardener should not inhale them! We settle on a diameter of 0.3 mm.

Producing Capsules

Now look at how we could make the capsules. The technique that we will use is called *coacervation* (Figure 11-6). It makes use of two different polymers: in this case *Arabic gum* and *gelatine*. Both are natural polymers: denaturated proteins. They are linear and contain large numbers of weak ionic groups. As a result, the polymers are charged, and their charge depends on the pH. At low pH they both have a positive electrical charge, at high pH a negative one. Over a small range of pH the two charges are different in sign. In this region the two polymers form a network, and they separate out of water to form a second aqueous phase that is polymer-rich.

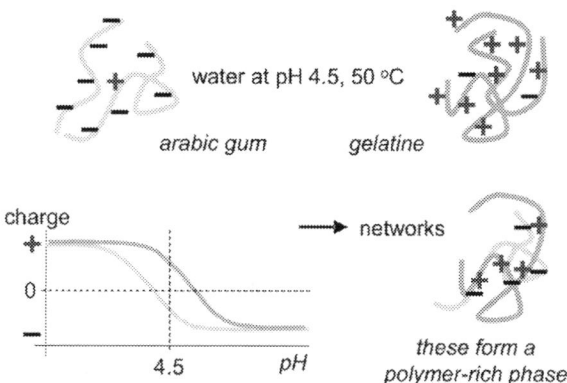

Figure 11-6 Coacervation using two polymers

The active material in our herbicide is a liquid that does not mix with water. It can be dispersed as droplets with a mixer – in our case the droplets have to be about 0.3 mm in diameter (Figure 11-7). If you then let a polymer-rich phase form by coacervation, the polymer spontaneously wets the drop surface. It forms a liquid polymer layer around the drop. Cross-linking the polymer gives a solid capsule.

The capsules are separated from the process liquid by filtering (Figure 11-8). The filter uses a *medium*: a flat material with little holes. Surprisingly the holes are usually chosen larger than the particles (capsules) to be retained. If the pores are not too large, particles form bridges

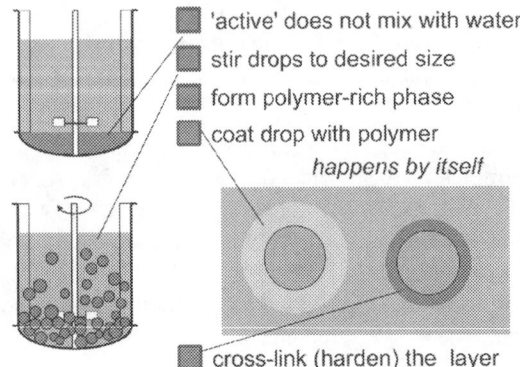

Figure 11-7 Forming drops with a polymer coating

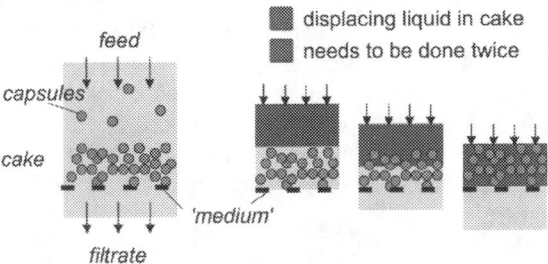

Figure 11-8 Filtering and washing the capsules

over them. These bridges then retain further particles, so that a *cake* is formed. There is a lot of liquid in the cake, with dissolved chemicals. You want to remove these. This is done by *washing*: displacing the liquid in the cake with clean liquid. The flow through a cake is not ideal: bits of dirty water stay behind. So more water is needed than the ideal amount: perhaps twice as much.

For our product we want dry capsules. This first requires blowing free water out of the cake, and then removing the remainder by drying with hot air (Figure 11-9). The remainder will be a few per cent of the volume of the cake; how much would again have to be determined by experiment. We will have more to say about drying in the lesson on Scaling Up.

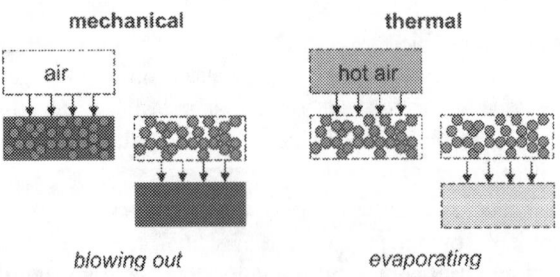

Figure 11-9 Drying by blowing out and evaporating

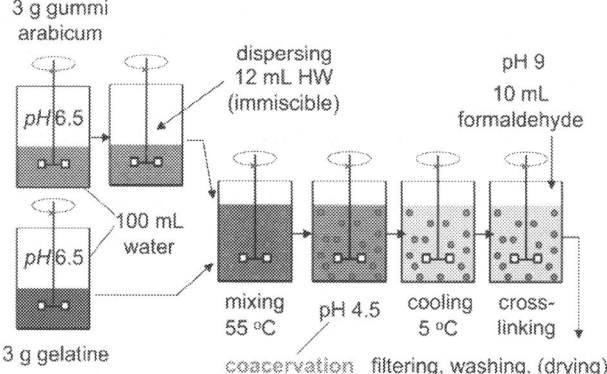

Figure 11-10 The laboratory recipe

Figure 11-10 shows the laboratory recipe for the process. We first form solutions of the separate polymers. Then the active material is dispersed as droplets of the desired size in one of the polymer solutions. The two solutions are mixed and the pH is adjusted to let the polymers precipitate. The polymer wets the 'active' drops and forms a weak layer around them. After cooling we cross-link the polymer with an excess of formaldehyde to obtain capsules with a good strength. These need to be filtered, and the process liquid washed out. The capsules can then be dried.

Flow Diagrams

We can now construct a process diagram showing each stage in the process, and where amounts enter or leave (Figure 11-11). Write the names of the main ingredient on the top of the page, and the main product at the bottom. A vertical line connecting these is the main line of the process: it is important to keep this line in mind. Put the steps from the recipe on this line in the right sequence. For a large process you may need several pages. You will be adding side lines for feed preparation, waste treatment and recycles. Don't let these disturb the main line of the diagram. Figure 11-11 is the diagram for our herbicide example.

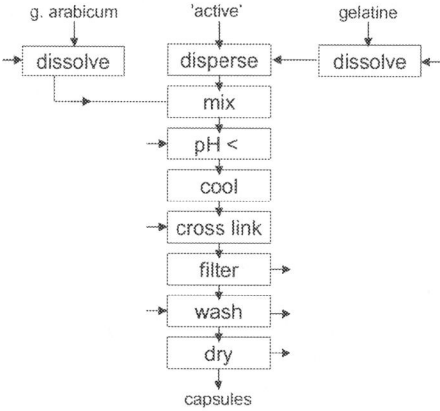

Figure 11-11 Flow diagram of the process

In the diagram we show the mass of the different chemicals entering and leaving each stage in the process. That in Figure 11-12 is for production of a *batch* of 100 kg of dry capsules. This is 3800 times the amount from our recipe. The electrolytes needed to adjust the pH in the different steps are left out. If the product becomes a success, we will be producing many batches, and possibly larger ones than 100 kg. We end with 55 kg of active material in capsules. To make this, we need 870 kg of water, 11 kg of the two biopolymers each, 46 kg of formaldehyde and some acid and base. Our plant is largely filled with water! The water leaves the process contaminated with 23 kg of formaldehyde (and traces of the other materials). We will not be allowed to discharge this.

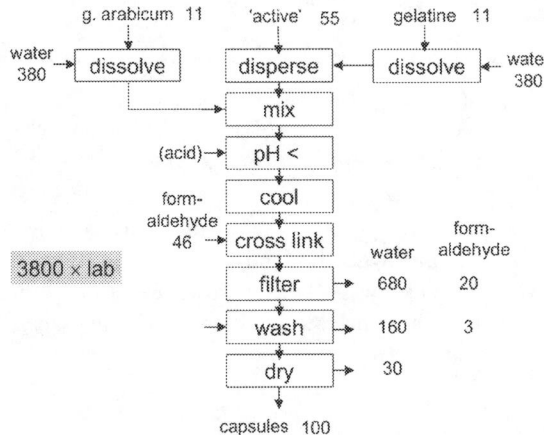

Figure 11-12 Flow diagram with kilograms per batch

At this point we can begin to look at the energy usage in the plant (Figure 11-13). We need to add energy to heat up the vessels for dissolving the biopolymers. We then have to cool before cross-linking, removing an even larger amount. This means that we must include heating and cooling facilities in our list of equipment. Finally we need a fairly large amount of energy to dry the capsules. We have not yet considered the energy for stirring and other operations. The stirring energy amounts to about 10 MJ per batch. Stirring and pumping usually do not require much energy compared to thermal processes.

This is a point to consider process improvements. One problem is that the biopolymers we can buy are not of constant quality. Would it be possible to get other materials that are more reliable? (This would mean a major redo of the work in the lab.) At this point you should also obtain a good idea of the prices of the ingredients and the energy used in the process. These may force you to go back to the lab to change the process. A fairly obvious improvement is to reduce the amount of water. This will reduce the size of equipment, the energy requirement and the amount of waste. However, you may be limited by a low solubility of the polymers, or by too high a viscosity of the solutions produced. The stream of waste water is a nuisance, especially because it contains formaldehyde. Could we separate the formaldehyde and recycle it? This might be possible with a membrane or with distillation.

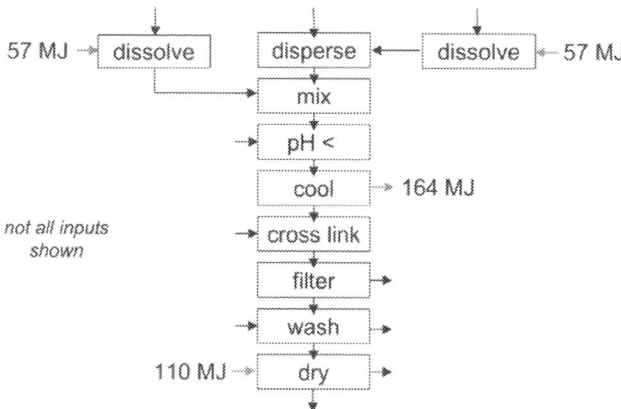

Figure 11-13 Energy requirements of the process

Figure 11-14 shows the process diagram with a formaldehyde separation and recycle. You will definitely want to test process changes in the lab before going into larger scale operations. Less water may make the process inoperable. The recycle may contain impurities that build up in the product.

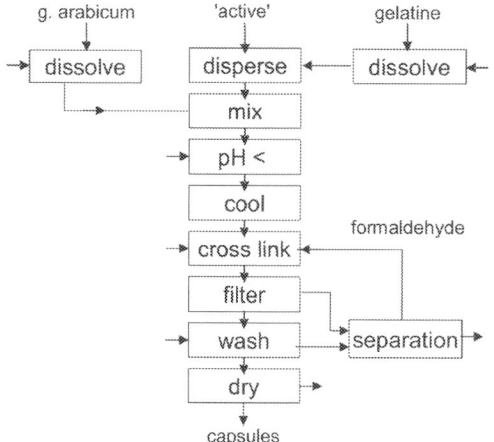

Figure 11-14 Diagram with process improvements

What Really Happened

A last word on the example: how did the project fare? It did not go well. We started fine: within a few months we had batches of capsules containing kerosene. We had spray-dried these in the staircase (!) of a high building. We had insight in materials consumption and problems in manufacturing. However, on our first meeting with marketing, half a year after the start of the project, we felt that interest was waning. The project was not continued after 1 year.

What have we learned from this? First that you have to be quick to solve a problem from marketing. We would only have had a chance if we had already been doing research on controlled release and capsulation. The second lesson is that we should have had marketing, applications and manufacturing people in the design team. Only then would we have any chance of getting things through. We also sinned against two other rules of product design: we did not analyse customer needs, and we only considered one solution.

Summary

This lesson has discussed the first – and important – step in designing a process to make your product.

1. Start with a recipe; from this construct a flow diagram (Figure 11-15).

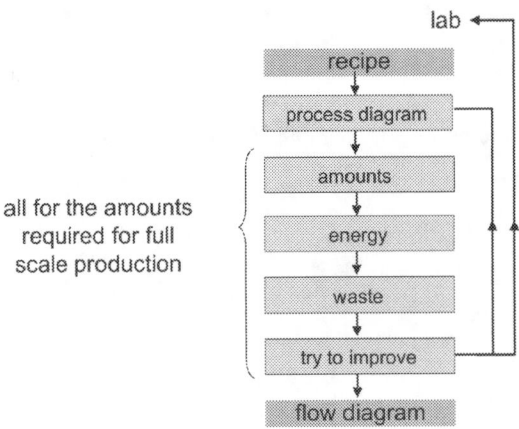

Figure 11-15 The method for flowsheeting

2. To get the amounts multiply the lab recipe so that you will produce what you will need for full scale production.
3. Then consider the amounts of energy this will require and the waste it will make.
4. Finally, try to improve the process. Some ways are by choosing cheaper ingredients, by separating and recycling waste streams and by increasing the concentrations and conversion rates in the plant.
5. After the last round of improvements, you will probably have to go back to the lab to test the changes made.

Further Reading

For more on flowsheets and balances:

Richard M. Felder and Ronald W. Rousseau *Elementary Principles of Chemical Processes*, 2nd edition, Wiley 1986.

Lesson 12: Estimate the Cost

With J. Abildskov and teams 1–12 (2004)

Below is a box of safety matches (Figure 12-1). The question is how much it would cost to make this. The only thing known at this moment is the price in the supermarket: about one and a half Danish kroner (or €0.2) per box. This is almost certainly an upper limit to the cost. But how much lower is it? You might be tempted to ring or e-mail Uddevalla (where the matches are made) to find out. Don't do that – you will only make a nuisance of yourself. Firms will not tell what their costs are: in doing so they would give away too much to customers and competitors. Even so, cost is important in product development, and you will have to build up experience. This is a frustrating thing to do, and not only from within the walls of a university.

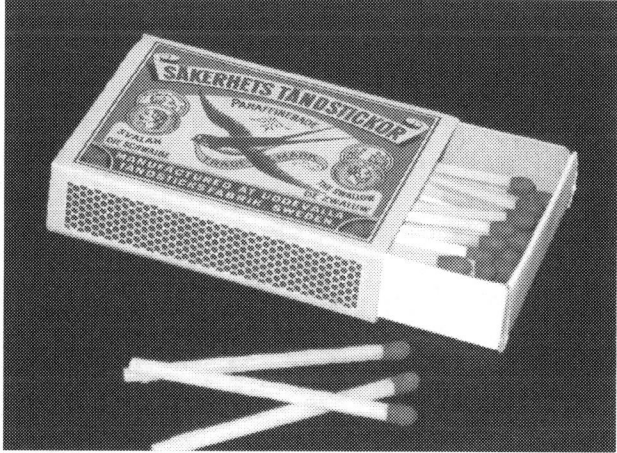

Figure 12-1 A box with matches

The Matchbox

The matchbox is an intriguing product. The design of the label indicates that it has been around for well over a century. You can only light a match when you also have the box. The matches alone do not ignite. This was a great invention at that time, which has prevented any number of fires and deaths. How does it work? The photos (Figure 12-2) show details of the head of a match (cut along its length) and of the side of the box where the match is to be struck. The match head contains potassium chlorate – a source of oxygen. It also contains colouring and a binder. On the sides of the box, a suspension of red phosphor particles has

Design and Development of Biological, Chemical, Food and Pharmaceutical Products   J.A. Wesselingh, S. Kiil and M.E. Vigild
© 2007 John Wiley & Sons, Ltd

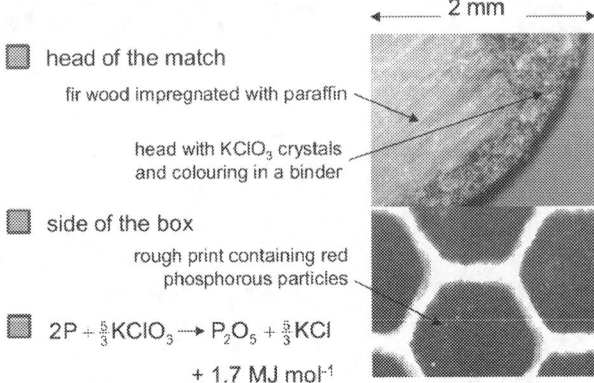

Figure 12-2 How a match ignites

been printed. When you strike the match, this gives friction and heating, enough to ignite the few phosphor particles that adhere to the match. (The combination of red phosphorus and potassium chlorate is very reactive.) This ignites the paraffin and wood in the match. The two reactants – chlorate and phosphorus – are separated, and only contacted for the milliseconds that you are striking the match.

There are many variations to the process for making matches, but most look like that in Figure 12-3. The main (central) line follows the wood that is to form the matches. This has to be cut, peeled, split and sorted into little sticks. The sticks are waxed (paraffinated) and then dipped into a $KClO_3$ suspension that is made separately. After drying, the matches are packed in boxes with sides printed with red phosphorus. There are many operations, and the figure shows only the main ones.

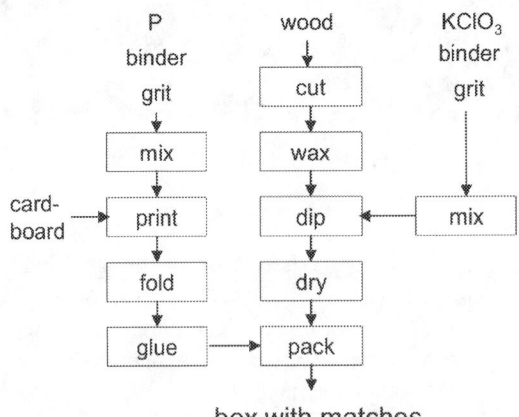

Figure 12-3 Flowsheet for match making

Organizing Expenses and Costs

There are many costs for such an operation. Figure 12-4 lists the important ones. Those dealing with materials, utilities, equipment and operators will be obvious, but there are others

BOM: bill of materials

materials	P KClO$_3$ wood binder grit cardboard
utilities	steam, water, electricity
equipment	to mix, print, fold, cut..., the building
operators	to run the equipment
hired-in	installation, maintenance, transport, marketing...
administration	personnel, finances, sales...
engineering	to develop
marketing	to market, sell
management	to supervise

Figure 12-4 Important cost items

that you should not forget. When you get involved in the management of any organization, you will be surprised by the huge number of transactions[1] happening. It is easy to lose sight of the forest because of the trees. In all organizations there are many activities, many products being developed, made and sold, and this further increases complexity. To avoid getting lost, the organization needs an administration – and ways of grouping of the costs and revenues that help retain an overview. In this lesson we look at two ways of grouping and organizing.

In the first grouping each cost is considered to belong to one of three groups:

(1) direct costs (which can easily be assigned to a single product),
(2) indirect costs (which cannot easily be assigned) and
(3) depreciation (to account for wear and ageing of equipment and development).

When you first see the administration of an organization it will probably be some variant of this grouping method. You will see the costs of your team or department, all subdivided into project accounts. You will probably not see the depreciation; this is handled by the bookkeepers. As we shall see, this grouping is not as sharp as one might wish; the division is a bit arbitrary.

Direct costs are those that can easily be assigned to a given product or activity. Examples are materials and parts. In processes consuming or producing large amounts of energy (oil refining and power stations) energy would also be in this category – for smaller operations energy is often taken to be part of the indirect costs. Personnel ('labour') that is directly connected to the production of a certain product is also booked as direct cost. So are costs related to equipment dedicated to that product. The costs of marketing and sales can usually also be assigned to a given product. Direct costs are easily traceable to a certain product or activity; direct costs can be influenced by the decisions of a design team.

---

[1] A transaction is anything that has to registered and be paid by somebody.

Indirect costs (overhead) are those that cannot easily be assigned to a certain product or activity. Examples are management costs of a company (not those of an individual product or activity), the administration, and the head office. Maintenance, shared equipment and utilities are often booked as overhead.[2] Overhead is shared by all products and activities via formulae using *cost drivers*. These are easily measured items such as use of raw materials, use of labour, or total sales. Each company has its methods for overhead calculation, and these often change. In principle overhead is calculated after the end of each fiscal year, but in practice most companies estimate it directly using experience. Overhead works much like a value-added tax; it can add substantially to costs. Development teams cannot influence overhead, so they are not motivated to minimize it, even though that would be in their advantage in the long term.

To make a product or provide a service, you need equipment. This includes buildings, plant, computers ... In most cases such equipment gradually loses value (an exception might be the value of the ground under the buildings). This happens over a number of years. The same happens to investments in development or acquisition of new products. In this situation, the cost of ageing and wear is often spread out over a number of years. For a computer, or the development of a product, this might be 3 years, for plant equipment 10 years, for a building 30 years. The simplest way of depreciating is to reduce the value of the asset or investment by a fixed percentage every year, until the asset has been 'written off'. There are more complicated ways of depreciating. You are usually not free to choose how to depreciate: this is determined by tax and financial authorities.

The second way of grouping costs is used to analyse the cost of manufacturing operations. Here we consider costs to be either:

(1) fixed costs, which do not depend on the size of the production, and
(2) variable costs, which are proportional to the production.

In our match factory, the cost of equipment and of management would be regarded as fixed: you cannot change these costs much on a short term. The cost of red phosphorus is variable: the more matches you make, the more phosphorus you have to buy. Costs are never truly fixed; you can increase the size of management if the company expands. Also they seldom rise in a completely linear fashion with production – if you expand production you may be able to get phosphorus with a discount. So, true variable costs do not exist either. Even so, the division is useful for discussing more-or-less stable operations.

Figure 12-5 shows the most important fixed costs.[3] These include depreciation of the part of the equipment and development that can be assigned to the product, the permanent personnel to operate the plant, and any long-term contracts for renting, supplies or maintenance. Overhead asked for fixed personnel is also a fixed cost.

---

[2] You will understand that everybody tries to book things on overhead, while management tries to discourage this.
[3] These are the fixed parts of the total cost, not those of a unit such as a matchbox.

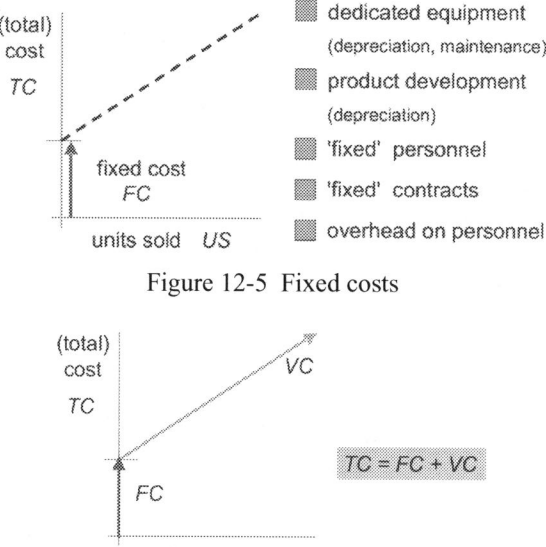

Figure 12-5 Fixed costs

Figure 12-6 Variable costs

Variable cost items (Figure 12-6) are materials and parts (where the amount required depends on the units produced). In a plant using large amounts of energy, this is often a variable cost – if you turn down production you need less energy. Personnel that can be hired at will, such as for maintenance or transport, can be seen as a variable cost. Marketing and sales costs that can be assigned to a product are also variable costs, as is most overhead.

The total cost is simply the sum of fixed and variable costs.

Of course the firm not only has costs, but also revenues from sales. The sales revenue is equal to the product of price-per-unit and number-of-units-sold (Figure 12-7). Here we consider the price for the manufacturer. This is not the price in the shop as we discuss further on.

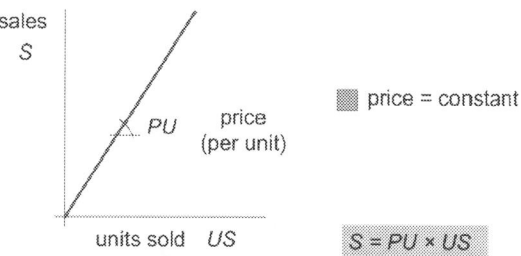

Figure 12-7 Sales

With the simple relations described above, you can analyse and understand quite a lot of the operation of a firm. You should, however, be aware of the limitations of this kind of analysis. Our Cost–Sales–Profit analysis assumes that a firm is working at a steady state (under stable conditions). It does not look at the effect of changing inventory (products in storage) – everything produced is taken to be sold. It assumes that the cost varies linearly with sales. None of these assumptions will be quite true. The model is best for analysing firms with a single product, but you can use it for multiple products with a bit of care.

Cost, Sales and Profit

To illustrate the concepts we have worked out the match factory using the parameters in Figure 12-8. These values are only (very) rough estimates: the results will be no better than our speculations. We can see match manufacturers grinning. We have taken the price of the plant to be thirty million euros; maintenance is 5% and depreciation 15% of this value per year. Match making is a mature industry, so we have neglected development costs. The personnel to run the plant consists of five shifts of five, with five extra. People cost 50 000 euros each per year. We have a fixed contract with a transport company, and our own company wants 25% overhead on personnel costs. The prices of the materials will be clear. Except for phosphorus they are bulk chemicals with a price of about €1 per kilogram. Energy is taken to be electricity, but the amount used is not important. Marketing and sales costs are taken as a fixed amount per matchbox, and overhead on materials is 25%.

fixed costs		**variable costs**	
price of equipment	€ 30M	price of wood	€ 1 kg^{-1}
maintenance	5% yr^{-1}	price of chlorate	€ 1 kg^{-1}
depreciation	15% yr^{-1}	price of phosphorous	€ 10 kg^{-1}
price of development	€ 0M	price of cardboard	€ 1 kg^{-1}
fixed personnel	€ 50k yr^{-1}	price of binder	€ 1 kg^{-1}
30 people		price of energy	€ 30 GJ^{-1}
transport	€ 500k yr^{-1}	hired personnel	none
overhead personnel	25 % yr^{-1}	marketing, sales	€ 0.001 unit^{-1}
		overhead materials	25% yr^{-1}

Figure 12-8 *Estimated* cost parameters

Figure 12-9 shows the results of the model calculation given separately in Appendix 12-1. The cost of some items is too small for drawing. In the lower part you see the fixed cost (where the equipment costs dominate). The upper part shows the variable cost: mostly due to materials and overhead. The top line is the total cost. Remember that this is using our guessed parameters.

All matchboxes produced are assumed to be sold and the price is taken to be constant (Figure 12-10). The price that the manufacturer gets is *not* the shop price. After manufacturing, the product is resold several times, and every reseller has to recoup costs and make some profit. The increase of the price is known as the gross margin. We have assumed that there are two intermediate steps with gross margins of 30% and 40%.[4] Together with a value added

---

[4] The difference between manufacturing cost and shop price will be larger if there are more steps.

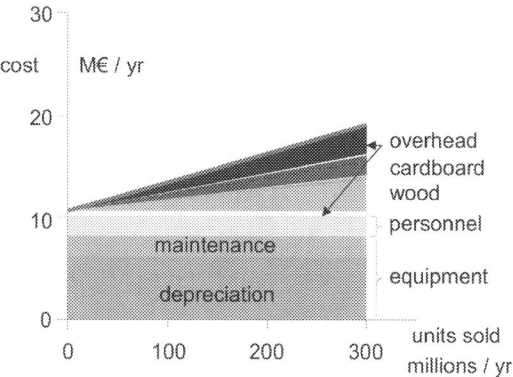

Figure 12-9 Cost versus production (sales)

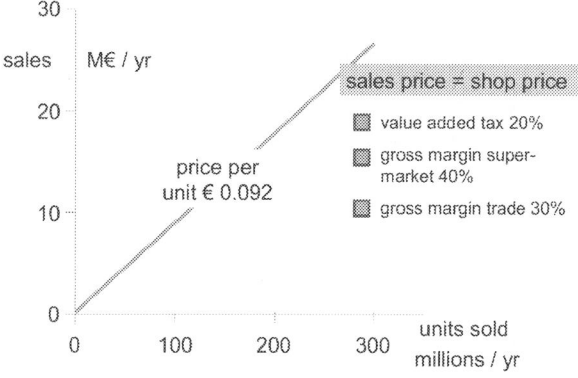

Figure 12-10 Revenue from sales

tax (VAT) of 20% this more than doubles the price for the final customer. From the known shop price (€0.20 per box) we have worked back to the sales price of the manufacturer, but you will understand that there is much uncertainty in the value.

Profit from sales should rise more rapidly than costs (Figure 12-11). If all is well, the two become equal at some number of units sold (the *breakeven* point). With our figures this is at 170 million matchboxes per year. Above this value the firm will make a profit on matchboxes. The difference between sales and cost is the profit before tax. We must say that our figures look too good; making boxes of matches is a mature industry, where profit margins are probably quite low.

Modelling for Analysis

The price per unit (matchbox) goes down rapidly with increasing production (Figure 12-12). This graph shows the situation for a single plant with our guessed parameters. If you have good parameters you can use your economic model to analyse all kinds of things. You can find out how sensitive your results are to changes in material prices, and to changes in

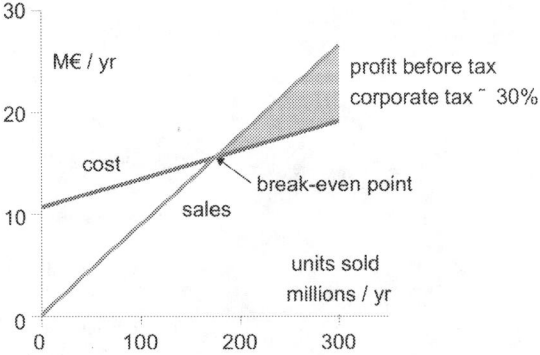

Figure 12-11 Breakeven point and profit[5]

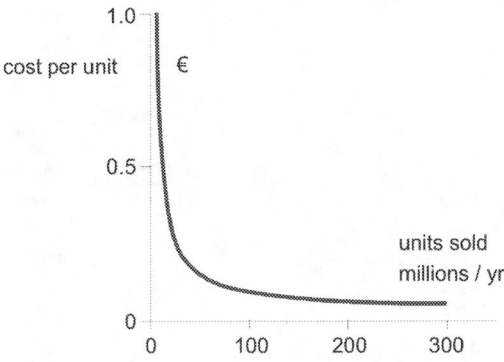

Figure 12-12 Cost per unit versus sales

personnel. You can find out how much it costs to take the plant out of operation for a month, and so on.

For cost modelling you need cost data. It is often difficult and time consuming to get good costs. And of course: they change all the time, depend on the quality you want, on the amounts you buy and on your negotiating position . . . There are several techniques that we have tried:

1. working back from prices (as in the matchbox example),
2. finding cost data in the firm (via the financial department),[6]
3. from external data on the web, or quotations from manufacturers.

The first method looks attractive, but can go badly wrong because you seldom know the number of trading steps and their gross margins. The second method is the most reliable, but not of much use for a student. The third often gets you somewhere, but the data will usually be incomplete. All in all: you need patience, you need to listen, to ask and to read, and to compare and check all the time.

---

[5] Taxes in this figure are corporate taxes, not the VAT mentioned earlier.
[6] It is usually not possible to do this well in a student project.

if you have **no idea**, start with

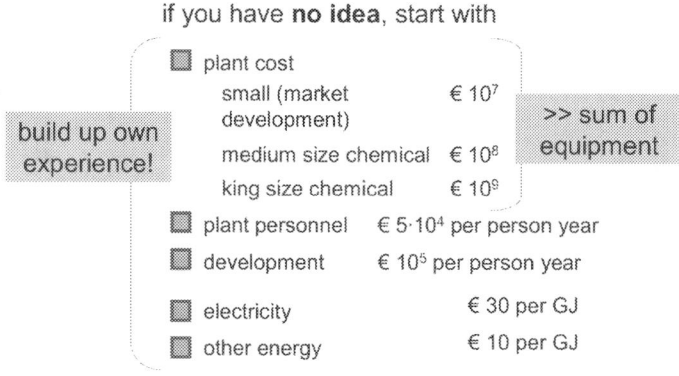

Figure 12-13 Costs of plant and operation

If you really do not know anything – and wish to get your financial model running in Excel – you might use the values in Figure 12-13 for the costs of plant. Beginners often assume that this is largely that of the important pieces of equipment. They forget the cost of infrastructure, transport, engineering, waste treatment . . . piping and heat exchangers . . . instrumentation. This can be many times that of the major equipment alone. If you have an idea of a similar plant you might use the formula in Figure 12-14 for a first guess.[7] It takes inflation and capacity differences into account – but there may be other variables. Fortunately plant costs usually do not dominate the overall cost of products. Costs of personnel are easier to estimate. The costs of energy are not fixed – they can vary greatly with the oil price. Realize that these figures are only orders of magnitude. Whatever you do, start to build up some own experience by reading papers and trade journals, from the Internet, by hearing from others *and noting the figures*.[8]

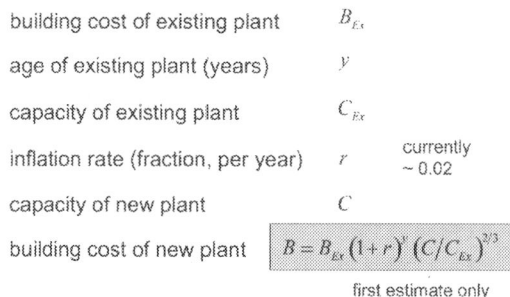

building cost of existing plant B_{Ex}

age of existing plant (years) y

capacity of existing plant C_{Ex}

inflation rate (fraction, per year) r currently ~ 0.02

capacity of new plant C

building cost of new plant $B = B_{Ex}(1+r)^y (C/C_{Ex})^{2/3}$

first estimate only

Figure 12-14 Guess cost from existing plant

The situation for materials is almost as difficult (Figure 12-15). Again, if you really have no idea, you might use these values. Beware of prices quoted for laboratory (analytical) chemicals. These are often ten to a hundred times higher than prices for technical chemicals because of high purification and distribution costs. Again, realize that our figures are only orders of magnitude. Good luck using them.

---

[7] If you use guessed figures, make a note in your spreadsheet!
[8] During an excursion: 'What would a plant like this cost?'

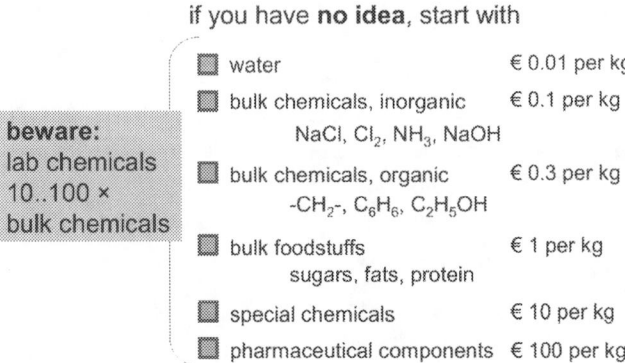

if you have **no idea**, start with

▣	water	€ 0.01 per kg
▣	bulk chemicals, inorganic	€ 0.1 per kg
	$NaCl$, Cl_2, NH_3, $NaOH$	
▣	bulk chemicals, organic	€ 0.3 per kg
	$-CH_2-$, C_6H_6, C_2H_5OH	
▣	bulk foodstuffs	€ 1 per kg
	sugars, fats, protein	
▣	special chemicals	€ 10 per kg
▣	pharmaceutical components	€ 100 per kg

beware:
lab chemicals
10..100 ×
bulk chemicals

Figure 12-15 Cost of materials for large scale production

Summary

It is time for the summary.

1. In any firm there are large numbers of costs and revenues.
2. To keep track of these, the firm needs an administration.
3. It also needs ways of grouping the costs and revenues, so that management can keep an overview.
4. We have discussed two ways of grouping costs:

   (1) as direct, indirect and depreciation costs, or

   (2) as fixed and variable costs.

   The first is most suitable to keep an overview of the firm; the second for understanding the operations for a certain product.
5. The firm also has revenues from the sales of products or services. These should – in the long run – exceed the costs.
6. We ended looking at how to start finding your way into the cost structure of an industry.
7. For the beginner it is difficult to get reliable cost data. It is even more difficult to get reliable estimates of future sales: not only for the beginner!

Further Reading

A good starting point, also for engineers, is

William H. Webster *Accounting for Managers*, McGraw-Hill 2004.

Appendix 12-1

This is the Excel file with our cost model of the match factory.

Costs in a Match Factory

Parameters

maintenance_factor	0.05
depreciation_factor	0.15
overhead_personnel	0.25
overhead_materials	0.25
personnel_number	30

Prices

equipment	€30,000,000.00
development	€0.00
person_per_year	€50,000.00

wood_per_kg	€1.00
chlorate_per_kg	€1.00
phosphorus_per_kg	€10.00
cardboard_per_kg	€1.00
binder_per_kg	€1.00
energy_per_GJ	€30.00
salescost_per_unit	€0.00
price_per_unit	€0.09

Materials (kg)

wood_per_box	1.10E-02
chlorate_per_box	1.90E-04
phosphorus_per_box	1.60E-04
cardboard_per_box	7.00E-03
binder_per_box	3.00E-04

Fixed Cost

maintenance	€1,500,000.00
depreciation	€4,500,000.00
personnel	€1,500,000.00
transport	€500,000.00
overhead personnel	€375,000.00
total fixed cost	€8,375,000.00

Units Sold	0.00E+00	1.00E+08	2.00E+08	3.00E+08
Variable Cost				
wood	€0.00	€1,100,000.00	€2,200,000.00	€3,300,000.00
chlorate	€0.00	€19,000.00	€38,000.00	€57,000.00
phosphorus	€0.00	€160,000.00	€320,000.00	€480,000.00
cardboard	€0.00	€700,000.00	€1,400,000.00	€2,100,000.00
binder	€0.00	€30,000.00	€60,000.00	€90,000.00
total materials	€0.00	€2,009,000.00	€4,018,000.00	€6,027,000.00
overhead materials	€0.00	€502,250.00	€1,004,500.00	€1,506,750.00
sales cost	€0.00	€100,000.00	€200,000.00	€300,000.00
total variable cost	€0.00	€2,611,250.00	€5,222,500.00	€7,833,750.00
Total Cost	€8,375,000.00	€10,986,250.00	€13,597,500.00	€16,208,750.00
Sales	€0.00	€9,000,000.00	€18,000,000.00	€27,000,000.00

Lesson 13: Equip the Process

With L.P.B.M. Janssen from the University of Groningen

You now have a formulation and a flow sheet for your process. The next step is to get equipment to do the job. Here there are two possibilities:

(1) you have to find everything yourself, or
(2) you have to use what is available.

The second is the most common situation. In either case you must look ahead. How are you going to do things on a production scale.[1] Should you modify the lab formulation before going on?

Process Operations

The starting point is again the formulation. Which operations are needed to make the product? There are many such operations: mixing, heating, cooling, separating, and – most important – the large group of operations for structuring a product. You must acquaint yourself with the operations that you will be using, and find out how they work. Analysing is essential, also here. This is also the point to find out whether there is already equipment available. Then you might consider combining operations, or leaving out steps. This will make your process simpler and cheaper, but probably also less flexible. Again, this means going back to the lab. Make a first design of the plant; set up a list of equipment, and try to get an idea of the price and operating costs. Finally you will have to *get* equipment for developing: borrow it, lease it, buy it, or find time slots in existing plant.[2]

There are many, many processing operations. In Figure 13-1 is a mind map showing some of those used for giving a product a structure. This is by no means complete. If you need any of these operations, begin having a look in 'Perry'.[3] Think of whether you might learn something from experiments in the kitchen. Have a look at manufacturers' web sites, and start talking with people who know about the equipment. Nearly every operation has its own Society, Working Party, or Institution, with meetings, courses and what have you. If possible, get involved in pilot or production runs with the real equipment.

[1] The lesson on Scaling Up also deals with this.

[2] This may be the plant of a contractor.

[3] For 'Perry' see Further Reading.

Design and Development of Biological, Chemical, Food and Pharmaceutical Products   J.A. Wesselingh, S. Kiil and M.E. Vigild
© 2007 John Wiley & Sons, Ltd

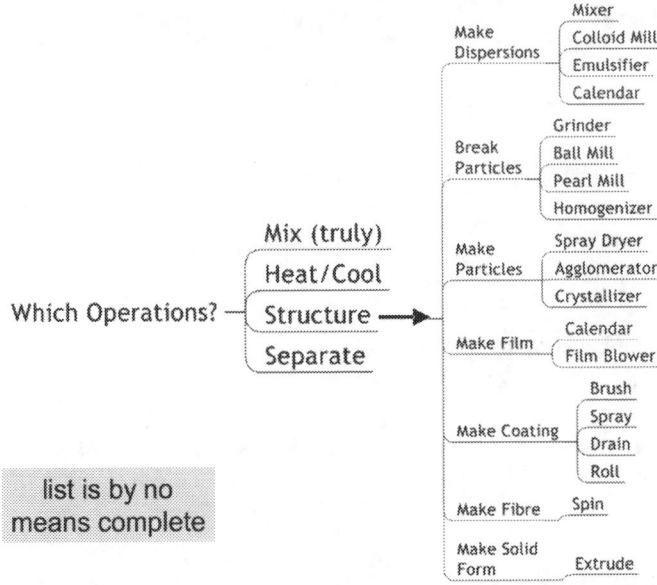

Figure 13-1 Some operations used for structuring

Wokkels: First Attempt

We illustrate the choice of equipment with the example of 'Wokkels' in Figure 13-2.[4] Nowadays this product is nothing special: you can find something like it in any supermarket. However, 30 years ago, this was a big hit for its developers. Try to think of yourself in their

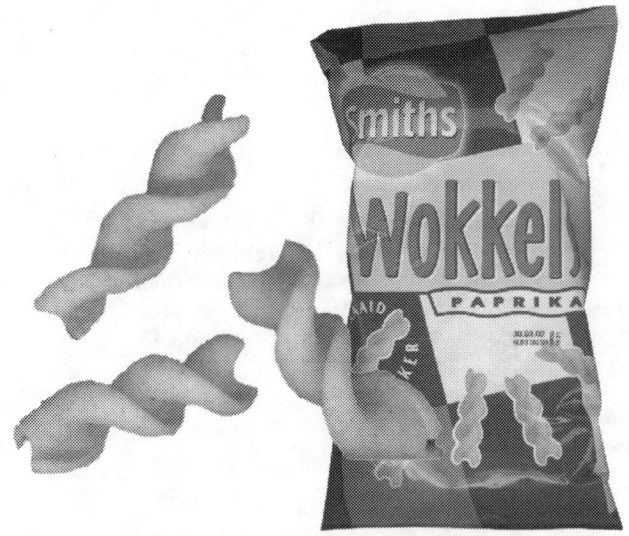

Figure 13-2 The example: Wokkels

---

[4] This is a combination of a number of stories.

situation. You are in the food business, working for a company that already produces snacks. You are wondering whether there will be a market for *light* snacks made of natural vegetable ingredients, and what these snacks should look like. A bright idea comes up. Wouldn't it be nice to be able to sell air ... Remember, at this point you do not have the picture above, and have little idea of what the product will look like.

You have gone through the whole rigmarole of getting customer needs, specifications, forming and selecting concepts. You have also developed a formulation, of which a shortened version is shown in Figure 13-3. The first three steps are batch mixing of potato starch and other ingredients with water, cooking under pressure so the mixture remains a liquid, and foaming by pressure relief. This will be followed by cutting, drying, toasting, seasoning and packaging.

① mix starch and water
② cook under pressure
③ foam by pressure relief
④ shape and cut foam
⑤ toast surface of foam
⑥ dry the snacks
⑦ cool the snacks

Figure 13-3 The formulation

The process will look like that in Figure 13-4. The first step is a batch mixer/cooker. It is followed by a heater, a cutter, a foamer and several other pieces of equipment. You try things out in an improvised manner: everything seems to work. You are making progress. However, because the mixer is operated batchwise, a lot of handling is required. Also the subsequent equipment is not utilized all the time. The proposal is put forward to the marketing department, together with an estimate of the cost. The response of the marketers is damning: the product is going to be too expensive. This is because of the high personnel cost, and the poor utilization of the equipment. You may be disappointed, you may be angry. But you have to go back to find a better formulation and process. This interaction between lab, process people and marketing is typical and essential.

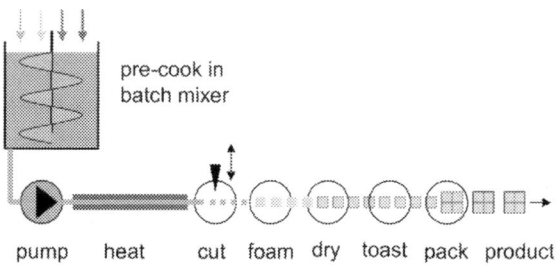

pre-cook in
batch mixer

pump   heat   cut foam dry toast pack product

Figure 13-4 First idea for the process

Wokkels: Second Attempt

In a second round, we consider the process in more detail (Figure 13-5). Starch is obtained from a number of plants (including corn and potato). It is in the form of small, hard micro-particles. These contain two kinds of material: about 20% of amylose (a linear poly-glucan) and the rest amylopectin (a branched poly-glucan). All particles have to be dissolved – the non-dissolved particles have a dull taste and are perceived as gritty. To dissolve the starch, we add water, which causes the particles to swell. Heating is enough to leach out the smaller amyloses, but to untangle the amylopectin the mixture has to be sheared.

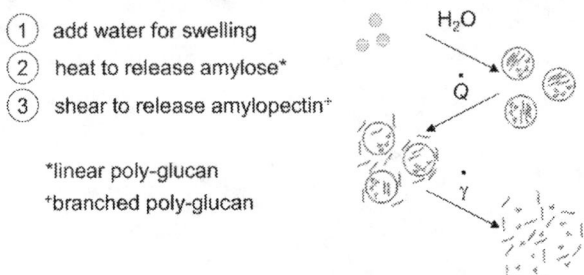

Figure 13-5 The dissolving of starch granules

The starch can be dissolved under different conditions. Figure 13-6 shows the results of differential scanning calorimetry (DSC): these show at which temperatures heat is taken up. A peak is an indication of a phase change. A high water-content gives a single peak at about 70 °C, where the starch dissolves. With lower water contents a second melting peak appears which shifts to higher temperatures as the water content is reduced. So there is quite some choice in the process conditions. The snacks should contain little water, so what you add will have to be removed. It looks as if high-temperature/low-water processing is the most interesting. Experiments indicate that the starch mixture then only needs a very short cooking time. These conditions have a further advantage: they degrade starch and make it more digestible.

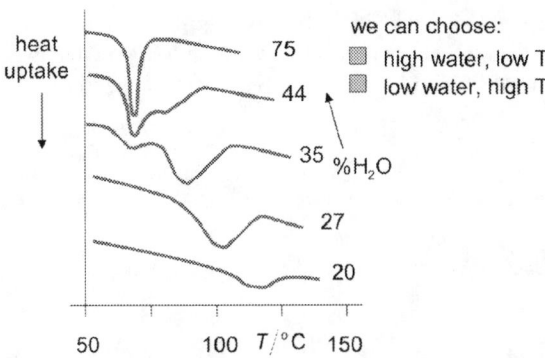

Figure 13-6 DSC measurements on starch and water

To foam the snacks, we might force the cooked fluid through an opening (a 'die', Figure 13-7). The fluid will contain about 20% water, at a temperature of about 150 °C. The vapour pressure

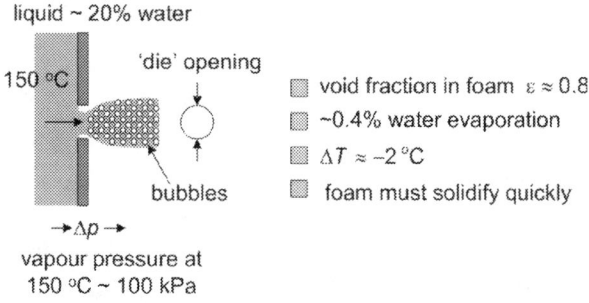

liquid ~ 20% water

'die' opening

150 °C

void fraction in foam $\varepsilon \approx 0.8$

~0.4% water evaporation

$\Delta T \approx -2\,°C$

foam must solidify quickly

bubbles

$\rightarrow \Delta p \rightarrow$

vapour pressure at
150 °C ~ 100 kPa

Figure 13-7 Foaming by expansion

of water will be about 1 atm under these conditions, so just right. A small fraction of this evaporates and forms the bubbles in the foam – we aim for foam with about 80% bubbles. The temperature goes down a little, as we find from an energy calculation. The foam must solidify before the bubbles collapse.

Figure 13-8 shows the required temperature and residence time of some possible reactors for your heating operation. The slurry reactor and corn cooker are classic and well tested pieces of equipment. The extruder has recently appeared;[5] it works at a high temperature, with a short residence time and high shear rates. This looks like what you need. High shear rates are required to dissolve the amylopectin, and they also reduce the size of the chains, and make them more digestible. The high temperature has the advantage that it kills all micro-organisms. It is, however, still below the browning line, so a separate toasting operation remains necessary.

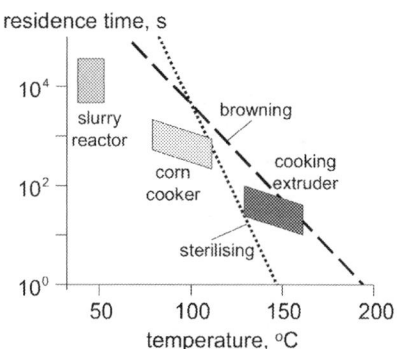

residence time, s

Figure 13-8 Three different reactors

Using an Extruder

The extruder might look like Figure 13-9. The feed, which is viscous and partly solid, enters at the left where it is picked up by the screw and thoroughly mixed. The screw causes the pressure to rise as the feed moves to the right. At the same time, temperature increases due to viscous dissipation. At the end of the extruder, the hot and cooked material moves through

---

[5] Remember: this is 30 years ago.

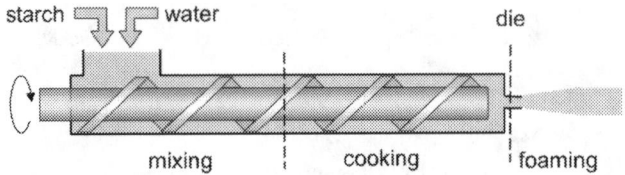

Figure 13-9 First idea for the extruder

the die. Water begins to boil because of the pressure reduction, and this foams the material. The extruder combines three important operations in a single piece of equipment. These are mixing, cooking and foaming. The difficult part is that the equipment has to be designed carefully to balance these operations.

During experiments with the extruder, you find spiral extrudates (Figure 13-10). The reason is that the die allows a flow larger at the outside than in the middle. The extrudate then must increase its circumference by spiralling. You like the shape. So do the marketers, and they find that consumers do too. With agreement from management, you decide to develop a spiral snack: a Wokkel. This does require going back to the design (phase 2) of the product . . .

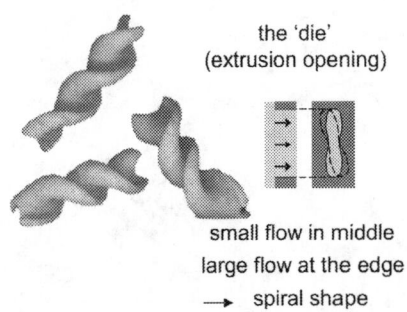

Figure 13-10 Spiral Wokkels[6]

You are expecting to produce 1000 kg of Wokkels per hour; the temperature in the extruder should go up to 150 °C, with a residence time of 20 s. This does not yet fix the dimensions of the extruder (Figure 13-11): the diameter, length, pitch and rotational speed and other details that we have not discussed, including the design of the die. One can model large parts of the behaviour of the extruder, and the manufacturer has experience. However, in the end, real development requires experiments with a real extruder.

---

[6] The shape of the Wokkel has nothing to do with the screw of the extruder.

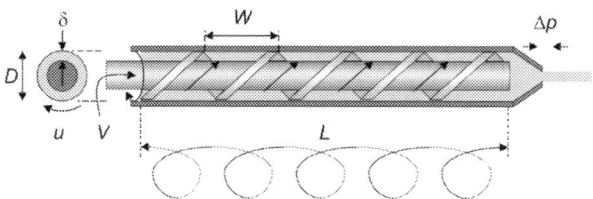

screw geometry	*from model and advice of manufacturer, experiment*
recipe	*starch + water; salt, milk powder, fat, spices*
moisture content	*natural: 11 - 14 %, 10 % added*
temp profile	$20\,^{0}C \longrightarrow 150\,^{0}C$
pressure profile	$0.1\ MPa \longrightarrow 20\ MPa$
residence time	*20 s*
feed	$1000\ kg\ hr^{-1}$
die head	*shape of product, enough resistance*

Figure 13-11 Final extruder parameters

Plant Designs

The first design of the plant looks like Figure 13-12. During trial runs, with an extruder from the manufacturer, you run into several complications. The feed contains too much water; part of this is removed in a vacuum section in the extruder. This also lowers the temperature before aromas and other volatile or heat-sensitive components are fed towards the end of the extruder.

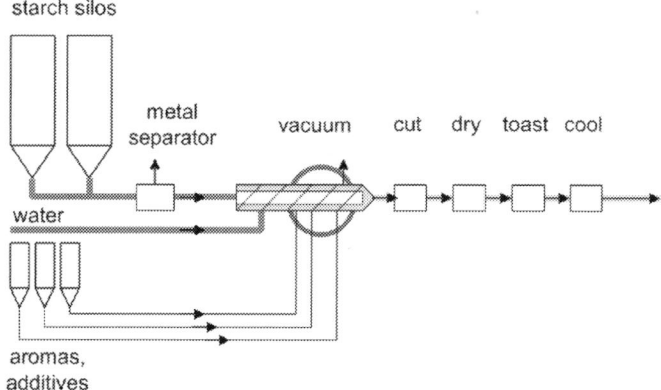

Figure 13-12 First plant design

A little later, the plant has been commissioned and now even upgraded. The throughput of the extruder has been increased by adding a pre-conditioner for swelling and partial dissolution of the raw materials (Figure 13-13).

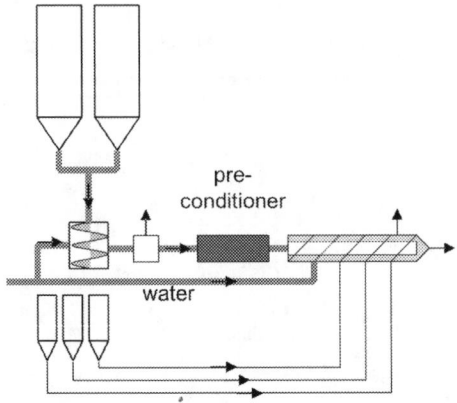

Figure 13-13 Improved plant design

Is this the end of the story? No. Any product needs further development, if only to keep up with the competition. Here is one of the ideas that remains to be worked out for the next version of the product. The foamed Wokkels have an extremely low density, especially with the way that they are packaged. This causes high transport costs, and requires large areas in supermarkets. Wouldn't it be a good idea to let the consumer do the foaming at home? This would have the additional advantage that the product could be 'home made' and 'fresher', possibly with less cost for the manufacturer. You convene a meeting of your colleagues . . .

Looking Back

We finish by considering how the flow of work compared with the original plan, where it would have flown from phase to phase (Figure 13-14). We have backtracked at least four times: when we decided to go for cooking extrusion, when we discovered 'wokkling', when we had to change the extruder, and when we installed the pre-conditioner in the already running plant. You might even regard looking at a new improved product as a fifth backtracking . . . The overall flow is towards the final product – but not in the orderly

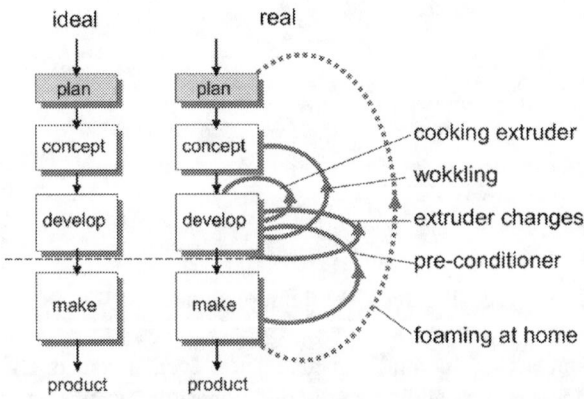

Figure 13-14 Ideal and real (tortuous) path of development

fashion that we had planned. Except in the simplest of projects, you must live with some back-tracking: it is unavoidable in the uncertainty of new development.

Summary

This lesson has introduced you to the choice of equipment for the plant.

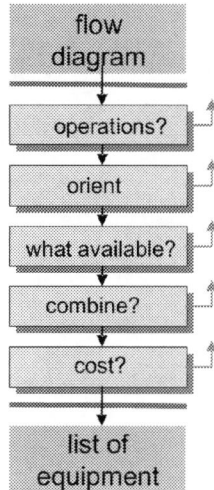

1. First consider the operations that are required in your flow diagram.
2. Then try to find out how they work.
3. When you have this, start finding what is already available in the firm, or can easily be hired, and what manufacturers of equipment can offer.
4. Consider whether you might be able to combine operations, so that you need less equipment.
5. Throughout the whole of this, you should be getting data on cost: that will largely determine your design choices.
6. You will end with a list of equipment.

Further Reading

Robert H. Perry and Don W. Green *Perry's Chemical Engineering Handbook*, 7th edition, McGraw-Hill 1997. This is the starting point for all process engineers, also those dealing with products. The 2500 pages of fine print may put you off. However, you do not have to read them in one go, and there is a searchable electronic version.

Lesson 14: Scale Up

An industry–university co-operation

Now comes a critical stage: learning to make large amounts of product. You need these for testing, both by yourself and by customers or potential customers.

There *are* differences between small and large operations. Consider a spray dryer. A laboratory machine might have a volume of 1 m^3. Suppose you are spraying a sugar solution, and something goes wrong. You end up with a kilogram of sticky, partly soluble sugar on the wall of the machine. Cleaning will be a nasty job. Now think of what happens if you do the same in a 1000 m^3 spray dryer, in which you deposit 1 ton of sugar ... #@&!! Believe us, this can happen. There are more differences between small and large operations, and you will have to learn to handle these.

The Method

Unless you have experience with related products, it is risky to scale up in one step. A method is shown below (Figure 14-1). Begin with the working lab recipe and a diagram with all process steps. Then design the equipment for each step in the large plant. Use experience (for example from equipment manufacturers). If they are available, computer models can also

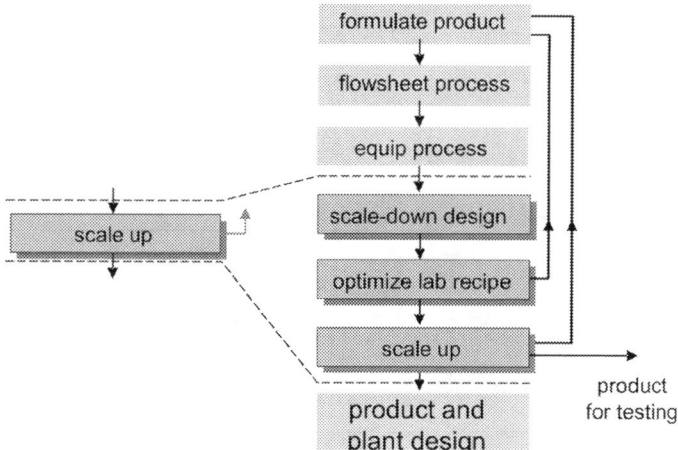

Figure 14-1 A method for scaling up

Design and Development of Biological, Chemical, Food and Pharmaceutical Products   J.A. Wesselingh,
S. Kiil and M.E. Vigild
© 2007 John Wiley & Sons, Ltd

help. Then start thinking: 'How could I get the same product from the lab and from the plant?' This should lead to a scaled down process, using lab equipment. Go back two stages and adjust the lab recipe for use with the new equipment, then optimize the recipe again. After you have the recipe working anew, scale up and start making product for serious testing. Perhaps you can do this on an existing plant; otherwise you may need some intermediate scale (which is expensive). When you have done it, you have the product and the plant design. This sounds easier than it is.

Pharmaceutical Tablets

An example: looking at a new application of *inulin* (Figure 14-2).[1] Inulin is a polysaccharide obtained from chicory roots. It is a foodstuff with the interesting properties: sweet, non-fattening and healthy. Although it sells well in the food industry, the company is looking for other markets. The question to be answered by a team of three students[2] is: could we use inulin as a filler–binder for pharmaceutical tablets?

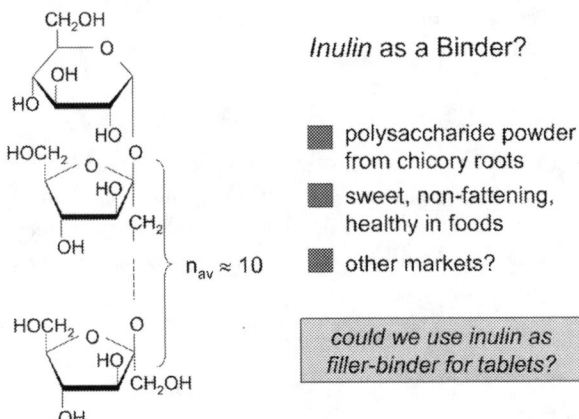

Figure 14-2 Properties of inulin

Inulin is produced on a 10 000 ton per year scale. This is much less than ordinary sugar, but still substantial. The extraction and purification are similar to those in beet sugar production (Figure 14-3). There is one important difference. Crystallized inulin is difficult to compress – we need an amorphous product. This is obtained by spray drying, where particles are formed so rapidly that they cannot crystallize. This is a critical step if you wish to make a good binder. There are more critical steps!

A tabletting machine makes hundreds of thousands of tablets per hour. The time available for filling the tablet cylinder is only a few microseconds, so the flow properties of the binder powder are important. In addition the tablet piston has to be lubricated, and the lubricant can

---

[1] Inulin and insulin have nothing to do with each other.
[2] The project was largely done by the Master's students T.P. Adrichem, R. Sepp and M. de Graaf, and sponsored by A. J. Mul from Sensus, a manufacturer of inulin. They were assisted by J.A. Wesselingh, H.W. Frijlink and G.K. Bolhuis from the University of Groningen.

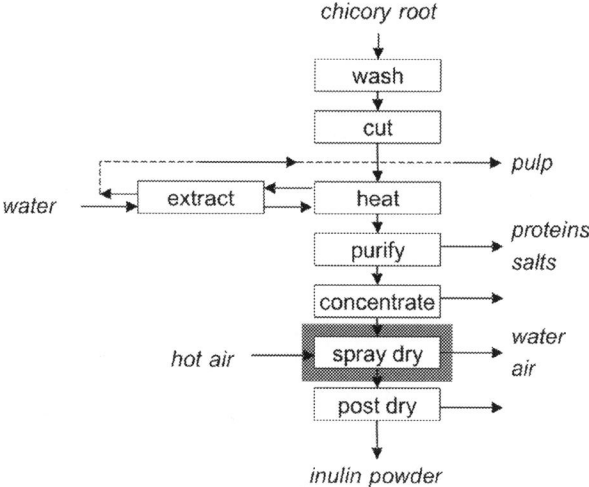

Figure 14-3 How inulin is made

binders →	Inulin	MCC	Dicalcium Phosphate	Mannitol
↓ property				
flow properties	0	—	+	0
binding strength	++	++	0	++
mixing properties	+	++	+	+
stability	++	++	0	+

Figure 14-4 Comparing inulin with other binders

impair the binding strength of the tablets formed. Figure 14-4 compares these two and some other properties of filler–binders that are thought to be important. It compares inulin with microcrystalline cellulose (MCC), dicalcium phosphate and mannitol (another saccharide). We see that inulin compares favourably on many points. Questions the students have to answer are: can we make a good binder on a small scale, and if so, can we make the same one on a large scale. We will only consider effects on the first two items: the flow and binding properties.

Powder Properties

Figure 14-5 shows a photograph of a good powder produced in a small (1 m^3) laboratory spray dryer. We see that it consists of spherical glassy particles, of which the largest have a diameter of about 50 µm. Many of the particles are hollow – we come back to that in a moment. The flow properties of spherical particles are expected to be good if:

(1) they are not too small and
(2) they do not stick together.

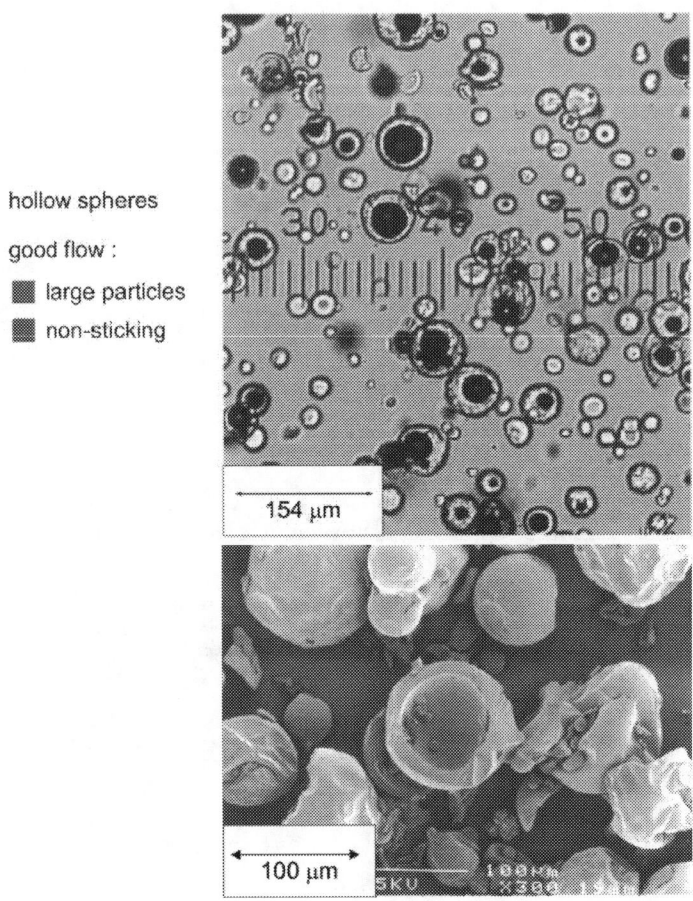

hollow spheres

good flow :

■ large particles

■ non-sticking

154 μm

100 μm

Figure 14-5 Hollow spheres made by spray drying

We can avoid sticking problems by keeping the particles cool and dry.[3] However, the particles must be large enough, both in the small and the large experiments.

We get particles of different sizes. Each has a mass equivalent diameter,[4] which is the diameter of a sphere with the same mass as the particle. One can characterize the sizes with a cumulative mass distribution such as in the upper part of Figure 14-6. This shows which mass fraction is in the particle with a diameter smaller than a certain value. The frequency distribution underneath is derived from the upper diagram: it gives an indication of which diameters are most common. We can try to characterize the drops with a single diameter; there are many different ways in which this can be done. They lead to parameters such as the d_{32} (Sauter diameter), d_{50} (mean diameter) and d_{max} (maximum

---

[3] Particles must stay below the glass transition temperature.
[4] This belongs to the subject of Particle Technology.

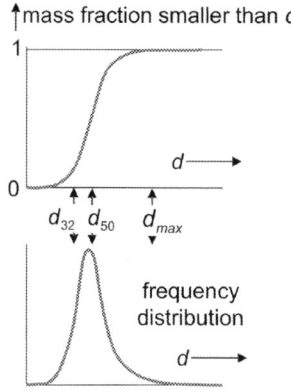

Figure 14-6 Particle size distributions

diameter). Each of these has its uses, but it would take too much time to discuss them here. The important diameter for us is the maximum diameter, which is just what its name suggests.

Figure 14-7 shows tablet data obtained by the students with their materials. It shows the strength of tablets against the compaction force used. We see that the strength of tablets of the inulin powder used here hardly depends on whether lubricant (magnesium stearate) is added or not. This is a desirable characteristic of such powders.

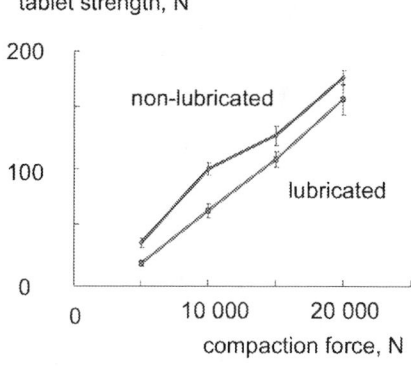

Figure 14-7 Tablet strength versus compaction force

The reason why hollow spheres are effective is shown in Figure 14-8. As said, lubrication is provided by magnesium stearate, which surrounds the particles. When solid particles are pressed together, the interfaces are covered by a lubricant film which gives poor binding. With hollow particles, fracturing forms fresh surfaces, which *do* give good binding. It is becoming clear what we need: well-dried spherical particles, with the same size and hollowness when they are produced on different scales.

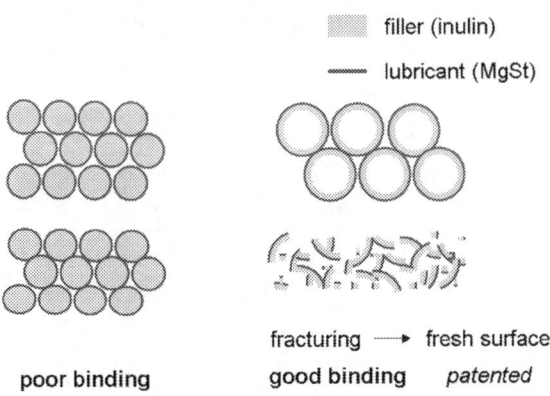

Figure 14-8 Why hollow spheres give good binding

Spray Drying

Figure 14-9 shows the spray dryer.[5] This is a large cylindrical vessel with a conical bottom. Hot air enters at the top via a distributor. A concentrated solution of inulin in water is dispersed as small droplets. These are flung outwards by a spinning wheel, and dry rapidly in the hot air. The dry powder falls down and is collected at the bottom of the machine. The air flow leaves the dryer via a tube in the conical section; powder carried by this flow is separated by a cyclone.

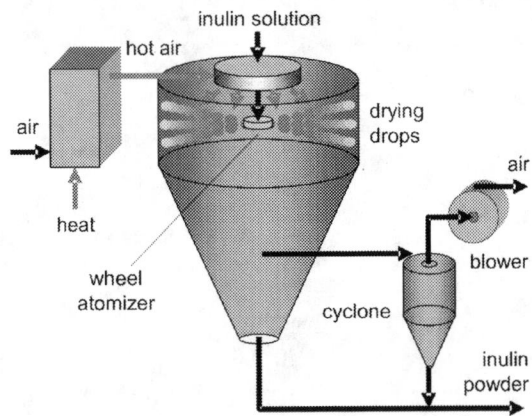

Figure 14-9 The spray dryer

Scaling Down

You want to use a small machine for development, and a large machine for production. The small machine should be as small as practical to allow quick and flexible experimentation. The size of the large machine is dictated by the required throughput unless (as here) it already exists. We shall see that this requires a different approach to the design of the atomizers. As

[5] This is not primarily a dryer, but a machine for making powders. The students used machines with diameters of 1.5, 3 and 12 m (full scale).

a result the two dryers will not have the same geometry. You *do* want the two machines to produce the same product. This means they should provide the same drop sizes, and the same drying conditions.

To understand the operation we need to look inside the dryer (Figure 14-10). Drops are ejected from the edge of the wheel with a velocity close to the rim speed (1). This might be a 100 m s^{-1}. However, the tiny drops are decelerated over a short distance by the surrounding air (2) and then carried on by the gas circulation (3). As long as their outside is wet, the drops dry at a more-or-less constant rate. Their outside has to be dry (4) before they hit the wall (5). Otherwise you will have to clean the spray dryer! The atomizer causes a large circulation flow. As a result, the bulk of the dryer has a more-or-less constant temperature and humidity (6). With temperature and humidity the same everywhere, the wet drops dry with a constant rate. Their drying time is roughly proportional to their diameter. They typically dry in a few seconds.

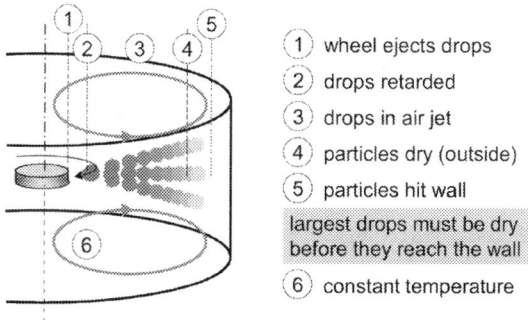

Figure 14-10 Inside the spray dryer

The drops are made by a vaned wheel (the atomizer, Figure 14-11). This forms thin films of liquid that disintegrate into droplets of the concentrated inulin solution. (In the drawing the wheel is open; actually the rim is closed except for slits to allow the film out.) Under suitable conditions, the vaporizing water carries inulin to the surface of the drop, where it forms a skin, and finally a hollow sphere.

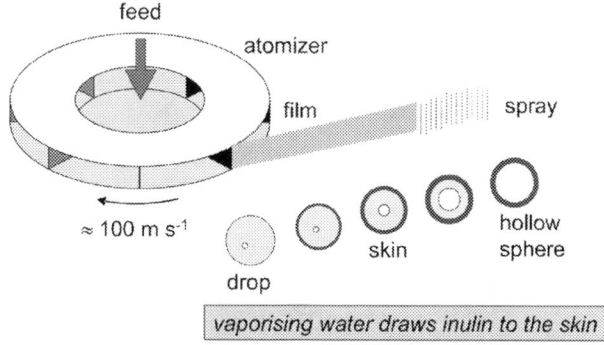

Figure 14-11 Formation of hollow spheres

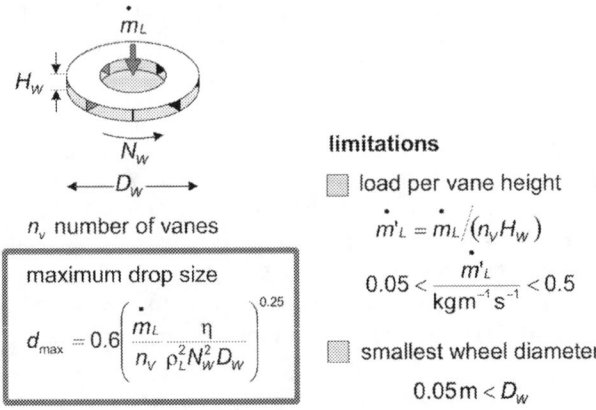

n_v number of vanes

maximum drop size

$$d_{max} = 0.6 \left(\frac{\dot{m}_L}{n_v \ \rho_L^2 N_w^2 D_w} \ \eta \right)^{0.25}$$

limitations

☐ load per vane height

$$\dot{m}'_L = \dot{m}_L / (n_v H_w)$$

$$0.05 < \frac{\dot{m}'_L}{\mathrm{kgm^{-1}s^{-1}}} < 0.5$$

☐ smallest wheel diameter

$$0.05\,\mathrm{m} < D_w$$

Figure 14-12 A formula for the drop size[6]

Figure 14-12 shows a formula for the size of the largest drops produced by a wheel atomizer. You can make the same drops with combinations of different variables: the mass flow of liquid, the number of vanes, the speed of rotation, the diameter and the height of the wheel ... There are practical limitations; two of these are shown. First, the liquid loading of the vane should neither be too low, nor too high. Too low values cause distribution problems; with too high values, flow in the wheel is no longer laminar. A second limitation (for small dryers) is that one can hardly make a good wheel smaller than about 5 cm in diameter.

Scaling Considerations

The time available for the drops to dry depends on their average velocity and the radius of the dryer (Figure 14-13). In the small machine you want a small radius; you get this by minimizing the velocity of the drops. This requires low ejection velocities and low air circulation velocities. (The two are related). In the large machine drops have to move away quickly from the atomizer to minimize collisions and agglomeration. This is a very different requirement.

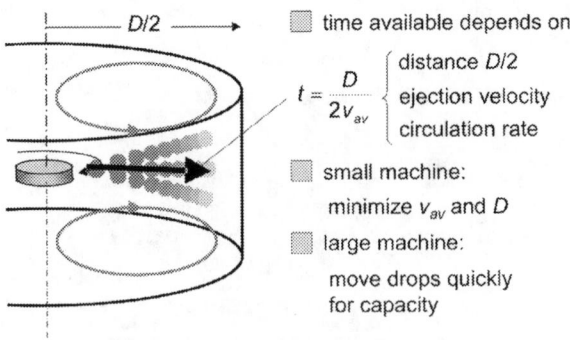

☐ time available depends on:

$$t = \frac{D}{2v_{av}} \quad \begin{cases} \text{distance } D/2 \\ \text{ejection velocity} \\ \text{circulation rate} \end{cases}$$

☐ small machine:

minimize v_{av} and D

☐ large machine:

move drops quickly for capacity

Figure 14-13 Drying time available

---

[6] This is a semi-theoretical equation assuming that liquid flows as a laminar film over slightly tilted plates.

To understand the behaviour of the spray dryers the students used a computer model that was put together for another occasion. It was based on the ideas from the previous figures. Figure 14-14 shows results of calculations for two sizes of spray dryer: a small lab machine (still with a diameter of over 2 m) and a large production machine. The two operate at the same temperature and humidity, and thus with the same drying conditions. Also they produce the same drop sizes. So you can expect them to produce the same product (well, roughly . . .). The dimensioning of the wheel for the two cases is different, as is the product load per volume. Scaling down required the installation of a new atomizer in our lab dryer – and a lot of tests.

	unit	small	large
maximum drop size	μm	60	60
number of vanes	-	2	16
vane liquid load	kg m^{-1} s^{-1}	0.05	0.5
throughput	kg s^{-1}	0.0005	0.5
height/diameter wheel	-	5	5
dryer diameter	m	2.15	13
wheel diameter	m	0.05	0.63
wheel speed	s^{-1}	59	18.5
centrifugal acceleration	m s^{-2}	3300	4200

these give *approximately* the same product

Figure 14-14 Results of scaling calculations

There are many other differences between lab and plant operations:

(1) In the lab, development often starts using standard lab chemicals. These can be of a much higher quality and price than what you will be using in the plant. If possible, the technical materials should be used in the later stages of development, also in the lab.
(2) The same applies to all kinds of auxiliary materials such as packings for separation columns, filter-media and -aids, and catalysts.
(3) Processes in the lab are mostly done batchwise. This is easier and more flexible than continuous operation. However, on a large scale continuous operation can be better. If you decide to change during the development, you will have to redo a lot of work.
(4) Finally there are many differences in procedures between lab and plant operations. You have to consider whether these might influence your plant and product design.

Other Equipment

We have only looked at the scaling down and scaling up of a spray dryer. Other equipment requires other rules. A few examples:

(1) Scaling up of a filter is relatively straightforward. If you do lab experiments with a Büchner funnel, and use the same feed, medium and pressure drop as on a large scale, you can expect the same cake properties.

(2) Scaling up of mixers is a bit more difficult. Most mixing operations are concerned with making dispersions. The trick is then to have the same level of turbulence on the scale of the dispersion. This requires not-too-small vessels, and the same level of dissipation.

(3) The same applies to a crystallizer, but here it is additionally important that nucleation (formation of new crystals) is controlled, for example by controlled addition of small crystals (seeding) and dissolving nuclei. Crystallization is often very sensitive to levels of impurities, so it is important to use the same materials on a small and on a large scale.

(4) As a final example: the extruder. This is a difficult machine in the lab. It operates continuously, and even the smallest extruders have a high throughput. So they can produce an enormous amount of waste. Small machines can be cooled easily, but this is not a good idea when you are going to scale up, as large machines cannot be cooled.

Summary

Our summary can be short.

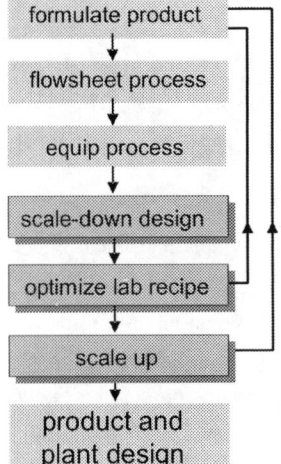

1. Before you make a product on a large scale, first choose your equipment.
2. Then try to learn how to make the same product in the lab.
3. Try to do as much as possible of the optimization in the lab, realizing the limitations (and advantages) that large equipment will provide.
4. Only start large production runs when you have a fairly good idea of what you are doing.
5. Failures in a production run on a large scale can be very expensive, not only because you lose product, but also because you have to dispose of the rubbish.

Further Reading

The standard text on spray drying is still K. Masters *Spray Drying Handbook*, Halsted Press 1985.

Part 4   **Exploit**

In these last four lessons we look ahead to when design and development of our product will be ready. We ask what is necessary to develop the market, try to predict the value of our project (how much money we can expect and when), and wonder how the product will be sold. We end looking even further: which products should come after this?

Lesson 15:
Organize the Market

With help from Thomas Heldgaard (Rockwool) and Sijmon van der Wal

You have developed a product, and want it bought by customers. This will not happen by itself: you will have to market and sell the product. This requires a marketing plan. Marketing is an integral part of any project and planning (well, speculating and thinking) has to start early. You have already been developing parts of this plan when you started thinking about customers and products in lessons 5–9 and about cost in lessons 12. Making a marketing plan is much like designing a product: you have to consider many possibilities and to make choices. Here we assume that a concept has been chosen, and look at the questions that you should then ask yourself.

'Live on Your Roof'

Our example is from the company named Rockwool. The company produces quite a number of things, but its main interest is in thermal insulation of buildings, using, not surprisingly, Rockwool (see Appendix 15-2).

Rockwool is made in several forms; Figure 15-1 gives an impression of types used in traditional house building. Most of the Rockwool materials are weak and not suited for loading mechanically. However, Rockwool has developed treadable insulation panels for flat

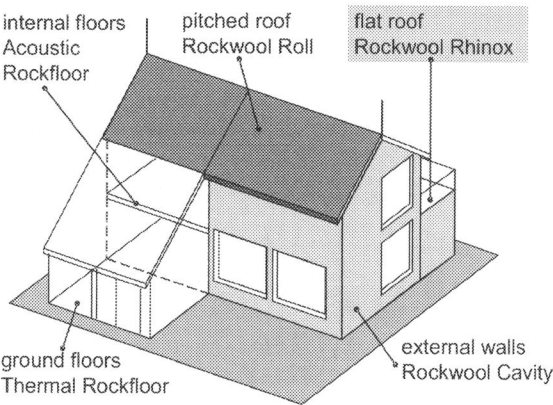

Figure 15-1 Some of the Rockwool products

Design and Development of Biological, Chemical, Food and Pharmaceutical Products   J.A. Wesselingh, S. Kiil and M.E. Vigild
© 2007 John Wiley & Sons, Ltd

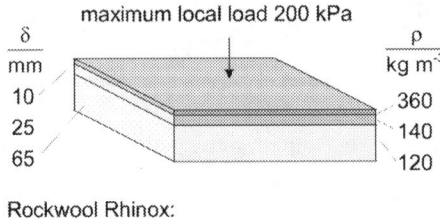

Rockwool Rhinox:
three-layer tread-resistant flat roof insulation

Figure 15-2 A three-layer treadable roof insulation

roofs. A recent type, Rockwool Rhinox (Figure 15-2), has a thin but fairly dense top layer, followed by a thicker but more open middle layer and a thick but weak bottom layer. The top layers spread the load over a large area, so that the bottom layer is hardly deformed by people walking on the roof. So we can build cheap treadable well-insulated flat roofs, and that is the beginning of the idea that we will explore in this lesson.

The idea is this. We can build cheap flat roof constructions on which one can do things; in summer people could *live* outside on such a roof. This is not new: in many countries living outside is common, also living on roofs. However, the fact that we can provide such roofs cheaply and with a good thermal (and possibly also acoustic) insulation may change the game. Could we market the *concept* 'Live on Your Roof' instead of the material? 'Live on Your Roof' will require that we understand and perhaps influence the lifestyle of our customers. It will mean that we get involved in selling design concepts and not just building-insulation.

One further idea that we are playing with is to find a first customer interested in the idea. We will get assistance from an architect and a construction engineer to work out the plans. They will have to develop ideas on living outside; on how to handle sun, cold, wind and rain. To entice the customer we may need to provide some guarantees or co-financing. In return we expect him to share experiences with us and further customers.

We are going to explore this by setting up a marketing plan. This is an exercise; we are not suggesting that it is a good idea. It is not the main way that Rockwool currently markets its materials.

The Method

With a complicated problem like this, it is not a bad idea to begin with a method. We will be using one called 'The HEMP' by its author. HEMP stands for Highly Effective Marketing Plan; it is described much better than we can do here in the book by Peter Knight (see Further Reading).

The HEMP consists of five groups of steps (Figure 15-3):

(A) Define your goal (product, turnover, profit).
(B) Look at your target audience (customers).

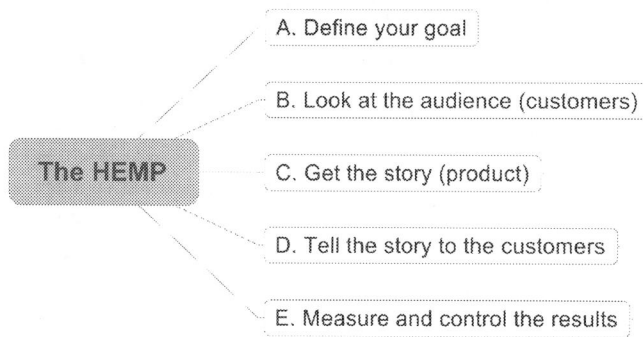

Figure 15-3 The five groups of questions

(C) Get your story (product) in order.
(D) Tell the story to the customers.
(E) Measure and control the results.

There are three steps in each group, so fifteen steps altogether. Groups (A) and (E) consider things that are important for your company (or yourself); steps (B), (C) and (D) consider things that are required for your customers. These are at least as important.

The HEMP is a general method, not only applicable to marketing of a product, but also to services and to non-profit activities. The author states that it is a linear method: one that goes forward step by step. This is not our experience; we have found that questions later in the sequence often send you back to an earlier point. For example, the goal and target may become clearer as you are working out the HEMP, causing you to go through the whole thing again. Not all steps are equally relevant to each project. Even so, we have found the HEMP to give a provoking set of questions that help you not to forget important things. There are few marketing publications of which that can be said.

In the following we work through the steps of the HEMP method and apply them to our example. In each paragraph we first briefly describe the step and then consider our situation, noting our ideas and impressions *in italic*.

Define Your Goal

We begin with a few questions that are important for you.

Step (1). What is the desired result? Begin your market plan by writing this down clearly. If you don't know, there is not much point in planning! Your goal has to be in measurable terms. A good plan has a single goal, and this goal must be worthwhile – for your company, and for you.

The goal is to evaluate whether 'Live on Your Roof' is a viable concept. This means that you are to have at least 500 customers and a turnover of one million euros 2 years after starting. You have 6 months to make a proposal.

Step (2). Estimate what the project will be worth. Which turnover could it generate? Could it give a profit, and when? You will need to have some idea if you want to get other people involved, perhaps as investors.

You must find out what your proposition is worth to a typical customer, how many customers you might expect, and the cost of materials and work. You may need some marketing research, but will have to keep it cheap at this point.

Step (3). Consider the consequences of your plan. There will be positive ones, but also negative ones. Consider what will happen if you do not pursue your plan. Will your competitors do so?

On the positive side: you expect 'Live on Your Roof' to be an attractive sales proposition. You may be able to draw customers away from other companies. 'Live on Your Roof' will lead to new learning in the company and perhaps to a different way of doing business. On the negative side there will be initial losses; you have to spend time and money in the first half year with no return. You may have the hassle of producing of prototype material that differs from the standard. And, as always, anything new will cannibalize existing sales.

The Target Audience (Customers)

This is perhaps the most important set of questions – it is unfortunately often overlooked.

Step (4). Here you consider the audience: the customers. Who will be buying the product? The better you know, the better your chances. The people buying are often not the end-users. Buying is often influenced by others as well, and this is handy to know.

Insulation material for buildings will seldom be bought by the house owner. It will be specified by the architect and the construction engineer in accordance with local building rules. The one to order and pay the material will be the builder, so this is the person to influence. The final choice is with the house owner, but he will be strongly influenced by the architect. So getting an architect and construction engineer involved early in the project looks like a good idea that you can add to the positives in Step (3).

Step (5). What are the buyers currently thinking and doing? They are undoubtedly spending the money that you hope to get, elsewhere on some other product. Why are they doing this? What do they think about the competition? Marketing research can help to find out. This is usually done by market research firms; it is difficult for insiders to be impartial. However, you can waste a lot of money on such research if you do not have clear goals.

Your buyers are currently having traditional roofs built, mostly pitched roofs. Many, but by no means all, will be insulated with Rockwool materials. If these customers do have a flat roof, they are probably not using it because it has not been constructed with that in mind. If they do 'live on their roof' the construction or insulation are not optimal. You might call ten customers to find out; after all, you are trying to define the 'customer's voice'.

Step (6). What do *you* want the buyers to think and to do? You may be able to change their habits by good communication and good products and services.

You want them to think of 'Living on Your Roof', and to lead to them buying your insulation materials and constructions.

Get the Story (Product)

The next questions consider what the story is that you wish to get across to your customers.

Step (7). What is the story? State what the products do and keep focused. What are you selling? You may think you know, but does the customer have the same idea? It is the idea of the customer that counts, not yours.

Your idea is: 'We will provide you (as customer) with a comfortable way of living outside on a well-constructed and insulated roof. This will not require ground space.' (It may turn out that the customer thinks of something else – for example the opportunity to 'show off'. You will then have to change your marketing strategy, but will only find out by doing.)

Step (8). The big thing. Can you tell what you are selling – quickly, clearly and convincingly? Could you get the main point over in 30 s? In 10 s? If you cannot, you still have something to work on.

You have already done this: 'Live on Your Roof' is about as short as you can make it.

Step (9). Is there a real benefit in your plan for your customers? If there is not, you are on a slippery slope. Is it a new technique, for the sake of the new technique? That will not be good enough. Reconsider?

'Live on Your Roof' will improve the lifestyle of customers; it will allow them to live outside even where space is short, such as in cities.

Tell the Story (to Customers)

The next group of questions is how you tell the story and communicate with your customers.

Step (10). Know yourself. There are always at least two in communication. One of them will be you (or your firm) and you should find out how the customers see the firm. Your firm must have an appropriate personality. If it doesn't, you will have to work on it, and it is easier to change *your* personality than that of the customers.

Rockwool is a reliable technically oriented provider of insulation materials for the building industry. It is a company mostly involved in business-to-business or B2B marketing, which requires a solid image (see Appendix 15-1). For the 'Live on Your Roof' concept a different image might be required, perhaps that of a life-style designer. It might be better to set up a separate little company under a different name to try the concept out. This new company can more easily make consistent noises on 'Live on Your Roof' than Rockwool as a whole can do. It may have to work in quite different ways.

Step (11). How to talk to the audience. There are many options to reach your audience: television, radio, press (including the trade press), cinema, telephone sales, folders, the Internet ... You must try to find those niches that reach and influence your target audience, but, as far as possible, not others. Otherwise you are sure to waste resources and make a nuisance out of yourself (see also Appendix 15-1).

What to do here? Your possible customers are only a small fraction of the people reached by traditional advertising. You are already thinking of getting an architect to make designs using Rhinox and to have a construction engineer to consider the technical problems. Via these people you might be able to get further customers, so a building firm can get experience with your product. Once you have built your first house, you could try to get coverage in architectural and home magazines. Before that you will need to have a web-site.[1]

Step (12). How much marketing budget? There is no real answer to this; you will have to find out by trying. You can set yourself a few limits. Step (2) will have given you some idea of how much profit you might expect from your project. Your marketing costs must remain below that amount and probably well below it. On the other hand, you have also planned a few things in Step (11). You can estimate how much these will cost.

In your case the first half year will have to be paid from this budget – there will be no income. What do you cost? What will a design by an architect cost? What will an advertisement in a trade journal cost? If this looks like costing more than you wish to spend, could you find other ways? You might be able to get an architect and a constructor interested if you could promise that further projects would be done by them. This would have the advantage for you that they would be motivated to do a good job.

Measure and Control the Results

The last group of questions considers how you are going to run the business.

Step (13). Other Resources. You are going to need resources to get your plan going and you have to know which ones before you really start. Especially people have to be brought on board early, whether they are your own employees or people you have hired or coaxed outside.

What are you going to need for 'Live on Your Roof'? Let us make a list starting at the beginning. It might look like this:

1. *Yourself*
2. *Office space and equipment*
3. *Your assistant (?)*
4. *The financial analysis (by Rockwool?)*
5. *Money (from Rockwool?)*
6. *The decision making people in Rockwool*
7. *The architect*
8. *The client who is willing to develop our ideas*
9. *The construction engineer*
10. *The builder*
11. *The people from Rockwool who make the prototype*
12. *The agent for getting the idea to further clients*
13. *The website . . .*

Have you got the important ones? Are your estimates realistic (not too optimistic)? Nobody likes extra expenses after a project has started. As plans always have to be adapted, you must

---

[1] The HEMP gives some worthwhile remarks on websites.

have a bit spare. Finally, you must have time and money commitments for your plans before you begin.

Step (14). How to Measure. You have to decide beforehand in which ways you will measure whether things are going well or not. This depends very much on the task which you have set yourself.

In this example you might set up a rough time schedule of the items to be finished (Step (13)). This involves getting the first ideas worked out, the prototype installed in a new building, getting communication material and getting the website in order. Your measurement will initially be whether you are more-or-less on schedule. At the same time you must keep expenditure under control, which should not be difficult in this example. After you have gone into publicity, you might start keeping notes on whether magazines are reacting, trying to find out whether potential customers are reading advertisements or articles, and following the response to your website. You will only proceed further if you see enough people seriously interested (and will have to think further on decision criteria). In most other HEMPs the problem will be to predict financial performance of a project, so that it does not run out of hand.

Measuring with a Website

A website is a good measurement tool. There are free monitoring tools that can give important information such as:

(1) How did customers find the website? If they found it via a search engine, which search items did they enter? Do these search items fit in your marketing strategy? Should you change the site or change the marketing strategy?
(2) How many visits do you have per day? Take action if the number of visits decreases in two subsequent months. Note that the number of visits is not the same as the number of hits. A page with 11 pictures may give 12 hits: one for the page and one for each picture. So hits are not the right parameters for assessing how much traffic your website generates.
(3) How long do visitors stay on your website? Do they come back? Those who come back are the ones that are interesting for marketing.
(4) Did you receive a request for information? What was the follow-up?

Step (15). What Next? Write your plan in your own words. Make a list of the first ten points or so that you are going to implement. If you feel better about completing stages of the plan than waiting till everything is ready, set out the stages.

You have already been doing this; you have been working on what to do in Step (13). It will be clear that the whole plan of getting a trial project working and publicized is only the first stage of the business (assuming that things work out well).

At the end: look ahead. After this HEMP you will need a new one, for the next stage of your business.

Summary

We summarize with a complete mind map of the Highly Effective Marketing Plan (Figure 15-4).

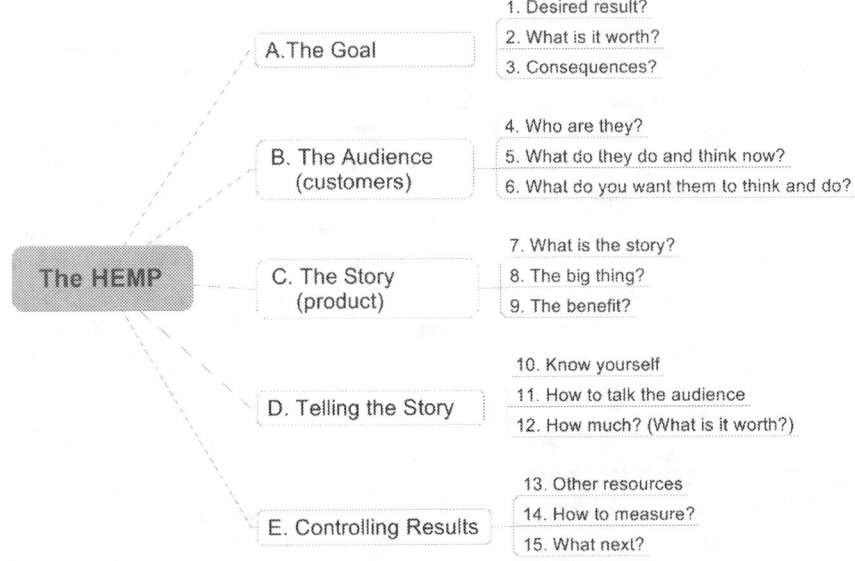

Figure 15-4 Overview of the HEMP method

Further Reading

This lesson is largely based on:

Peter Knight *The Highly Effective Marketing Plan (HEMP)*, Pearson 2004.

On marketing in general: Alexander Hiam *Marketing for Dummies*, Hungry Minds 1997, 2001.

The business-to-business market: Steve Minett *B2B Marketing*, Pearson 2002.

Appendix 15-1
Two Markets and Advertising

You may get involved in two different kinds of market (Figure 15-5). The one you know from the supermarket is the 'B2C' or business-to-consumer market. Here there are huge numbers of small transactions, which are mostly anonymous (via a cashier for example). This is a market for end-users and it is important. This is the market commonly considered in MBA courses and in all the advertising you see around you. The other 'B2B' or business-to-business market will probably be even more important for you as an engineer. Here the number of transactions is smaller, but the money involved per transaction is orders of magnitude higher.

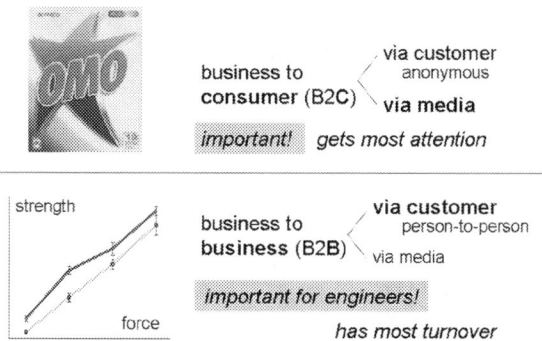

Figure 15-5 The two kinds of market

Because of this person-to-person contacts are much more important as we shall see in lesson 17. B2B companies communicate with customers in ways that are quite different from those of B2C companies.

For a B2B company, it is important to be seen as technically and economically competent (Figure 15-6). The firm has to be trustworthy. In addition, it must show interest in the customer – not so much in itself. The result can look a bit boring compared with the 'personalities' of B2C companies, where fashion and emotion play a much larger role in promoting products. However, we will see that selling in the B2B market is at least as exciting as the stakes are much higher.

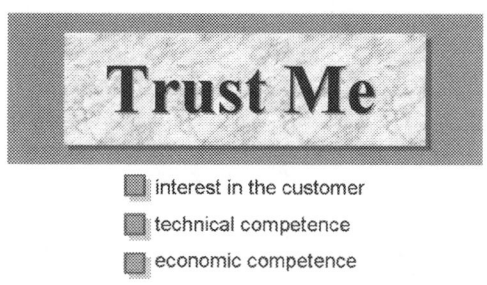

Figure 15-6 The desired business-to-business image

The difference between B2B and B2C marketing also shows in advertising. Important media in B2C marketing are TV, radio and billboards; these are seldom used in B2B marketing. There, advertising is strongly targeted. Getting trade magazines to publish stories on your good and reliable products (with experience from customers) is effective, but cannot be controlled. Direct mail to, or contacts with selected customers is effective – if you have a good list of possible customers. Advertisements in trade journals are more expensive; they are also different from those in consumer media, focusing more on performance. Trade fairs are very expensive: you have to seriously consider whether they are worth the trouble. Finally, advertising on the Internet, via the firm's own or other websites, is increasing rapidly. B2B sales on the Internet still have a much higher value than B2C sales.

In your marketing plan you will have to decide what to spend on the different items. A good marketing advisor may help, but such people do have an interest in promoting more advertisements.

Appendix 15-2
The Design of Rockwool

Rockwool is made of thin fibres spun from molten rock and bonded with polymer at their crossing points to give a very open random mat (Figure 15-7). The fibres have a diameter of about 7 μm; they appear to be straight and cylindrical. The void fraction of the most common type is 0.94. You might wonder why the values have been chosen so. This is probably a result of trying out and chance. However, a few calculations largely explain these dimensions.

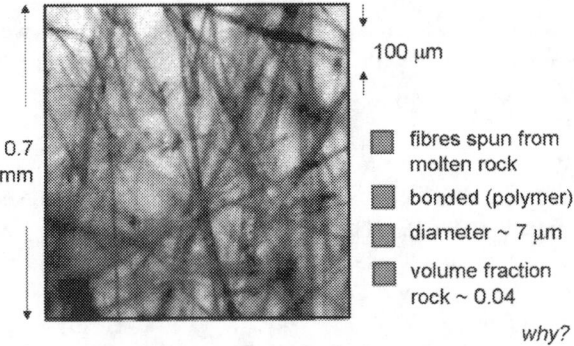

Figure 15-7 Microphoto of Rockwool

Why are fibres so thin?

Under the microscope we see fibres that are straight and cylindrical, with a diameter of about:

$$D := 7 \cdot 10^{-6} \cdot m$$

You might wonder why the fibres are so thin. The thickness does not appear in the equations for the heat transfer or the mechanical properties. A probable reason is that the fibre has to be pliable to allow handling of the material. This is only so if it is thin enough.

Properties of materials are often given in gigapascal: we have to define this unit because Mathcad does not know it:

$$GPa := 10^9 \cdot Pa$$

The stiffness (modulus of elasticity) of the fibre is roughly:

$$E := 50 \cdot 10^3 \cdot GPa$$

For the yield stress in tension we guess:

$$\sigma_{max} := 10 \cdot GPa$$

When a fibre is bent, stresses develop in the fibre. When the tension stresses on the outside of the bend exceed the yield stress in tension, the fibre will break. This happens when the bending radius becomes smaller than a critical value:

$$R_{crit} := \frac{1}{2} \cdot \frac{E}{\sigma_{max}} \cdot D \qquad\qquad R_{crit} = 0.018 \text{ m}$$

We see that we must have thin fibres to allow bending.

The Fraction of Fibre

Why does Rockwool have a volume fraction of fibre of about 0.04? We can try to understand this with a few calculations.

For the pure rock we assume the parameter values

density	$\rho := 3000 \cdot \text{kg} \cdot \text{m}^{-3}$
stiffness	$E := 50 \cdot 10^9 \cdot \text{Pa}$
thermal conductivity	$\lambda := 1.5 \cdot \text{W} \cdot \text{m}^{-1} \cdot \text{K}^{-1}$
	$\lambda_{air} := 0.021 \cdot \text{W} \cdot \text{m}^{-1} \cdot \text{K}^{-1}$

One third of the fibers will be oriented in the transport direction. As a result the thermal conductivity becomes:

$$\lambda_W(\varepsilon) := \frac{\varepsilon}{3} \cdot \lambda + 1 - \frac{\varepsilon}{3} \cdot \lambda_{air}$$

Here ε is the volume fraction of rock.

You might think that something similar would apply to the stiffness (or modulus of elasticity), but this is not so. The fibres are only bonded where they touch each other. These touching points lie at a distance from each other of about:

$$L = \frac{D}{\varepsilon}$$

Here D is the diameter of the fibre.

The stress on the fibres is proportional to the average stress on the mat and inversely proportional to the fraction of fibres:

$$\sigma_{fibre} = \frac{\sigma}{\varepsilon}$$

The deflection of a fibre is proportional to the stress and to the third power of the length between supports:

$$\delta = \sigma_{fibre} \cdot \frac{L^3}{E \cdot D^2}$$

The relative change in length of the mat under stress will be proportional to:

$$\frac{\delta}{L} = \frac{\sigma_{\text{fibre}}}{E} \cdot \frac{L^2}{D} = \frac{\sigma}{E} \cdot \varepsilon^{-3}$$

So the stiffness decreases rapidly when the fraction of fibre is lowered.

The results are plotted in Figure 15-8. To get a low thermal conductivity we would like to have a low fibre fraction, but if we choose it too low, the mat is so flexible that it can stand no stresses. The value $= 0.04$ is probably a compromise.

The mechanical theories used here are from J.E. Gordon *Structures or why things don't fall down*, Da Capo Press 2003.

Lesson 16:
Forecast Money Flows

A spreadsheet exercise

This lesson is on forecasting how money is spent and received during a development project. This is speculation, certainly early in the project and when you do not have experience. Hence the results are not reliable.[1] However, you will see that they teach you things that are useful in making decisions in development work. Here even a rough idea of the cost and revenue of a decision is much better than *no* idea. You can best follow this lesson by putting the example in a spreadsheet and playing with it. This is not at all difficult, and it is fun.

Your Ballpoint Project

Money is both spent and received during a project. The top part of Figure 16-1 shows how money, received from sales, increases in time. In the bottom part we see the amounts spent on development, on preparing the production, on marketing and support, and on production. All amounts are accumulated. Most of the expenses are made *before* we start receiving money from sales.

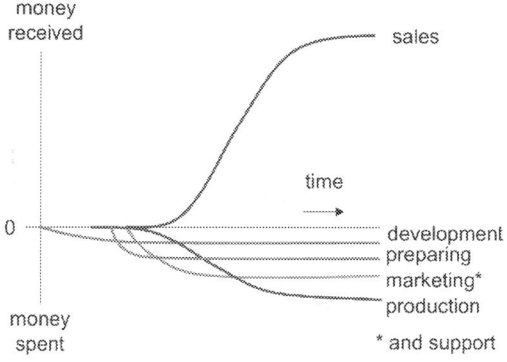

Figure 16-1 Money spent and received in a project

Companies will seldom tell you the financial history of their projects, so we are going to make up an example. Assume that you have invented the

[1] The relation between these financial estimates and those in Lesson 12 is discussed in Appendix 16-1.

Design and Development of Biological, Chemical, Food and Pharmaceutical Products   J.A. Wesselingh, S. Kiil and M.E. Vigild
© 2007 John Wiley & Sons, Ltd

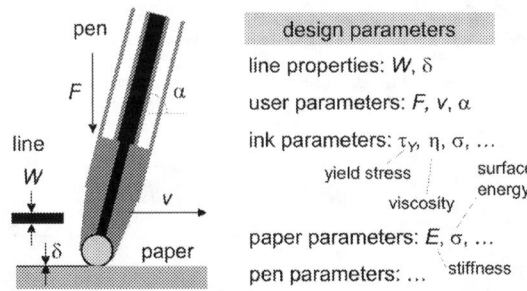

Figure 16-2 Some technical parameters of the pen

ballpoint. You have managed to find a need, set specifications, create concepts (and select one), make a prototype, get a patent, and you have even got a small trial production and sales going. The engineer in you has learned to understand the technicalities and relations between design variables (Figure 16-2). Now you want to improve your product and expand operations: Project Ballpoint 2. To do this you will need to have an idea of what will happen with money in your project.

The Economic Model

For this money out/in analysis, we use a four-step method:

1. We first build a model in a spreadsheet, in its simplest or base form.[2]
2. We use the model to do a *sensitivity analysis*: to see which changes in our project have a large effect, and which ones do not.
3. We use the results to help make decisions.
4. Some important factors cannot be included in the model; we consider these separately.

Back to the Ballpoint 2 project. You think further development is going to take 5 person–years of work, which costs €500 000. For preparing of the production you expect to spend €200 000; during production, on marketing and support €100 000 per year (Figure 16-3). Marketing research suggests you will be able to sell the product up to 4 years from now: it will then be overtaken by other products, either from you or from the competition. In the sales period you

	k€	
development	500	*about 5*
production prep	200	*person-years*
marketing	100	per year
production	0.004	per unit
sales price	0.008	per unit
sales	200000	per year

Figure 16-3 Costs assumed in our project

---

[2] Keep the model simple. Simple means using only a few categories and large time steps. The uncertainties in development do not warrant much more and complexity may confuse.

hope to sell 200 000 units per year, at a price of €8 (the ballpoint is at this moment still a novelty). The cost per unit is €4, estimated as in the lesson 12.

In your spreadsheet, use one quarter of a year as the unit of time. Spread out the different activities over the 4 years (Figure 16-4). Take development to require 1 year, or four quarters. Preparing production takes two quarters, of which one can overlap with the end of development. Marketing and support activities begin in earnest one quarter before production begins and go on for the rest of the 4 years. Assume that sales follow production immediately. There are many assumptions: experience with similar projects is desirable to be able to make reasonable ones. When your report such calculations you must also report the assumptions!

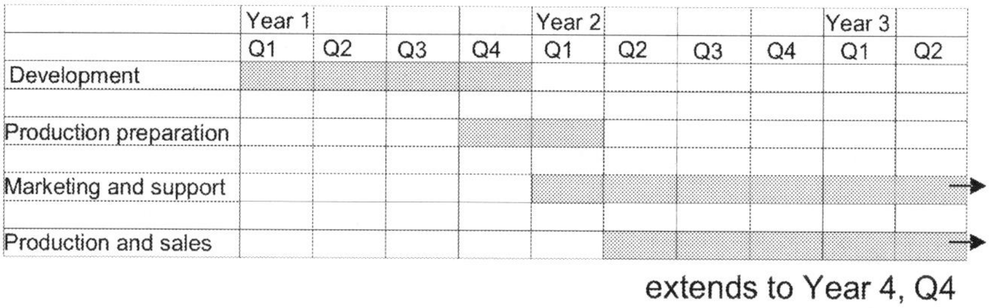

	Year 1				Year 2				Year 3	
	Q1	Q2	Q3	Q4	Q1	Q2	Q3	Q4	Q1	Q2
Development										
Production preparation										
Marketing and support										→
Production and sales										→

extends to Year 4, Q4

Figure 16-4 The spreading out of the activities

Divide the amounts of money between the different periods as shown in Figure 16-5. Money-in is positive, money-out negative. All amounts are rounded to thousands of euros or k€. If you do not agree with the choices made, you can change these later. For example, sales will not be constant: they increase at first, and then go down gradually as competing products enter the market. If you have an idea of how this will happen, you can put it in your model.

Money out per Quarter
Development: -500 / 4 = -125   and so on...
Preparation: -200 / 2 = -100
Marketing: -100 / 4 = -25
Production: 200 000 × (-0.004) / 4 = -200

Money in   Sales: 200 000 × (+0.008) / 4 = 400   all in k€

Figure 16-5 Amounts of money per quarter

The sum of the money in or out in each period is the money received or the period cash flow. Your spreadsheet will calculate this (Figure 16-6).

	Year 1				Year 2		
	Q1	Q2	Q3	Q4	Q1	Q2	Q3
Development	-125	-125	-125	-125			
Preparation				-100	-100		
Marketing					-25	-25	-25
Production						-200	-200
Sales						400	400
Received	-125	-125	-125	-225	-125	175	175

(money received) = sum(column values)

Figure 16-6 Money received per quarter

Model Results

You can plot everything with your spreadsheet. Figure 16-7 shows the money received in the different quarters. That is *using your assumptions*. Remember that you have assumed that sales only last into quarter 16.

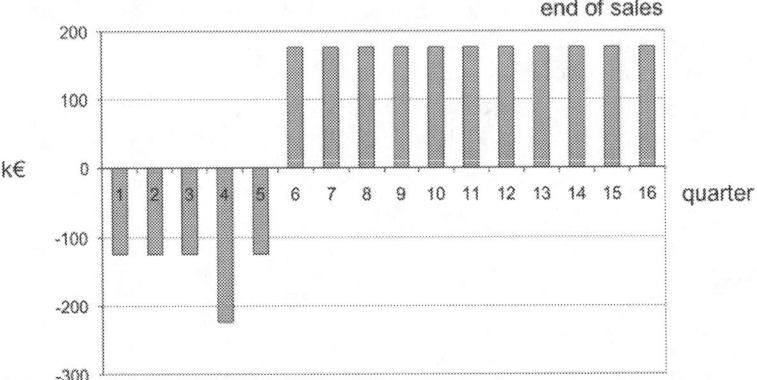

Figure 16-7 Plot of money received per quarter

Figure 16-8 shows the accumulated amount of money. This first decreases as you spend, but have no income. It then starts increasing, and in a good project it will end well above the zero line. The value at the end – after the last sales – is the *value* of the *project* or VP.[3] *With your assumptions*, you get a value of k€800. An important parameter for each product is the required *investment*. This is the amount of money you must have available in the dip of the diagram, here k€700. You must have certainty of getting this amount *before* you start the project.

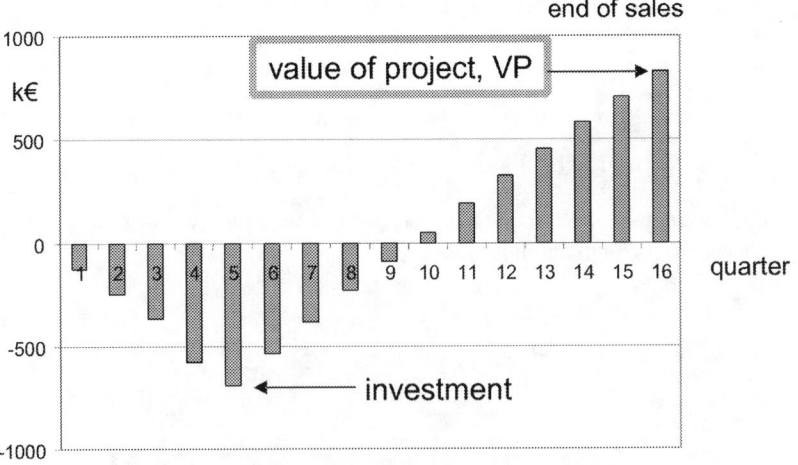

Figure 16-8 Money received accumulated

---

[3] Most value calculations use a more refined method (the NPV method discussed in Appendix 16-2). However, this is not recommended for development projects where all team members have to understand and use the model.

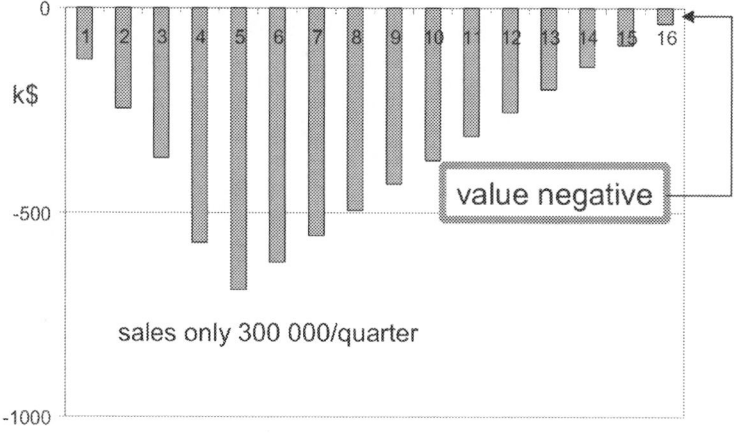

Figure 16-9 What if the sales are lower …?

If sales are less than expected, the value of the project may become negative (Figure 16-9). If you think the value will be negative, you should either terminate the project or find ways of improving it sufficiently.

Model Sensitivities

Now the second part of the exercise: the model lets you find out how sensitive the value of the project is to your assumptions. Unless your assumptions are terribly bad, the results can be very useful in deciding on alternative development paths. Factors that are usually considered in the sensitivity analysis are the effects of development time, sales volume, product manufacturing cost and development cost. Calculating their effect may seem a lot of work, but the spreadsheet gives results quickly.

Here is one example: the effect of development time on the VP (Figure 16-10). We have assumed the development cost to be independent of the time, so we can halve the development

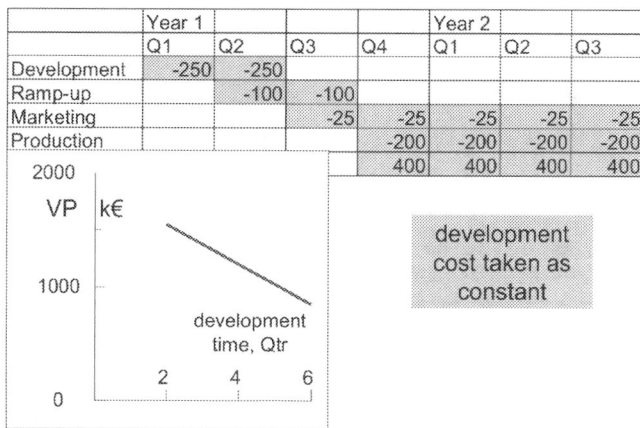

	Year 1				Year 2		
	Q1	Q2	Q3	Q4	Q1	Q2	Q3
Development	-250	-250					
Ramp-up		-100	-100				
Marketing			-25	-25	-25	-25	-25
Production				-200	-200	-200	-200
				400	400	400	400

Figure 16-10 The value of the project (VP) versus time required for development

time by putting twice as many people on the project.[4] Also, we keep assuming that the product can be sold up to 4 years from now. You see that there is a large effect of the development time: the shorter, the higher the VP. This is because we get into the market earlier, so our sales last longer.

A second example (Figure 16-11) shows the effect of sales volume on the value of the project (again, according to our assumptions). We see that the effect is large. Below about 250 000 units sold per year, the value of the project becomes negative; for sales above the base case it becomes very profitable. Unfortunately sales are the least predictable part of most product development projects. About three quarters of the projects that fail do so because sales are lower than expected.

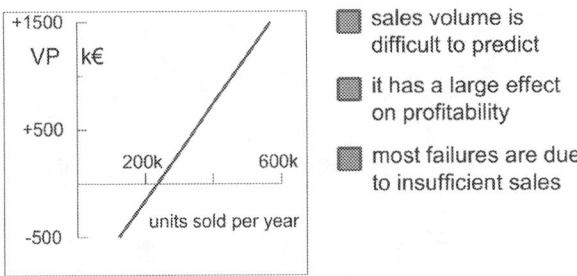

Figure 16-11 The value of the project versus the sales

Using Sensitivities

Figure 16-12 shows the four sensitivities that are usually calculated: the effects of changes in development time, sales volume, manufacturing cost and development cost. Experience shows that changes are usually more or less linear in these variables, and that the estimation of changes is more reliable than that of the value of the project.

factor	VP increase
development time	k€ 60 per month reduction
sales volume	k€ 200 for 10% more sales
product cost	k€ 5.5 for $ 1 lower per unit
development cost	k€ 50 for 10% lower cost

Figure 16-12 Four calculated sensitivities of the project

As a development team you use the sensitivities to help make decisions. Suppose you are considering the production of two kinds of pen with different colours of ink. You expect this to require an extra quarter for development, and that it will increase sales by 10%. What should you do? Postpone the launch of the product? Do the development after launching the

---

[4] It may not be possible to cut development time in half. You may not have the people. For a discussion see Smith and Reinertsen.

first product? Forget about it? A quick calculation using the sensitivities will immediately tell you.

Economic analysis of what a team is doing should go on all the time. However, it is especially important at *gates*: points where decisions are taken to go on or to stop. It is also important when large decisions have to be made on the direction of design and development. At these points earlier studies must be updated.

Sunk Costs

This is a place to point out two mistakes that are easily made in project decisions. Suppose the project has run according to your model through the fourth quarter (Figure 16-13). You have then made the expenses in the first four columns. When people see these figures you can expect two kinds of reaction, both irrational:

(1) We are only spending, not earning. We should stop!
(2) We have spent so much that we must go on.

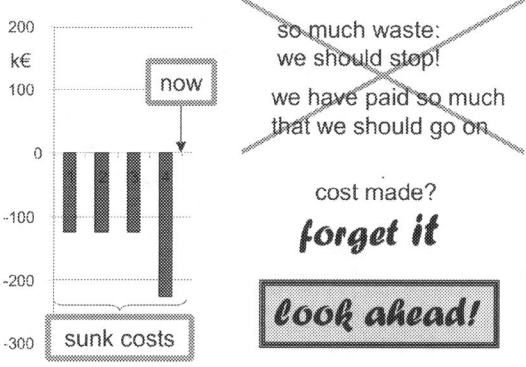

Figure 16-13 Forget sunk costs: look ahead

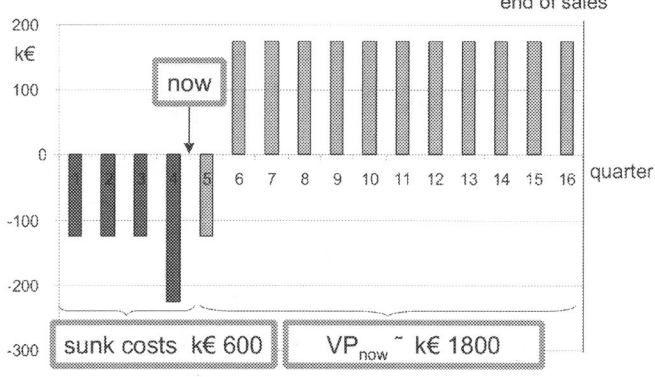

Figure 16-14 The VP has risen!

The important thing to realize is that there is nothing that can be done about the expenses so far. You cannot get them back: they are *sunk costs*. When making decisions you should calculate the VP *from now onwards*. You should only look at what you can gain or lose in the future.[5]

Because the sunk costs do not count any more, the VP in your example has increased to a value of about k€1800 (Figure 16-14), making it even more attractive to finish the project. This is not because 'we have already spent so much', but because *you expect to earn €1.8 million more when you go on than when you stop*. This does not mean that the profit of the project increases – you have already spent k€600.

Limitations of VP Analysis

VP analysis is useful, but it has drawbacks. First of all, it only counts measurable quantities and disregards all others. This means, for example, that it does not consider the advantages of learning and development of knowledge in the company.[6] This is a serious deficiency. A second criticism is that the results are only as good as the assumptions and the data. It is tempting to fiddle with these, either to keep a project going, or to kill it. Both you and management have to be aware of this danger. A third problem is that too much analysis leads to a bureaucratic atmosphere, retards product development, and stifles ideas. This is less of a problem when a team uses VP analysis for internal team decisions. These problems can be partly solved by adding a fourth step: a *qualitative analysis* ('looking around' in ordinary speech).

In this looking around (Figure 16-15) we consider how the project interacts with the rest of the firm, the market and the world. Is the firm learning anything important from this project? How will the project be influenced by actions of competitors, customers and suppliers? You should consider all of these. The world interacts with the project and the project with the world. Points to consider are shifts in the economy, government regulations and social trends. The team should discuss these things, and let them affect decisions. Don't fall into the trap of not considering important effects because you cannot quantify them.

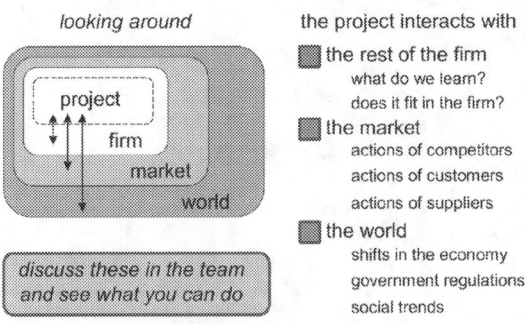

Figure 16-15 Looking outside the project

---

[5] It can be difficult for the people who made the plans to accept sunk costs.
[6] VP analysis will tell you that this course has a negative value as there are no sales!

Summary

Our summary can be short.

1. Forecasting is not reliable, but you had better try anyhow.
2. Forecasting helps to estimate the value of your project. You should try to know this at any time.
3. Sensitivity analysis helps you understand which changes influence the project value most.
4. Sensitivities are a great help in deciding whether and how projects can best be changed.

Further Reading

This lesson owes a lot to:

Karl T. Ulrich and Steven D. Eppinger *Product Design and Development*, 3rd edition, McGraw-Hill 2003, Chapter 15

and

Preston G. Smith and Donald G. Reinertsen *Developing Products in Half the Time*, 2nd edition, Wiley 1998, Chapter 2.

The second reference goes much further than we do.

Appendix 16-1
Relations between Financial Models

Lesson 12 considers two money models: the bookkeeping model (1) and the operational or Cost–Sales–Profit model (2) (Figure 16-16). Here we have the Value-of-Project method (3). Is there any relation between these models? Obviously they deal with the same flows of money, but there is a difference. The first two deal with current costs and revenues, and perhaps extrapolate these a bit. The VP method deals with *future* costs and revenues. If the prediction were to be accurate, the results would be the same. Our VP method looks at how the money flows develop in time (item (3) in Figure 16-17). In a normal business there is

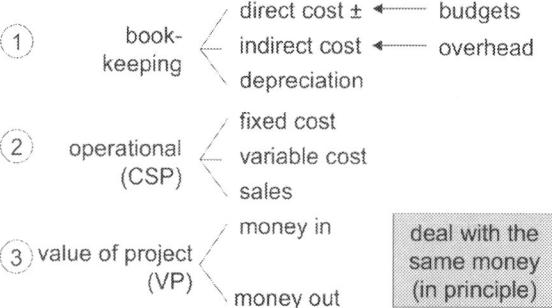

Figure 16-16 Three financial models

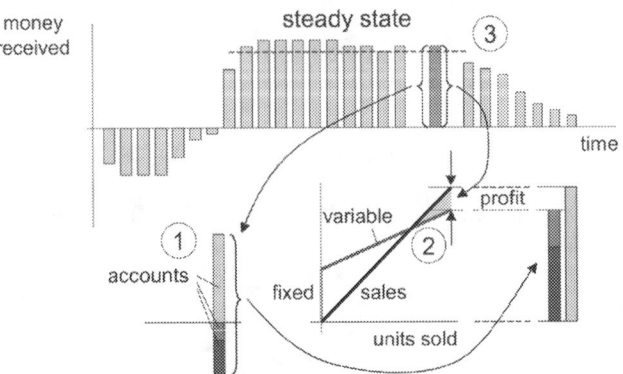

Figure 16-17 Comparing the three financial models

usually a more-or-less steady period after development and starting up. This is the domain of the bookkeeping (1) and Cost-Sales-Profit (2) methods.

Appendix 16-2
The NPV Method[7]

Most investments are judged using a model that is similar to the VP model used here, but more sophisticated. The starting point is that money is expected to deliver a certain return r (Figure 16-18). For the purpose of this explanation we give r a value of 0.1 per year ('a 10% return'). As a result, €100 at this moment will have become €110 in a year, €121 in 2 years and so on. Conversely €100 in a number of years will be worth less at this moment. So amounts of money that we pay or receive in the future are worth less in current terms than they would be otherwise. Note that PV (Present Value) is not the same as VP (Value of Project).

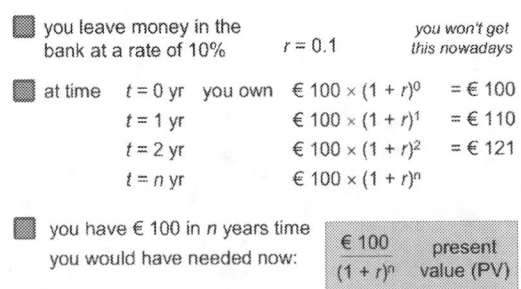

Figure 16-18 The value of money in the future

It is easy to take this into account in a spreadsheet (Figure 16-19). Excel even has a set of functions to do that, but you can also program them yourself.

Over not-too-long periods the differences between the VP and the NPV method are not large. Figure 16-20 shows how things work out for the example from this lesson.

---

[7] NPV stands for Net Present Value.

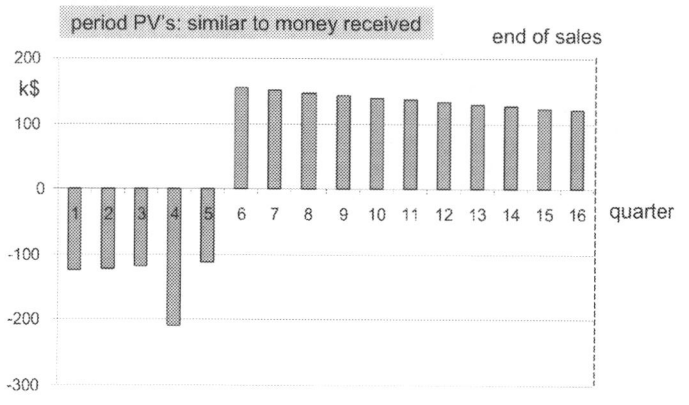

Rate	0.1						
	Year 1				Year 2		
	Q1	Q2	Q3	Q4	Q1	Q2	Q3
Development	-166.6	-166.6	-166.6				
Ramp-up			-100	-100			
Marketing				-25	-25	-25	-25
Production					-200	-200	-200
Sales					400	400	400
Cash Flow	-166.6	-166.6	-266.6	-125	175	175	175
Years	0	0.25	0.5	0.75	1	1.25	1.5
Present Value	167	-163	-254	-116	159	155	152

$$(PV) = (sum)/(1+r)^t$$

also called *discounted cash flow*

Figure 16-19 Present Value calculation in Excel

Figure 16-20 To be compared with Figure 16-7

Rate	0.1						
	Year 1				Year 2		
	Q1	Q2	Q3	Q4	Q1	Q2	Q3
Development	-125	-125	-125	-125			
Ramping-up				-100	-100		
Marketing					-25	-25	-25
Production						-200	-200
Sales						400	400
Received	-125	-125	-125	-225	-125	175	175
Years	0	0.25	0.5	0.75	1	1.25	1.5
Present Value	-125	-122	-119	-209	-114	155	152

present value of the project = NPV = sum(PV)

here: NPV = k€ 820

Figure 16-21 The project value in the NPV method

Here the project value calculated by the NPV method is smaller (Figure 16-21). However, realize that differences caused by uncertainties in development projects are usually much larger. The simpler VP method is more suitable for following what is going on in a development project. This is discussed in detail in the book of Smith and Reinertsen.

Lesson 17: Learn to Sell

The product will only be a success if you are able to sell it. We spend this lesson on selling, to help you see how selling can influence development. Everybody is a seller sometimes in life. Even scientists have to sell their ideas to people who fund their research. Many of us do not like selling – it always brings the risk 'I may be turned down'. That hurts. Even so, selling can be a rewarding experience – both for the seller and the buyer – when the product and the price fit.

Buyer–Seller Interaction

The simple products you use at home are mostly sold in retail stores, with little interaction between customer and sales personnel. You pick up things and pay at the cashier. The same applies to Internet selling which is now rapidly taking off for selling of commodities between companies. Pricing and conditions are set beforehand by the seller.[1] The decision is in the hands of the customer (where it should be). However, even in these simple-product sales, firms try to keep the sales a bit personal to get feedback from customers. For more complicated products – manufacturing equipment, materials with performance specifications, services, and houses – there is always at least one salesperson involved, and sometimes there are many. Here prices and conditions are not set beforehand, but are the result of negotiations. Most large business-to-business transactions fall in this category, and those are what we consider here.

Let us begin looking at the traditional way of selling. The salesman gathers knowledge on the product and learns technical details and features so they can be told at the touch of a button. He shows the product to the customer (or *prospect*), and pushes by demonstrating features, answering objections and overwhelming the customer. A successful skirmish ends with the *closing* of a sale, and the customer wondering what she has done.[2] This way of selling comes naturally, but it has its problems. For one thing: this method creates distrust between seller and buyer. The salesman leads; this makes the buyer defensive. The result is not a constructive dialogue, but the buyer trying to 'break in'. She will use any opportunity for asking: 'What does that cost?' Unfortunately this brings price into discussion at the wrong point. You have not yet established whether there is any value for the customer in your proposition, and then everything is expensive! Neither does this way easily lead to repeat sales, which are the most profitable. This way of working gives sellers a bad name. It is also

---

[1] The seller can and will change prices depending on the market situation. However, at any given moment, the buyer should be able to reckon on certain prices and conditions.

[2] In this lesson the salesperson is a 'he' and the customer a 'she'.

Design and Development of Biological, Chemical, Food and Pharmaceutical Products   J.A. Wesselingh, S. Kiil and M.E. Vigild
© 2007 John Wiley & Sons, Ltd

bad for the self-image of the buyer (who feels 'sold'). Finally it puts off those people who could be the best salespeople: professionals who really could know what the customer needs. There are better ways.

The trick is to change the way you look at selling. You should regard it as *helping customers* to achieve their goals and solve their problems.[3] This may sound naive, but if you manage, the dividends are impressive, both for seller and buyer. You must regard the customer as a *person* – not just somebody. You need to *care* about this person – which is difficult because the caring has to be real, not pretended. You must find ways of building trust, to allow exploration of problems the customer needs to solve, and to find whether you can help.

In this interaction, it is mostly up to you to find if *you* can get enough out of the problem. You may benefit not only from the sale, but also from learning new things and getting a reference.[4] Unless you can see ways to satisfy both parties, you should stop. Note that the parties can reach this conclusion together; this is different from 'being turned down'. The chance of working together later is left open, and probably improved. Also customer-centric selling has its problems, but they differ from those of the traditional selling method.

Contacting the Customer

Before you can talk, you must have contact with a customer.[5] This is the first difficulty in selling: getting attention. If you have managed to get interesting reviews of your product in the trade press, or have the right way of advertising, the customer may come to you. This is the best starting point. If not, you will have to approach potential customers. Doing this directly by telephone or e-mail is possible, but reckon on many negative responses. It is easier to start with a reference: a person (possibly an earlier customer) who recommends you. You have to prepare every possibility, and try to find out a bit about the customer and why she might be interested. You will need to know more about this in the next stage.

Most organizations have a hierarchy with different levels. In one of these your product will actually be used. If possible, do not aim first at this level, but one or two levels higher (assuming you can find out). If you find interest there, it will be easier to find your way through the organization. Also these people may have the authority to buy things, which you should not expect from users.

At some point, you hopefully will get in contact with your prospect, probably by telephone. In this first contact, you only have a short moment: reckon on half a minute. In this fleeting moment you must get the customer to become curious, to get the idea that you may have

---

[3] You may find that this way of looking at things is also useful in daily life.

[4] A reference is a customer who is prepared to tell new customers about her good experience with you.

[5] In selling terms: you must find a prospect (prospective buyer).

something that helps her attain goals or solve problems. If you think you have a contact, you may be able to talk longer, but it is probably better to arrange a further telephone call at a predetermined moment when more time is available.[6] At some point you may want to see each other face-to-face, but realize that this takes *a lot* more time.

And if things go wrong? Don't worry too much about that beforehand.[7] You will stress yourself and become defensive. Yes, you will often not be able to make a contact. However, realize that you are not turned down as a person – at least if you have been well-prepared. What is being turned down is your product or your presentation. You may have to work on that for the next time. Also, if the customer really has no interest, *getting turned down early is good news*. It saves a lot of wasted time. Weeding out the wrong contacts early is a bit like weeding out poor concepts in product design. In the beginning you may not like it, but it is essential. In the long run you will be proud of your 'garden'.

Selling a Catalyst

Let us take an example. Suppose you are a catalyst manufacturer. The standard catalyst in the branch consists of spherical particles. However, you have realized that other shapes have a better surface to volume ratio (Figure 17-1). In reactions that are diffusion limited, this means a higher reaction rate. This will allow to make reactors smaller, or to increase the production in existing reactors. You have developed and patented catalyst particles in the form of hollow cylinders.[8] These give a lower pressure drop than spherical particles with the same diameter, but their surface area is more than 80% larger. The price of the old catalyst is €30 000 per m^3 of catalyst. You will need a higher price for the new one, but how high can you go?

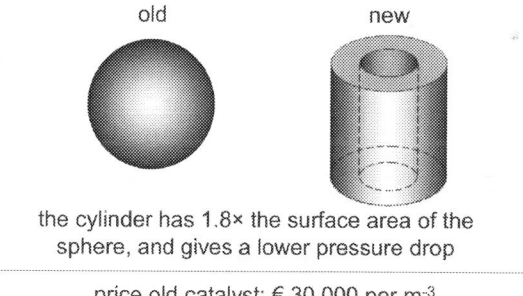

old　　　　　　new

the cylinder has 1.8× the surface area of the
sphere, and gives a lower pressure drop

price old catalyst: € 30 000 per m-3

Figure 17-1　Old and new catalyst shapes

One of your customers is a manufacturer of methanol. Her firm has several plants, with a huge production capacity. A methanol plant converts methane and water into methanol in two steps. In the first 'reformer' reactor methane is converted into carbon monoxide and hydrogen (Figure 17-2). In the second 'synthesis' reactor the carbon monoxide and part of

---

[6] Which clothes will you wear? Better over-dress than under-dress for the first time.

[7] You will be less stressed if you start with prospects that are not promising and regard these as an exercise.

[8] The effects of catalyst shapes were explored a long time ago: most patents will have expired. However, they are still a good example.

reformer reaction

$$CH_4 + H_2O \rightleftharpoons CO + 3\,H_2 \qquad 1\ MPa, 1000K$$

considered here

synthesis reaction

$$CO + 2\,H_2 \rightleftharpoons CH_3OH \qquad 10\ MPa, 600K$$

raw material CH_4: € 200 per ton CH_3OH variable cost

catalyst replacement: M€ 7.5 per year   ⎫
capital and personnel: M€ 50 per year   ⎬ fixed costs
  ⎭

sales price: € 300 per ton CH_3OH

full production: 1 Mt per year

Figure 17-2 Data for the methanol process[9]

the hydrogen are converted into methanol. Here we look at the reformer reactor, which is run at an intermediate pressure, but at a very high temperature. We have also given a few cost figures that you will need in a moment. You see one variable cost for methane and two fixed costs. One of the fixed costs is the replacement of catalyst, which has to be done every 2 years. The firm gets its revenue from the sales of methanol; at full capacity the plant can produce 1 000 000 tons per year. In this example, contacting the customer will not be difficult. The worlds of methanol producers and catalyst manufacturers are not that large.

The reformer reaction runs at a high temperature in the tubes of a huge furnace. The burner chambers are about 10 m high (Figure 17-3). The burner chambers have walls consisting of steel tubes about 10 cm in diameter (Figure 17-4). The catalyst particles, with diameters of the order of 1 cm, are in the tubes. The reacting gases flow through the tubes, around the catalyst particles.

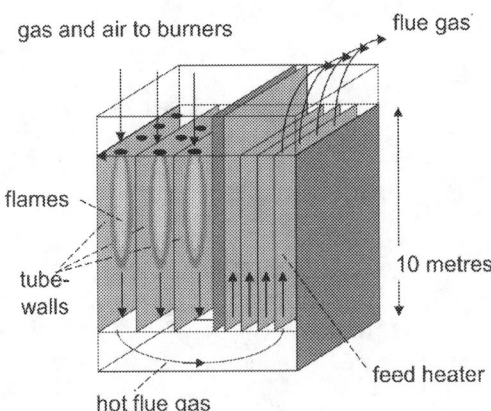

Figure 17-3 The reformer furnace

---

[9] The figures are not the real ones.

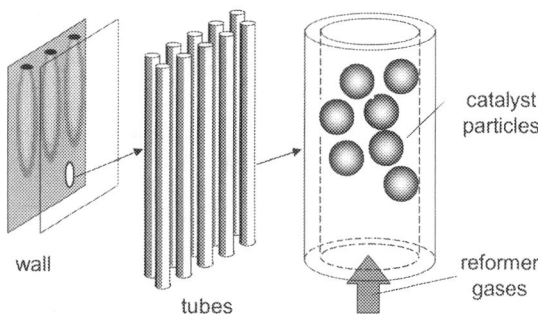

Figure 17-4 The tube walls of the furnace

The Sales Meeting

So you have arranged an appointment. Before you go, try to find out who the customer is. Place yourself in her shoes! Try to get an idea where your product may help your customer.[10] However, realize that you can only anticipate and may have to change your ideas during the appointment. Then prepare a number of questions, of which most should be open, as you have been told in 'Interview Your Customer'. In our example you should already be getting the information together that we have discussed *before the appointment*.

Consider the appointment as an interview. Ask questions. Listen and summarize answers to show they have been understood, and to allow corrections where they have not. Point out the difference between what the customer has and would like. Only if the customer *feels* a need should you go further. Somewhere you will have to tell the customer about your product and firm. However, be careful – you can overwhelm the customer with features that she does not understand, or which are irrelevant. A good sales talk is a conversation, not a product presentation. You may need to discuss product details later, probably with people on a lower level. If you cannot get the customer to feel a need: stop. If you find needs, but cannot satisfy them, refer the customer to someone else. If you do find offerings that interest the customer, discuss who else needs to be involved and get her to help you get appointments with these people.

While talking with your customer, you find out that she wants to increase the throughput of the plant (Figure 17-5). This is currently limited by the rate of reaction in the reformer. A further problem with the reactor is that the activity of the catalyst decreases in time, probably due to fouling. You discuss that an increase in throughput should be possible with your new catalyst. She thinks perhaps by 10% – then other parts of her plant will become limiting. Then you will not be using the full capacity of the catalyst, so you think it will keep sufficient activity for a 50% longer period. Also this is attractive to the customer. A rough calculation tells that the increase in gross revenue will be about €7 000 000 per year. This looks attractive enough to start working on a proposition.

---

[10] This looks suspiciously like the interviewing exercise in 'Find Needs'. It is! Selling is one of the best places to get hold of customer needs.

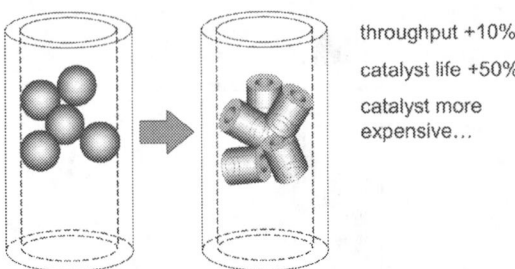

throughput +10%

catalyst life +50%

catalyst more expensive...

Figure 17-5 Effects of the change of catalyst

Negotiations

This is a point to review what the advantages and disadvantages are of the new proposal, compared with the current situation.[11] Try to do this both for the seller and for the buyer (Figure 17-6). The advantages for yourself are that you should be able to sell the new catalyst at a higher price than the old one. Another one is that, assuming all works well, you may be able to get your customer to serve as a reference. That will improve your chances for further sales. The disadvantages are that there will be less catalyst replacement in the new situation (yes, that is good for the customer, but not for you). Also, you run a risk that things will not work out as expected. Finally, you will have to spend time on the proposal. The advantages and disadvantages for the buyer should be clear. You do not have to share these with her; she should know herself. However, knowing each other's position may make things easier.

	pros	cons
seller: **catalyst** manufacturer	higher price get reference	less replacement higher risk time spent
buyer: **methanol** manufacturer	less replacement higher sales	higher price higher risk time spent

Figure 17-6 Positions of seller and buyer

In a firm of any size, you will need to convince more than one person to make a sale: perhaps a whole committee (Figure 17-7). This means further talks with people with other functions in the organization. These will be people who are to use your product, people who are to implement your solution, financial people and so on. The idea remains the same as in your first appointment, but each interview must be prepared separately and aimed at the person who you are meeting. During these interviews you will be building up ideas of how to meet the goals of your customer, so that you can come up with a proposal. In our methanol example this will require developing a technical model of the plant to allow comparison of

---

[11] Try to convert the advantages and disadvantages for both sides into money. This may give the best baseline for profitable negotiations.

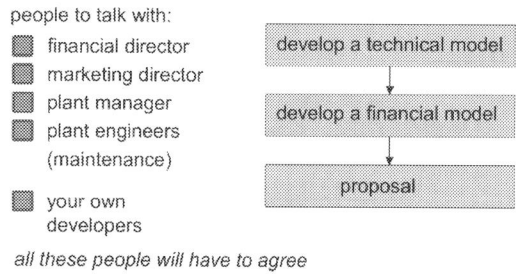

people to talk with:
- financial director
- marketing director
- plant manager
- plant engineers (maintenance)

- your own developers

develop a technical model

develop a financial model

proposal

all these people will have to agree

Figure 17-7 Things to be done

the situation before and after the change. You will also need a cost model such as discussed in lesson 12. These will give a more accurate picture of what can be attained, and what is necessary for implementation.

While working out the proposal, you know that at some point you will be negotiating a contract. So note the strengths and weaknesses of your customer and yourself (Figure 17-8). The customer will be doing the same! You can both gain from the new catalyst, so you want to reach an agreement. Your customer can try to get competing bids. If she manages, she can put you under pressure. However, you have a patent, which makes it difficult for competitors. Also, you have got into the race earlier, so you know more. The moment of the sale is not so important for you, but your customer has to plan for the next maintenance shutdown and is under time pressure. She will play out that she runs a higher risk than you do. Finally you both want to keep a good relation, as you may need each other in the future.

	strong	**weak**
seller catalyst manufacturer	gains by sale has patent timing not so important	competitors want to keep relation
buyer methanol manufacturer	gains by sale competitors higher risk	needs replacement at certain moment want to keep relation

Figure 17-8 Positions of seller and buyer (2)

How these negotiations work out depends on many things, but you might expect the larger part of the seven million to go to the methanol plant (perhaps two thirds). To get your part you must double the price of the catalyst. You may get commitments for references and further catalyst deliveries.

After the sale call the customer to hear whether everything is in order. Don't wait until you hear that something is wrong! If it is, try to get things in order. If everything is in order, and the customer is happy, tell her that it was a pleasure to work with her. You don't have to buy her flowers, but tell her which things ran very well. Then try to get new ideas from her on how you might improve your product. You may both be able to profit from that. Finally ask whether she would mind being an *active* reference for a next client.

Summary

What does this lesson on selling tell you about product development?

1. You see that your product must address needs of the customer, as we have stressed from the beginning.
2. The product must be able to catch the mind – be new, better or cheaper.
3. You have to be able to explain the product to a customer in half a minute, and quickly connect it to customer goals and problems.
4. You must find ways of reaching customers.
5. You must know the technical parameters of your product.
6. Then you must build an economic case for your customer. If the price you need to ask allows the customer a good return, you have a good chance of getting the sale.

Remember that this applies to fairly large sales in the professional business-to-business world. In sales to consumers, emotion and fashion considerations often dominate.

Further Reading

On selling:

Spencer Johnson *The One Minute Sales Person*, Harper Collins Publishers 1985, 2004.

Michael T. Bosworth and John R. Holland *Customer Centric Selling*, McGraw-Hill, 2004.

Improving your negotiation capabilities:

Roger Fisher and William Ury *Getting to YES*, Penguin 1991.

Lesson 18:
Plan Future Products

In this last lesson we discuss the initial phase of product development (Figure 18-1). This phase is also known as *product planning*. A little thought will tell you that this phase considers *what* you are going to develop. Actually, we were vague about this: if you look back you will see that the project scope appears out of the blue in lesson 5. The decision had already been made for us.

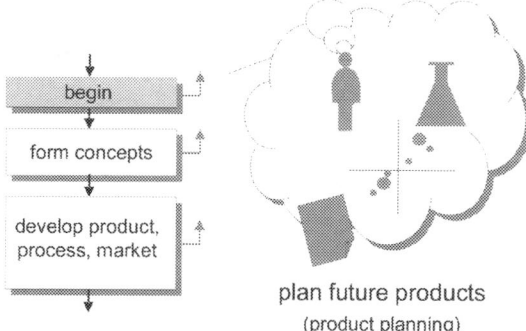

plan future products
(product planning)

Figure 18-1 The begin phase of innovation

There are three reasons why the beginning is covered at the end of these lessons:

(1) Where you begin is not as important as it might seem. In the sustaining development of successful products, there is neither a beginning nor an end in sight. Development just continues. We explain this further on.
(2) Product planning is perhaps the most difficult part of innovation. It requires overview and experience – which you are only starting to build up.
(3) Young, inexperienced engineers seldom begin at 'the beginning'. However, there is one important exception: in developing of disruptive products that we discuss at the end of this lesson.

The Planning Process

The planning process for a not-too-small firm might look like that in Figure 18-2.[1] In many firms it is done once a year, but this may cause the firm to lose too much time so more

[1] Small firms use simpler procedures.

Design and Development of Biological, Chemical, Food and Pharmaceutical Products   J.A. Wesselingh,
S. Kiil and M.E. Vigild
© 2007 John Wiley & Sons, Ltd

planning cycles are needed. Product planning starts with gathering of ideas, which we discuss further in a moment. Just as in concept development (lesson 7) you should be getting far more ideas than you can handle. You need bits of time to analyse the situation (lesson 3) and to form an impression of what these ideas might mean for the firm. This may be spread out over a number of people. However, you only want to spend a little time and money on each idea in this stage. Assessing and ranking is similar to what you did when selecting concepts (lesson 8). You end with a ranked list of ideas.

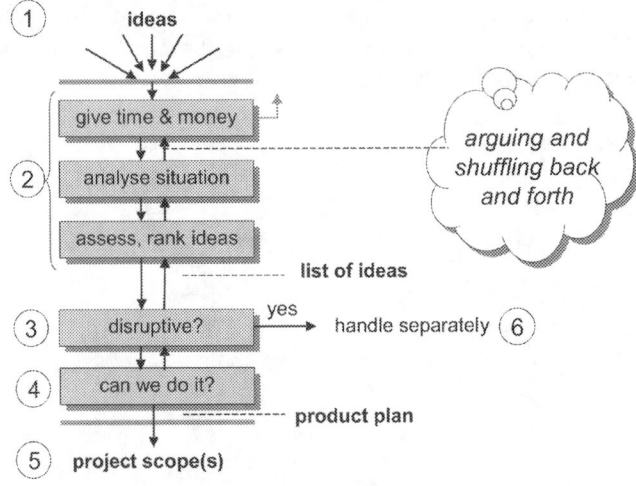

Figure 18-2 The method for product planning[2]

At this point you should consider whether there are any *disruptive* ideas on your list. We introduced this term under the finding of customer needs (lesson 5). Disruptive ideas require the customer to adopt new working habits. The strong and weak points of the ideas can be quite different from existing ones. All too often disruptive products do not look promising on a short term – and you have to be sufficiently sensitive not to discard them too early. In the long term they may have the potential of disrupting the field that you are working in. They require a way of handling different from that for sustaining ideas; set them aside for the moment.

You will notice that the arrows in Figure 18-2 go up and down. Product planning is not straightforward; it involves a lot of arguing. And as the engineer tends to see it: 'politics'. Different projects compete with each other for limited resources and so do the people involved.

Sustaining Developments

The great number of ideas will usually be sustaining. These are for improvements or extensions of existing products. Note that the ideas do not have to concern the product

---

[2] The numbers in the figure will reappear in other connected figures.

only; they can also consider the manufacturing process, or the marketing and distribution channels – anything that might lead to an improvement for the customer or for you. The last step in the method (a difficult one) is to consider how much development capability you have. How many and which kinds of people do you have available for development? What about the other resources? There are many uncertainties here, but you will have to form an idea of which projects you will be able to handle. This leads to the *product plan*, which then has to be worked out in project scopes (which is where we started in lesson 5).

You should collect ideas from many sources (Figure 18-3). Obvious ones are your marketing and sales people, your colleagues in research and development teams, but also outsiders such as suppliers, customers and university contacts. This collecting requires a bit of prodding – people have to be encouraged to help. Somebody has to do this, has to keep people informed that something is being done with their idea, and has to administrate the ideas.

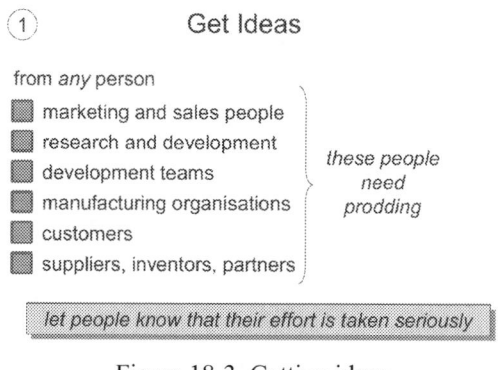

Figure 18-3 Getting ideas

The ideas need to be assessed and ranked (a bit like the customer needs in lesson 5). Figure 18-4 gives a list of criteria that are used for such rankings. The first is whether the idea fits in the *competitive strategy* of the firm; we discuss this separately in the following paragraph. The second question is whether the idea fits in the *market segments* that you are interested in. These might be the professional-, the consumer-, the low-end, or the high-end

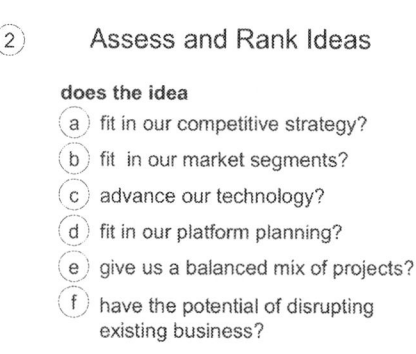

Figure 18-4 Assessing and ranking of ideas

segments. A third one is whether you are going to learn something from the idea – whether it will *advance* your *technology*. We discuss this further on. A fourth is whether the idea fits in your *platform* planning. Platforms are again discussed separately. Then you have to consider whether your set of projects covers both the near future (improving existing operations) and a further future. Finally you do want to know whether there are disruptive ideas around.

Remarks on the Steps

Most firms have a competitive strategy: an idea of how they do things and what they want to be. Figure 18-5 shows four typical strategies. You might think that a firm should aim at all good things simultaneously, but experience shows that that does not work. A firm has to make choices.

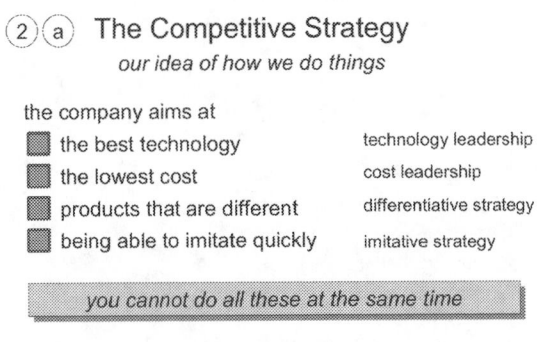

Figure 18-5 Four common strategies

Technology is improving all the time – also the technology of your suppliers. It is a good idea to try to include a limited number of improvements in each new product; to try them out and learn how well they work. The problem is that a new technology usually starts with a lower level of performance than the old one (Figure 18-6). You have to start thinking about using the new technology when you see that it is beginning to make progress, and you think

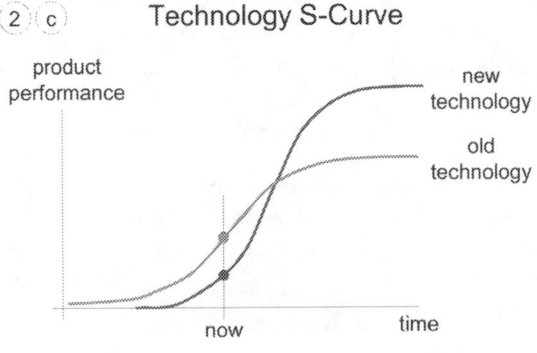

Figure 18-6 Technology S-curves[3]

---

[3] The S is sheared.

it is going to overtake the old way of working. This is often an act of faith. You can develop a new product with new technology, but with old technology as a fall-back. However, this does require more resources.

Many firms use product *platforms*. The idea is most obvious for companies producing devices. You may have noticed that a company like HP (Hewlett Packard) has new printer models every few months. They manage this by having a basic technology that is modified each time to suit new customers. Car manufacturers use similar tricks. Modifications (add-ons) can be made much more quickly and cheaply than a new platform – and such renewals are important for marketing.

A technique used by large firms to show whether they have a *balanced set of projects*, covering both the near and the further future, is the portfolio map (Figure 18-7). The axes of this diagram show how fundamentally the project is thought to change the *product* (this is the vertical axis) and the *process* (the horizontal axis). These changes vary from no-change to disruptive. Each project is ranked on these two axes and plotted as a circle with an area proportional the expected expenses in the year considered. This is a lot of work. A firm should try to have projects distributed around the diagonal. The box no-change/no-change represents a dying product: there should be no projects there. You might think that disruptive projects should be the most important in development. However, as we discuss a little further on, there are reasons to keep disruptive research on a not-too-high level of expenditure. So in a balanced portfolio the most important expenses tend to be in the middle of the diagonal.

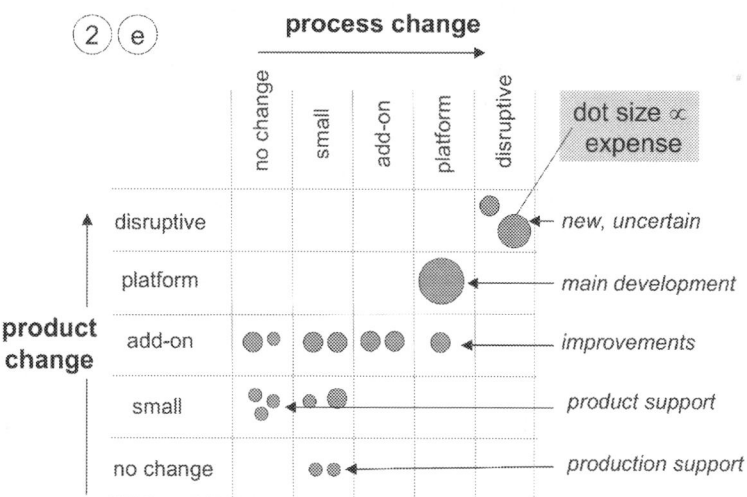

Figure 18-7 Balancing with a portfolio map

The Product Plan

We are then at the last question: can we do it? (Figure 18-8) Do we have the right kind of people? Chemists, chemical engineers, mechanical engineers, marketing people . . .? Do we

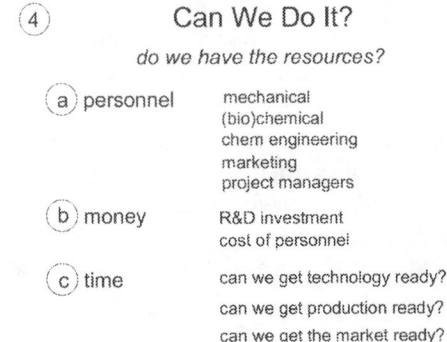

Figure 18-8 Setting up a product plan

have people who can and want to manage the projects? Do we have enough of them? What about the other resources? Answering these questions and combining the ideas and resources in a good *product plan* is usually the job of the R&D director. It is difficult and outside the scope of this text. We can only note a few of the difficulties:

(1) There is always a strong pressure to do more development than the available capacity allows.
(2) This can lead to overloading of development departments, and to projects being finished too late or not at all.
(3) It also means that there will be insufficient time for playing and learning: activities that are essential for any research or development organization.
(4) Most firms set aside some resources for disruptive developments. These have to be kept outside the main planning scheme for reasons we discuss further on.

When we have a coherent (and not overloaded) product plan the last step is to write the project scopes (Figure 18-9) and to form project teams. You already know the rest.

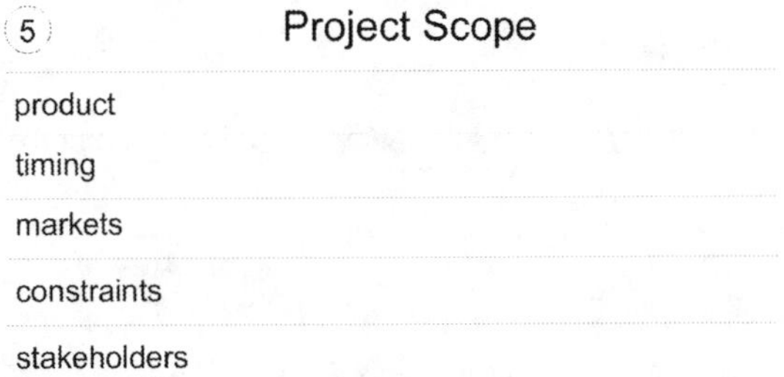

5   Project Scope

product

timing

markets

constraints

stakeholders

Figure 18-9 The items in the project scope

A last remark in this section: many of the ideas for sustaining product development come from the market – from customers. This is why product development often looks like a continuous cycle (Figure 18-10). Of course there is an end to the cycle (most products eventually die), but often only after a long series of developments.

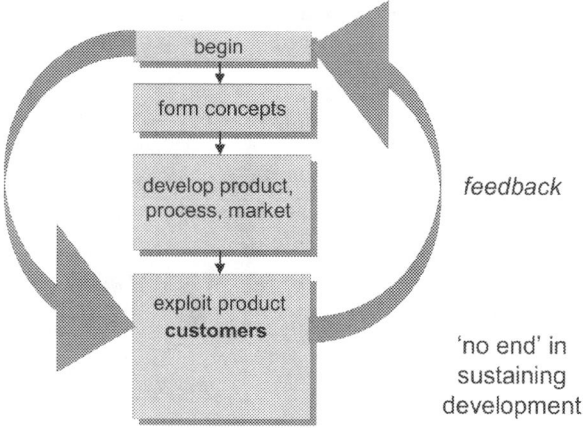

Figure 18-10 Sustaining development is cyclic

Disruptive Developments

Back to disruptive ideas (Figure 18-11). These are the ones that should give industrial leaders nightmares; they are the ideas that may wipe out complete industries. They always start with disadvantages; their success is not assured. They often need long lead times, and cannot be planned. For them, NPV calculations are useless ...

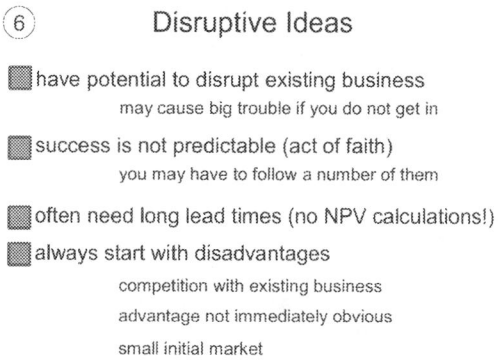

Figure 18-11 Disruptive ideas

Let us take an old example to show some of the problems: the transition from gas lighting to electric lighting in the last decennia of the nineteenth century. Gas, made by gasifying coal, had become a common energy carrier early in the century. Every city had its own municipal gas manufacturer, and there was a complete infrastructure for piping gas around the place. Gas lamps were to be found everywhere, both in buildings and in the streets. There was a large organization for lighting the street lamps every evening, with lamp-lighters going around with fire and small ladders. Then came electric light, using incandescent bulbs with glowing wires. In the first instance this was hardly competition for the gas companies. Electricity had to be produced locally – there was no infrastructure to transport it. The first lamps had an extremely low light-efficiency and a short life-time. They were used to decorate shop windows.

Now put yourself in the position of the research director of a gas firm. Your firm is extremely busy running gas factories (chemical plant!), seeing to it that they do not explode, that they do not smell too much, that they do not poison employees, and that they deliver a constant quality of gas in sufficient amounts so that you never run out. Your external people are busy keeping the piping infrastructure in order, attending to leaks, teaching people how to use gas and not to blow up their houses. There is any number of things that need to be maintained and improved, and everybody is very busy. Ask yourself three questions:

1. Does the gas firm have the electrical engineers in house to develop an electrical lighting system?
2. Will the owners be interested in putting large parts of their profits into the development of decorative lighting for shop windows and fairs?
3. How do you think the plant engineers will react if the owners take away their facilities for plant maintenance and improvement?

With hindsight you can see that electric lighting has large advantages over gas lighting. Transport of electricity is safer and cheaper than that of gas, and electricity is more easily switched on and off. Once the electric lighting technique had developed to a certain point, gas lighting was doomed – but the gas companies hardly had any chance of getting into the new market.[4] The lesson: it is difficult to develop a disruptive idea in an existing organization. If you do so you must separate it from the daily business, otherwise it will be swamped.

Now the other side of the story: you are a young engineer living one and half centuries back and having the vision of electrical lighting in every house.[5] How do you begin? You have little money compared with the gas companies; there are no power stations; there is no electrical grid; and you only have half an idea of how to construct an electric lamp with a glowing wire. One thing is clear: you must *learn* or *discover* many new things. How to make electricity, how to transport electricity, how to make proper wires in lamps, how to make glass vacuum bulbs ... You will have to learn *cheaply*: in your garage (well, they didn't have garages in the nineteenth century) or in a tolerant university department. You will be borrowing bits of equipment and be grateful for gifts. Friends and family, or government subsidizers, interested research directors, or venture capitalists may have to help keep you alive. You will have to develop a good story to get and keep that help. At some point you will no longer be able to do things alone: then outside help really becomes important.

You get over the first technical hurdles and can make lamps that will give a yellowish light for perhaps 20 hours. Now you must find customers with applications where the disadvantages of your product are not that important, but the advantages are. Ah! Decoration of shop windows

---

[4] Gas is still doing well for heating: gas transports energy more efficiently than electricity. Coal gas has been superseded by natural gas: a change that gas firms have managed to accommodate.
[5] Your name is Thomas Alva Edison.

in the Christmas season. You only need a small local generator, and it does not matter if a few bulbs burn out. You earn a little bit of money from this experience, learn a lot and get free publicity. It is time to find new markets – and to keep on learning.

Handling Disruptive Developments

Are you beginning to get the idea (Figure 18-12)? If you have a vision of something very worthwhile (and disruptive) you will be the one who has to do it. You will have to behave as a *product champion*. Begin with playing, learning and discovery. This has to be done cheaply – large investments in this stage can easily become a millstone around your neck. Keep the cost down so it does not become too important. Don't try to plan things strictly: if you use project planning and NPVs only regard them as ways for focusing your mind. Develop your story so you can get bits of help from your surroundings. Then find customers and applications to try out your ideas, earn a bit of money and learn further. You will need new customers: people who are not tied up to the old ideas and appreciate the advantages of your idea.

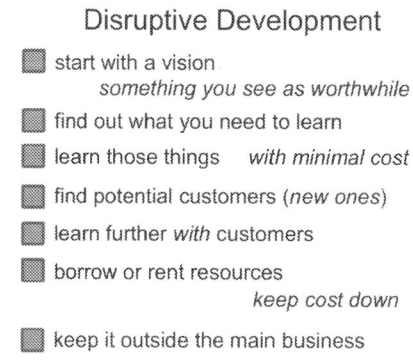

Disruptive Development

- start with a vision
  something you see as worthwhile
- find out what you need to learn
- learn those things   *with minimal cost*
- find potential customers (*new ones*)
- learn further *with* customers
- borrow or rent resources
  keep cost down
- keep it outside the main business

Figure 18-12 How to do disruptive developments

Somewhere in between you will no longer be able to do everything on your own and will have to start building an organization. You must have developed a convincing story before this point!

There are examples of firms that have managed to survive a disruptive development by doing it themselves – but not many. One that comes to mind is HP (Hewlett Packard). HP pioneered the use of laser printers for personal use and managed to become market leader. It later picked up the idea of inkjet printers – a truly disruptive idea. It is now also market leader in this area, with two divisions competing with each other. HP even kept the development of the new device separated from that of the regular business – by thousands of kilometres. There are other ways: remember the story of the NovoPen?

Many disruptive ideas get developed in a pattern like that of electric lighting. Many end as a deception, but they don't necessarily kill the developers. Even failures often lead to people and firms learning things that they can use later. Those ideas that do get through can be very rewarding.

From Disruptive to Sustaining

This lesson has considered disruptive and sustaining developments as separate. However, a successful disruptive product will eventually become mainstream, and its further development is then a matter of sustaining. The transition is gradual.

The type of research changes during development (Figure 18-13). Disruptive ideas are often found by exploring the outside world – for example by encouraging and discussing university research. Sustaining development is mostly done by professional organizations, and at least partly inside the firm. In the last phases of product life, development is limited to product maintenance and process efficiency improvements.

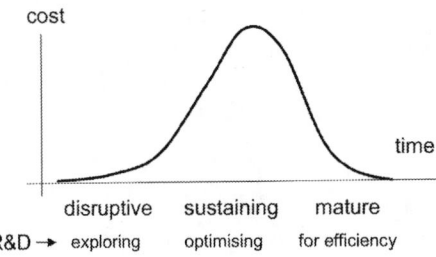

Figure 18-13 Different phases in R&D

Summary

This lesson introduces how development plans for new products are set up (Figure 18-14). This starts by collecting ideas from many sources, then analysing and ranking the ideas. Disruptive

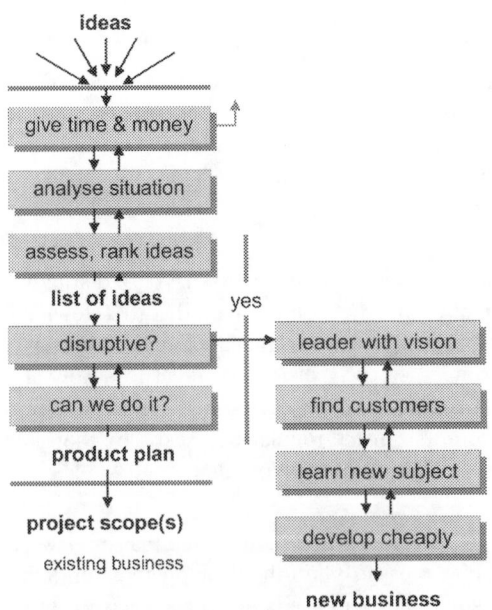

Figure 18-14 The planning process

ideas (which may lead to new business) are routed separately; the ideas for sustaining existing products remain. We decide for which projects we have sufficient development capacity: those form the product plan.

Disruptive ideas have to be developed outside the mainstream of the organization. They require their own leadership, which has to develop a product vision, find customers and applications, and learn what has to be learned. The development has to be done in a cheap and flexible manner, often together with customers.

This ends our lessons.

Further Reading

Product planning of Xerox in the nineties:

Karl T. Ulrich and Steven D. Eppinger *Product Design and Development*, 3rd edition, McGraw-Hill 2003, Chapter 3.

The dilemmas for firms facing a disruptive competitor:

Clayton M. Christensen *The Innovator's Dilemma*, Harvard Business School Press 1997.

Conclusion

Let us look back one last time. We have divided development into four stages: Begin, Design, Develop and Exploit. In each of these there were four or five lessons as is summarized in Figure 1. In development these lessons follow each other roughly. There is nearly always some backtracking – and sometimes a lot. Just to recall, we summarize each lesson in one or two sentences.

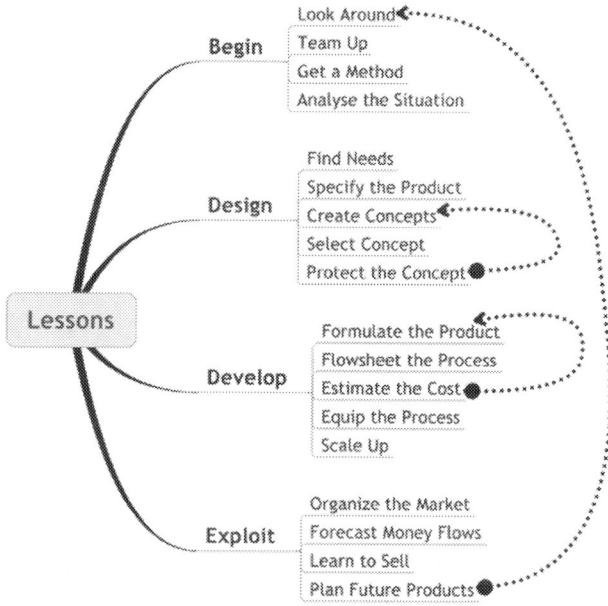

Figure 1 Summary of the course

Begin

1 Look Around. Look at the many different products of the biological, chemical, food and pharmaceutical industry and wonder.

2 Team Up. Get ready to work in a firm and to develop products in a team.

3 Get a Method. Use a method in your development work.

4 Analyse the Situation. Look at the why and how of a product: the surroundings, the people that use it, and the effects.

Design and Development of Biological, Chemical, Food and Pharmaceutical Products   J.A. Wesselingh,
S. Kiil and M.E. Vigild
© 2007 John Wiley & Sons, Ltd

Design

5 Find Needs. Ask questions to find out what others (especially customers) think about the problem and which needs the product should serve.

6 Specify the Product. Specify what the product will have to do; look at how it will do that separately.

7 Create Concepts. Create many concepts for better products.

8 Select a Concept. Select one (or a few) from the many concepts, quantify the behaviour of the product, and set better specifications.

9 Protect the Concept. See to it that you are allowed to produce and sell your product, while others are not.

Develop

10 Formulate the Product. Make the product in the lab and describe the ingredients and procedure in a recipe.

11 Flowsheet the Process. Draw a flow diagram of the process showing the materials (and energy) entering and leaving the process. Consider process changes and recycles.

12 Estimate the Cost. Make a cost model of the manufacturing process.

13 Equip the Process. List the steps in the process and the equipment needed. Get to understand the equipment.

14 Scale Up. Try the process out on a scale sufficiently large to finalize the product and begin market development.

Exploit

15 Organize the Market. Make a plan for the project: consider the expected turnover/profit/loss, the customers, the story around the product, how that will be communicated, and the distribution channel.

16 Forecast Money Flows. Forecast the costs and revenues of the project to find whether it has value.

17 Learn to Sell. Make sure that you have the right material for selling the product. You must be able to form an economic justification of your product for the customer.

18 Plan Future Products. Look ahead at what the firm is going to be doing after this product. Consider product improvements but also new business.

We hope that you will find this structure of innovation helpful in your career. Perhaps you will be part of a big company, perhaps somewhere on your own creating something new. Whatever you will be doing, we hope that you will fare well.

Projects

The projects in our course change every year – this is a set to give you and your teachers an idea of how we do things.

We typically have four projects:

1. Understanding Products (40 hr)
2. From Needs to Concept (40 hr)
3. Making a Product (40 hr)
4. Your Own Product (80 hr)

The times are what are expected from each student. The first project uses lessons 1–4; the second lessons 5–9; the third lessons 10–15, and the fourth requires everything. Projects are done by teams of four or five students, and end with a presentation or a report.

Project 1: Understanding Products

In this first project you are to learn how to do two things:

to organize work done in a team, and
to analyse a simple product or a part of it.

Read This First

We are expecting you to do a number of things:

(1) Find your assignment and make a plan of the project: who is going to do what (and when).
(2) Collect information on your problem.
(3) Set up simple experiments to study the subject.
(4) Set up theoretical models to quantify the subject.
(5) Report the results in a presentation of 8 minutes.

You have only a few weeks, so we cannot expect the results to be perfect. The job is too large to do it all together: you will have to divide the work. How you do this is up to you. We give suggestions, but feel free to experiment. The goal of this exercise is to learn, not to show that you have mastered everything.

Find and Plan the Project

Your project will be marked in the 'List of Assignments'. When you have read it – which should take only a moment – you will have to divide the work, and this requires planning and coordination. We suggest that you choose a chairperson who has this as a main task. Small teams can work without a 'chair', but it is usually easier when somebody does take responsibility for keeping an overview of the project.

Read the note 'Plan Your Project'; then discuss what you think has to be done. A blackboard, or a big note-block that everybody can see, does help in the discussions. Make a first division of the tasks. (You will probably have to change this, possibly several times.) The chair sees to it that times for the next meetings are agreed on, and everybody goes off to do their job or jobs.

The chair puts the plan in Excel before the next meeting and perhaps does other things as well. Possible items for the others are setting up and doing experiments, finding information, setting up a model (theory) of the phenomena, and preparing the presentation. You can *start*

Design and Development of Biological, Chemical, Food and Pharmaceutical Products   J.A. Wesselingh, S. Kiil and M.E. Vigild
© 2007 John Wiley & Sons, Ltd

to model your product and *prepare* the presentation before the other things are ready, but can only finish them when the other things have been done. The plan will have to be updated as the project advances: don't try to make a perfect plan in one go. Your mentors would appreciate getting a copy of the last version of your plan, which should show more or less what has happened. This is so that we will have a more realistic idea of the times required for the next course.

Collect Information

Don't spend too much time on this! Read lesson 4 'Analyse the Situation'. Then chat with other people, look up a few things in your own textbooks, and Google a bit. A visit to the library to see whether there is any book on your subject may be useful. Do see to it that you have notes or copies of anything that looks worthwhile.

Set Up Experiments

The assignments require simple experiments to find out what the structure is of the product, and what the rates are of processes in the product. Read the note 'Experiment at Home' before starting. The problem is to devise experiments that are simple, but from which you can learn something. This requires some creativity.

You will have to find equipment for the experiments. You may be able to borrow a few things, such as a simple electronic microscope, a multimeter and a digital weighing scale. If you use any of these, let one person sort out how they work – don't do everything together! However, the actual experiments are often best done with two people: four hands can do more than two. Remember to report your results. We are not asking for a proper report from this project, but you need the experimental data when putting the presentation together.

Model Quantitatively

You are expected to set up a simple theory of the structure of your product, and of what happens with your product. You may need to set up balances and transport equations as you have learned in Transport Phenomena or Process Engineering. For some assignments the Notes on Colloids may help. Our experience is that many teams find this job difficult, so start early.

Present Results

First read the note 'Present your Results'. You only have eight minutes, plus two minutes for discussion of your presentation. So it is essential that you have *timed* the presentation beforehand.

Everybody has to prepare him or herself for the presentation. One team member will deliver the presentation. In the discussion all team members are allowed to participate.

Evaluation

For the evaluation we expect copies of the sheets used in the presentation and would appreciate getting the final project plan if you have made one. Copies of the final project plan if you have made one would also be useful.

Summary

The summary is a mind map of this note, constructed in the program MindManager (Figure P1-1). You may find it useful to structure discussions and planning in the team. MindManager is easy to learn.

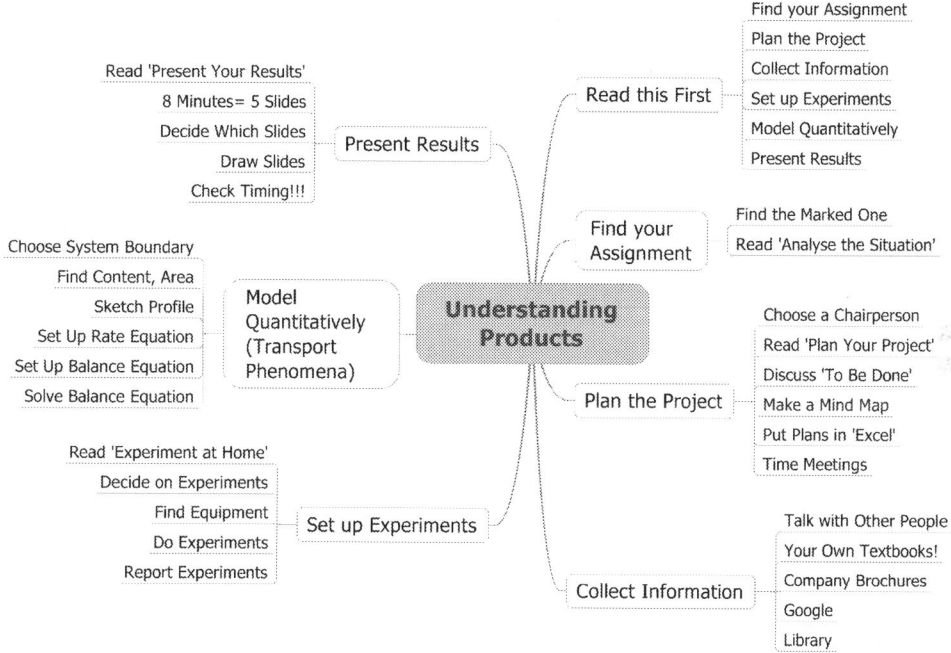

Figure P1-1 Mind map of Project 1

List of Assignments

1 Water Absorption by Tissue

Determine how much liquid kitchen tissue can take up, how quickly it does this, and develop quantitative models to describe this.

2 Water Absorption by a Towel

Determine how much liquid a towel can take up, how quickly it does so, and make a quantitative model of these processes.

3 Battery

Take an ordinary battery (not a lithium-ion one!) apart, find out how it works, and make a quantitative model of it. (The contents are poisonous and corrosive, so wear glasses, do not eat the battery, and do not wear your best clothes.)

4 Paintbrush

Form a quantitative idea of how a paintbrush works.

5 Centrifuge
Find the important technical parameters of the centrifuge in your washing machine and make a quantitative model of the machine.

6 Cleaning of Syrup
Dream up mechanisms for cleaning a plate with corn syrup (or a similar liquid) on it.

7 Raincoats
Determine how much different kinds of textile, a cheap impermeable raincoat and a breathing (Gore-Tex) raincoat reduce evaporation. Make a quantitative model of breathing/cooling/transpiration through a raincoat.

8 Dissolving
Determine the rate of dissolution of a number of household particles in water and construct a theory. Rates of dissolution are important in many pharmaceuticals and feedstuffs.

9 Draining
Measure the rate of draining of water from a towel and construct a theory.

10 Drying of a Towel
Determine how quickly a towel dries and construct a theory.

11 Drying of Paint
Determine how quickly paint dries, and construct a theory.

12 Melting of an Ice Cube
Find out how quickly an ice cube melts and construct a theory.

13 Freezing an Ice Cube
Find out how quickly water freezes into an ice cube and construct a theory.

14 Mechanical Properties
Determine the modulus of elasticity and yield strength of a number of household materials. You are to present both measurement results and the models you have used to derive these.

15 Fountain Pen
Find out how a fountain pen is constructed and make a quantitative model of how it works.

16 Ballpoint
Find out how a ballpoint is constructed and make a quantitative model of how it works.

17 Permeability
Determine the permeability of textile, and estimate the rate at which water percolates through textile in a washing machine.

18 Permeation
Determine the permeation and filtration characteristics of a coffee filter.

19 Rheology
Measure the rheological parameters of a number of household fluids, and think about why they have their values.

20 Spraying
Learn how the atomizer of a spray dryer for milk works by analysing a plant spray.

21 Wetting
Develop simple models and experiments to determine the wetting properties of a number of household materials.

22 Candle
Develop simple models and experiments to find out how a candle works.

23 Wicks
Develop simple models and experiments to find out how a wick works. (A wick is a string that transports liquid, such as in a candle. However, a wick can also transport liquid downwards.)

24 Sponge
Take a sponge, determine its water uptake and release under different conditions and make a quantitative model of its behaviour.

25 Vacuum Cleaner Filter
Have a good look at a vacuum cleaner filter, try to find or measure its technical parameters and make a quantitative model of its behaviour.

26 Rinsing of Textile
In a washing machine, detergent chemicals are to enter the textile, dirt is to leave, and remnants of the detergent are to be rinsed out again. All this requires water to enter and leave the textile. An important 'pumping' mechanism is thought to be due to the bending and straightening of the textile. Try to measure how much water is released and taken up in a bending cycle, and make a quantitative analysis of the problem.

27 Ignition of a Safety Match
Determine which factors govern the ignition of a match when you light it. Make a quantitative model of the phenomena.

Project 2:
From Needs to Concept

In this project, you will be going through the design phase of product development. You are to create many new concepts and make a choice out of these. Some problems are more psychological than technical, but also this is part of product development.

Links with Project 1

Remember that what you have learned in the first project is also applicable to this one. In particular, you may find it handy to:

Choose a chair (you might change roles!).
Make a plan for the new project.
Estimate whether concepts can work.
Do some experiments around the final concept.

There are differences between the first and second assignments. Here, much of the work has to be done by all people in parallel, perhaps excluding the chair. A fair number of items will have to be worked out together in meetings. Notes may have to be taken (by the chair?). Plan when you can get together, using the course timetable.

Find Your Assignment

Your assignment is given on a separate list at the end of this document. In addition, you will find an assignment for another group who will be interviewing you as *customers*. It is up to you whether you want to prepare yourself for that.

Sit Down with the Team

Sit down with your team and consider how you want to start the process. You will find that the assignment is no more than a brief description of an undesirable situation. It is up to you to make sense of it and to form a plan on how to improve the situation. This is not easy: you must reckon on feeling uncertain when you begin, but you should get through this as your plan unfolds.

Analyse the situation and discuss it in the team. Find out how much you know, what you don't know, what you would like to know. Generate ideas and generate questions for customers. Write them down. Be careful not to corner yourself in this early stage – keep an open mind.

Design and Development of Biological, Chemical, Food and Pharmaceutical Products J.A. Wesselingh, S. Kiil and M.E. Vigild
© 2007 John Wiley & Sons, Ltd

Find Needs

In the next course block, 2 hours will be reserved for interactions between project team and customer. In one of these hours you will be a customer and will be interviewed by another team. In the other hour you will be interviewing somebody from another team, who will play to be customer. It will be all the better if you manage to interview people outside the course.

To prepare yourself, read:

Lesson 5 on 'Find Needs' and
the Note on 'Interview Your Customer'.

You are expected to be prepared when you arrive in the lecture room. Try to discuss not only the traditional way but also other ways of looking at the problem.

After the interview, interpret, tidy up, order and rank the needs. You may find it handy to use mind maps for this exercise. You can instead use tables in Word if you find them easier. The team will need a single ranked list of needs in the next set of lessons.

Specify the Product

Before the next lectures, it might be an idea to try to orient yourself on what the competition in your product is up to (although you will not have enough time to do this well). After Lesson 6 'Specify the Product', the team is to form metrics and target specifications.

Create Concepts

The next step in the program is to create a large number of concepts of your product. How many is difficult to say beforehand, but aim at tens. We hope that all of you will have been collecting and noting ideas before. These can be existing products, but also new ones. If you do not have enough ideas, you might set up a brainstorming session. Try to increase the number of concepts using splitting techniques (looking at the problem from different viewpoints) as described in Lesson 7. At the end of this exercise the team should have a list or mind map with concepts.

Select a Concept

We are expecting you to try out both the top-down method and the concepts-criteria matrix method from Lesson 8.

Set up a tree diagram of your ideas and try to rank them according to level. Set ideas on details aside. Eliminate nonsense ideas, or those that you think will not work anyhow. Divide the work for collecting more information on each high-level concept between the team members. You can get information from many sources: from books, the Internet, by consulting experts, from the experience of team members and so on. Present and discuss the results in the team. Improve your diagram by rearranging. Use the diagram in discussions to prune the number of concepts to perhaps five or ten before trying the matrix method.

Construct criteria and use the concepts-criteria matrix to decide which concept to develop further. Realize that this part of the project takes two or three meetings, so you must plan time for this. Here we are expecting you – as engineers – to do some 'back of an envelope' calculations to try to get a better quantitative understanding of some of the design problems. (There are examples of such calculations in the appendices of Lessons 4, 6, 7, 8 and 15.)

After this step you should not have more than two concepts left – preferably one, but potentially also zero. Conclude by updating your specifications.

To Be Handed In
We are not expecting a well-designed report of this exercise, but we do want the following:

A tidied up, grouped and ranked list of needs
Lists of metrics and specifications (updated)
The original list of concepts
The tidied up list of high-level concepts (with a tree diagram)
The list of criteria
The concept–criteria matrix
A brief description of the final choice, with a sketch and calculations where appropriate.

This is a lot of work; you will need some careful planning to get it done in the two and a half weeks available. Good luck!

Assignments for Project 2
The assignments are given in a separate list. Your assignment will be marked with a '1'. You will be interviewed on the assignment marked '2'; for you this is only important on the second day of this project.

Project Planning
In Figure P2-1 you will find a mind map with the main items that need to be done. You may find this handy for planning your work. This is the last time that we will be helping you in this way – after this project teams should look after the whole of their own planning.

List of Assignments
1. Beach towels take up too much space for cyclists, and sand sticks to them.
2. Milk usually turns sour within a few days.
3. A punctured tyre is a great nuisance when one is cycling.
4. In the heat of the summer children often stain their clothes with molten ice cream.
5. Current packs of snacks take up a lot of space.
6. The plasticizers used to soften plastics in toys are toxic.
7. Soft drinks damage teeth.
8. During the night it often gets damp in a camping tent.
9. The paper towels used in the university toilets are difficult to pick up one by one, they get too wet and they often get left on the floor.

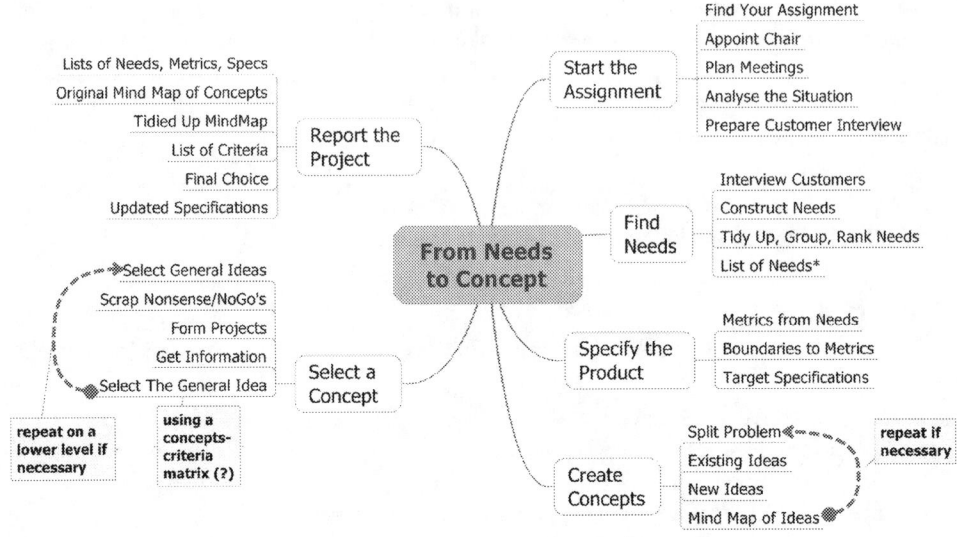

Figure P2-1 Mind map of Project 2

10. Oil is a limited resource; we need other energy sources for transportation.
11. Corn Flakes rapidly loose their crispness when milk is poured on them.
12. Ice formation on car windows is a nuisance, and can be dangerous.
13. Chewing gum remnants on the streets are a nuisance.
14. Cyclists get wet during rainy weather: either due to the rain, or due to their own sweat when they wear rain clothes.
15. Solvent-based paints are being replaced by water-based (latex) paints. They often dry too quickly (and sometimes too slowly), so working with them is difficult.
16. Military people wear protective clothing, also in warm countries. However, this can easily cause them to become overheated.
17. Plants need water depending on temperature, wind, and sun, also when the owners go on holiday.
18. We use chalk to write on 'blackboards'. Chalk causes dust, which is bad for many things, including computers. Instead of blackboards, whiteboards have come into use. However, all markers around are too thin (compared with chalk).
19. If marker pens are left open, they dry out.
20. The fresh taste of chewing gum only lasts a few minutes.

Project 3: Making a Product

Making a product on a commercial scale involves many people, and requires money and time. Doing it really is out of the question in a student project. However, you can learn much by trying to find out what the production would look like.

Read This First

Read Lessons 10 through 14 (at least those parts that we have not yet introduced). Realize that you are to consider something similar to what is described there, but for a different product.

Look up your product in the list behind this assignment. You may find it old-fashioned and uninspiring, but you will need to find or guess a recipe for your product. It is *essential* that you start with a good recipe with all the major components, their amounts and the processing steps (such as shown in Figure 11-10). For a new, challenging, product you would have to do that yourself (as shown in Lesson 10). For these old products you can find a lot in cooking books or in other literature.

Now read Lesson 11 (on Flowsheeting) a second time, because that lesson will form the backbone of this project. Your main task is to construct a process with good flowsheets.

Make estimates of the product required for a country with ten million inhabitants (not necessarily customers). This number is arbitrary: if you have a reason, you may choose a different one.

Set up a process diagram, with amounts of materials and energy.

Get estimates of the cost of ingredients and energy.

Improve the process diagram by considering recycles of materials and energy, by considering cheaper ingredients, or by reducing the number of steps.

If you have time, we would appreciate if you consider part of the following items as well, but we understand that this will often be superficial:

Analyse which operations are needed in the process.

Orient yourself on the equipment required.

Discuss which problems are to be expected on scaling up.

Make an estimate of equipment cost.

Give recommendations for scaling down.

Make a cost model of the production.

Estimate the price required to break even.

Design and Development of Biological, Chemical, Food and Pharmaceutical Products   J.A. Wesselingh,
S. Kiil and M.E. Vigild
© 2007 John Wiley & Sons, Ltd

You can easily spend weeks on the Internet looking for price data – don't do that. Set aside a limited amount of time, and use the guesses from the book if you have not found good data.

As before, we recommend that you read the assignment of Project 1 and 2 again, and keep in mind that you can use the techniques from both earlier projects. Remember that it is not forbidden to do experiments!

Evaluation

For the evaluation we expect (in the form of tables, or short paragraphs – less that a page each)

A table of contents
The recipe that you have decided upon (and how it was obtained)
Your estimates of the market size
The final process diagram with amounts entering and leaving
If relevant: a separate diagram for energy
A short discussion how you tried to improve the process

Only if you have time:

Estimates of the cost of ingredients (with references and remarks on reliability)
For which operations you would need data for scaling up
A cost model for production (with an Excel spreadsheet)
Estimate of required sales prices for breakeven (with discussion)
Recommendations on what would be needed to really go on.
An appendix with copies of anything you would have liked to have at the beginning of the project.

Your Product

Your product is marked in the list below. Some assignments will be easier than others, so we do not expect all teams to report with the same level of reliability.

List of Assignments

You are to consider the marked product from the following list.

Shampoo
Paint
Powder Coating
Capsulated Herbicide
Chewing Gum
Bread
Pressure Sensitive Adhesives
Matchbox
Ink

Paper
Ice Cream
Car Tyres
Beer
Concrete
Soap
Margarine
Enzyme Granulates for Detergents
Drugs (Tablets)
Chocolate Bars
Headache Pills
Insulin

Project 4: Your Own Product

Instructions

During the last month of this course you will be working on your final project. This will be in a new team that the course leaders are putting together in the coming weeks.

In the schedule below we are assuming that your team will plan a meeting twice a week (this can be very short).

All teams should have decided which product they are going to develop after their second meeting.

You are to present a first version of your plans to mentors and other teams on the fourth meeting. This is a discussion meeting, not a 'sales' meeting, meant to look at what you think and the problems you are expecting. It is up to you who will present the plans. We reckon on 8 minutes per team, but this will be followed by discussions between the mentors and the teams separately.

The mentors expect to see you regularly, say once a week. This will normally be on appointment during the hours assigned to the course.

These instructions for the project are minimum requirements – you are free to try other things.

Choice of the Product

As a team you should identify a product that you wish to design or to improve. We have already tried to help you to find ideas, by provoking you to look somewhere where you might not have otherwise. We expect the team to begin with many ideas, but to make a choice together. Don't be too formal on this – you want something that looks challenging and interesting, but also feasible.

Planning and Organization

We are expecting you to set up a project documentation system. After your first analysis of the situation, you should begin to plan which tasks you think should be done. These plans will be discussed and modified after each project meeting.

The project meetings are to be prepared and chaired by one of you (this is not the responsibility of your mentors). Your mentors will be available, but will try to behave as *consultants*: not as teachers and not as chairmen.

Design and Development of Biological, Chemical, Food and Pharmaceutical Products   J.A. Wesselingh, S. Kiil and M.E. Vigild
© 2007 John Wiley & Sons, Ltd

Analyse the Situation

Your orientation on the problem area may include:

reading: Internet, folders, articles, parts of books, patents . . .
interviewing people who might know about the area (both inside and outside university, face-to-face, by e-mail, by telephone . . .)
trying to split (decompose) the problem area in different ways.

Please try splitting: this often gives rise to more interesting ideas that the other techniques do. Realize that you should be working on your project while you are gathering knowledge: analysing will go on during the whole project.

If you think you need to know more about specific parts of science and technology, your mentors may be able to help you. We may be able to help with a discussion of – say – one hour on subjects that we know about. We can only handle a few of such activities, so think about this early. If we do not know ourselves, we may be able to help by getting you in contact with others.

Experiments

Whether you can or should do any experiments in the project depends on the subject that you choose. There are many products where you can learn a lot from simple experiments, but experiments do cost time and they need planning. If you include experiments, we expect you to follow the guidelines that we have given for 'Experiments at Home'.

Prices

In a real project price data are important, but you do not have the time to get everything right. Set aside a limited amount of time for searching prices, and use the guesses from the book if you have not found good data in time. (Of course, in the improbable case that you have time left at the end of the project, we would appreciate further research.)

Contents

The design project should include the phases (described in the course notes) and addressed in the first three reports in this course. These are:

(1) Needs. Which needs should the product fulfil?
(2) Specifications. Metrics, units, limitations.
(3) Concepts. Which working principles might do the job?
(4) Selection. Which idea is the most promising?
(5) Protection. Do we need it, how could we do it? Briefly!
(6) Product Recipe
(7) Process
(8) Equipment
(9) Cost. Make a cost model.

In addition, we expect you to consider the last lessons of the course:

(10) Forecast. What is the value of your project?

(11) Market. What is your goal? What is it worth? Turnover, profit, when? What are the positive, what the negative consequences? To whom will you be selling? Who are your end-users? On what do they spend their money now? The competition? What do you want them to think about you? What is your story? The big thing? Benefit for the customer? How will you communicate the product? *This may be a good starting point for your summary.*

(12) Have you thought about sales material?

(13) What will you do next if the product is a success?

Report

The design project should be described in a well-structured technical report. We expect proper references. The report is to be handed in 1 week before the final presentation. We want to see your documentation, but do not need a copy. You then still have a week to prepare your presentation.

Your report should not be too long. We are not interested in having 300 pages from each of you. Think in terms of 30 or 40 pages (we can hardly be specific as it depends . . .). Remember that making a report concise takes time!

Final Presentation

The final presentation is on the last half day scheduled. You will have 20 minutes per team. We leave it up to you how the team structures the presentation, and who does it. We do expect everybody to participate in the preparation. Keep the guidelines in mind that we have given you for presentations. Realize that a report and a presentation are quite different things: figures and tables in a report are seldom good for a presentation.

Hints

This is a large job. Neither you nor we can expect it to be done perfectly. The thing is to try to make a beginning with everything – and then to improve upon this later.

If you think about it, you will realize that the goal of the project is not 'developing a product'. (Much as we would like it to be.) The goal is 'write a report'. When writing a report, people often make the mistake of first getting everything ready: all ideas, all data, all theories, all experiments . . . and then writing it up at the very end. This is asking for trouble, as the writing nearly always requires more time than planned, and it turns out that you have forgotten things.

A better way is to start writing almost immediately. Set up a plan which things have to be done (you could even copy parts of this assignment). Put these in MindManager. When you are satisfied, export the plan to Word as an outline. Word automatically generates chapter and paragraph titles. Then start filling in the paragraphs, first provisionally. Keep separate copies of the parts: Word sometimes makes a hash of things when you put them together. Expand, improve, correct, and shorten as you go on. If you want to change the sequence of chapters and paragraphs: you can drag whole chapters to a new position in the outline view of Word. You can also add or delete chapters. Always re-read what you have done, looking especially at references. Don't delete a chapter unless you have a copy!

While you are busy, you will find that certain things are missing, or not yet done well enough. This will cause you to change plans, possibly several times.

In this way, you always have a working document that shows the position at the moment. Just before time is up, you tidy it up as well as you can, and that's it. You can even let Word generate a table of contents, but do practice on a separate file. Good luck!

Notes

Here are four notes on things to do in your projects:

1. Experiment at home
2. Plan Your Project
3. Present Your Results
4. Interview Your Customer

Behind these, you will find a separate set of notes on Colloids.

Note 1: Experiment at Home

Occasionally, one has to learn a totally new part of engineering. You almost certainly will during this course. The best way is usually to start reading a book. However, a book alone may not convey a 'feeling' for the subject. You then look around whether you can find something useful, usually in the kitchen or the garage, to play with. Our experience is that we can often learn a surprising amount with simple and cheap experiments, and comparing the results with what we are told in literature.

During the course on innovation, we will ask you to do some experiments at home. These will require ingenuity; doing reliable experiments with household equipment is not easy. Below are a few guidelines.

Document Your Experiments

You must write down everything necessary to allow your experiment to be repeated. So:

Note the dimensions of your equipment (glasses, spoons, hole sizes of sieves and so on).

Describe the materials that you use. If you are looking at a detergent powder note the trade name, and anything on composition given on the box. If you are working with water or air, note the temperature.

If you are dealing with liquids or gases, try to find the viscosity (or other rheological parameters).

If you are dealing with particles, try to give a diameter. You can determine the size of sugar or salt particles on graph paper under a magnifying glass. Take averages of a reasonable number of particles. You can get an idea of the diameter of very fine particles by letting a small puff of them settle in stagnant air and using Stokes' law for the settling of a sphere. This is most easily done in a sun ray in an otherwise shadowy room. Particles usually have a distribution of sizes and shapes, and you have to think beforehand which is the limiting particle size or shape for your experiment.

Report amounts! Even a rough measure such as a flat spoonful is better than nothing.

Learn to estimate times. For example when determining the number of revolutions per second of a stirrer, you can count the seconds as twenty-one, twenty-two, twenty-three etc. Check with a stopwatch!

Always try to check the reproducibility of your measurements.

Design and Development of Biological, Chemical, Food and Pharmaceutical Products   J.A. Wesselingh, S. Kiil and M.E. Vigild
© 2007 John Wiley & Sons, Ltd

Find Measuring Equipment

Start looking around what you could use for measuring things, and make a little collection. You will find a surprising number of instruments in the home if you look around well:

Mass: you will probably find several balances in the home. The smallest are used for measuring weights of letters; they have an accuracy of a few grams. Those in the kitchen typically go up to a kilogram; in the bathroom up to 100 kg. You can construct a primitive balance from almost anything, and coins or even snippets of paper and cardboard can be useful weights.

Dimensions: ruler, calibrated tape, millimetre paper with a magnifying glass ..., taking the length of a person as a little under two metres ..., the width of your thumb as 25 mm (check!), the span of your hand (21 cm, check!). A hair has a thickness of about 50 μm; the thinnest line in a 600 dpi printer is 1/600 of an inch, or again 50 μm. You cannot see things that are much smaller: 20 or 30 μm is the limit.

Small dimensions: you can borrow a simple electronic microscope. Realize that even learning to work with a 'children's microscope' takes time, and that software always has its frustrations. Let one person try this out first. You will find that preparation of the sample, the lighting you use and a critical attitude to what you see are all important in microscopy. Do not expect wonders immediately.

Time: your watch (most digital ones are also stopwatches), counting seconds as twenty-ONE, twenty-TWO, twenty-THREE and so on. Noting hours and dates when the times are long.

Velocity: remember that your walking velocity is about 1 m s^{-1}, a car or train around 30 m s^{-1}, a jet plane about 300 m s^{-1}.

Forces: you can measure small forces using the extension of a rubber band, larger ones using springs.

Temperature: you will probably find several thermometers in the home. High temperatures can be estimated from the colour of the radiance as seen in a dark room.

Moisture: there may be a barometer with a hygrometer in the home.

Electricity: you will be surprised how handy it is to have a modern multimeter. Be careful not to overload the multimeter (especially in its resistance and current measuring modes).

Light: modern cameras usually have lighting instruments built in. However, there are still separate instruments around which can be handy.

Many houses have a water meter, an electricity meter and a gas meter.

Nowadays many digital instruments can be obtained cheaply on the Internet. These can often be coupled to a computer, allowing real-time registration. You might have a look at www.vernier.com, but there are other sites.

Get Properties

Try to get an order of magnitude feeling for all common properties of gases, liquids and solids. Properties such as density, thermal capacity, enthalpy of vaporization, thermal conductivity, viscosity, diffusivity . . . Both countries where we have worked have little books for secondary schools with a nice collection of data. (Denmark: Databog Kemi og Fysik; the Netherlands: Binas).

Final Remarks

Don't make a mess of the kitchen just before cooking.

Tidy up after your experiments!

After reading this, you may think we prefer primitive experiments to good ones. However, this is only so when you can learn more quickly from the simpler experiment. The trick is to start in a simple manner and to improve as you go on. There is nothing wrong with good laboratory equipment, and with 'proper' experiments. However, setting these up often requires much more time than doing a creative household experiment, and you often learn as much from the simple experiment.

Note 2: Plan Your Project

'Start at the beginning' the boss said.
'Then proceed to the end and finish.'

Have a look at the assignment above, and grin. That does not happen, does it? Well, think again. If you have a good boss, *you* (as a team) will be the ones who have to sort out the details of what you have to do. That is just as well; things are not made better if other people (your boss ...) keep interfering. So you may expect instructions that are quite broad. You will have to define what has to be done yourself, but keep your boss informed while you are doing that. He has to know what is happening; also he may know things that you do not.

Let us consider one of the assignments for Project 1. Your team is to do this:

'Make a hot cup of coffee and measure the temperature as a function of time. Develop a quantitative model that describes this.'

There are five of you: Alexandra, Bernard, Charles, Debbie and Edward. The start of the project is on Monday, August 30th; you are to present your results on Thursday, September 16th.[1] You have 8 minutes for the presentation, and two and a half weeks to prepare it.

Before you set off, a word on terminology. We talk about 'project planning'. This is an unfortunate and misleading set of words – but everybody uses them. You can *plan* when you know what you have to do – to follow lessons from two to four, for example. You *cannot* plan when you do not yet know what to do: you cannot 'plan' in the beginning of a development project. You can only think of what you must learn and discover – perhaps speculate would be a better word. Because this is important, it is repeated in Figure N2-1. We will try to help a little with this first assignment, but realize that every project is different, and that it remains *your* problem. These notes are not instructions.

Starting the Project

A first thing you might consider is to choose a 'chair'. Small groups (say up to three, but it depends) do not need a *leader* or *chair*. However, in larger groups it usually helps if one person takes on this role.[2] The chair should focus on keeping an overview of the project, and

---

[1] Your time schedule may be different...

[2] The chair and others have different roles. You should learn to play both, perhaps by changing roles in different projects. There is no single 'best' way of chairing – each person has an own style. However, autocratic styles seldom work well in designing.

Design and Development of Biological, Chemical, Food and Pharmaceutical Products   J.A. Wesselingh, S. Kiil and M.E. Vigild
© 2007 John Wiley & Sons, Ltd

Planning = Speculating

■ you can plan when you know what to do

   when you are following a course,
   that someone else has planned…

■ you **cannot** plan when do not yet know

■ you **can and must** think (speculate) about
   what has to be learned and discovered

'planning' is an unfortunate word in development

Figure N2-1 Planning is speculating!

on coordinating the different activities. In a small project, it can be handy if the chair takes notes and works them out. Depending on the workload, the chair can do some other activities, but they should not dominate. The chair does not have to be the person who knows most about the problem. It is more important that he or she can maintain an overview, get on with all team members, and delegate work. It is all too easy to end up with one or two people being overloaded, and the rest having little to do. This can happen even when all people really want to be involved.

Back to our assignment: the cooling of a cup of coffee. When you do not know what to do, you might first try to get some ideas. What could you explore? Which things are interesting? Which things can you tackle? Where could you have fun? Where is adventure?[3] And if you try out all the ideas you get, will you finish on time? Back to Earth: what are you going to do? 'I want to go back home on time.' 'Who is going to look after the thermometers?' 'Couldn't we get a cup of coffee…?' This can go on for some time, and it may help if the team tries to bring some structure into the discussion.

Mind Mapping

A technique that often helps is shown in Figure N2-2. It goes under the grandiose name of *mind mapping,* but it is quite effective – and also simple. Start by stating the problem with a simple title in big letters on the middle of a sheet of paper. Then add a few legs (not more than five to seven) and start jotting down the ideas that come out of the meeting on the legs. Somebody may ask 'when is coffee too hot?' followed by 'when too cold?' and 'how quickly

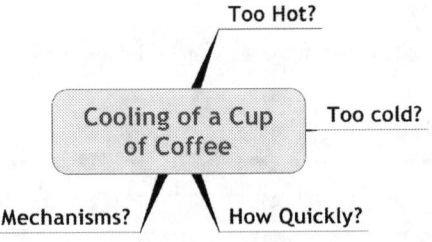

Figure N2-2 First mind map of the project

---

[3] There are limits to adventure with a cup of coffee.

should it cool?'. You might then get 'what are the cooling mechanisms?' Just summarize the remarks on the legs. We have drawn Figure N2-2 using the program MindManager, but you can also do it with a big sheet of paper and felt pens, or on a blackboard, so that everybody can follow the discussion.

You will quickly get down to adding sub-questions, or grouping earlier questions (Figure N2-3). Then you may have to start rearranging, which will require redrawing if you do it on a sheet of paper. Don't let the branches run out of hand – five to seven items per branch are enough. Try to keep the names of the items short (certainly of the main items). Once you get the knack of it, you will be surprised how such a structure helps to form an overview of a problem.

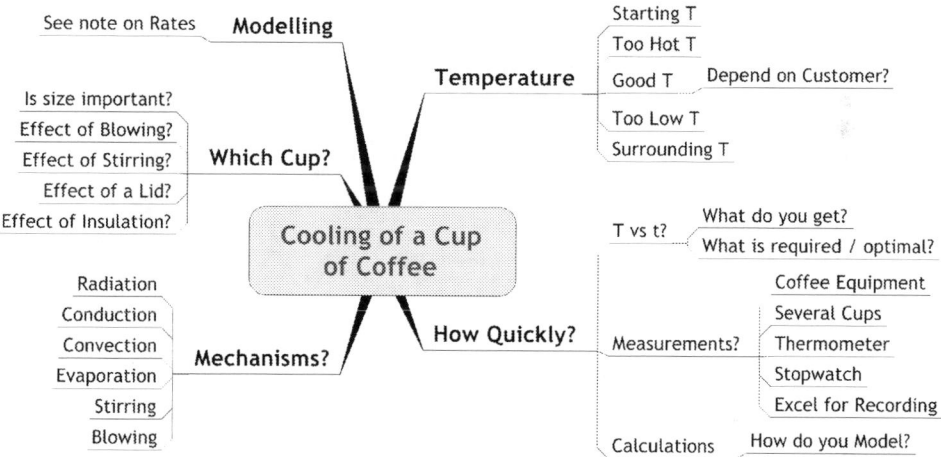

Figure N2-3 The mind map a bit later

Figure N2-4 shows where you might be at the beginning of the second meeting, when the chair has tidied up things a bit. The plans are getting clearer, although the item 'Improving the Cup of Coffee' has not yet been worked out. The mind map will keep on changing during the project, as your ideas evolve. Even so, you should start (or already be) working on the items that are getting into the plan.

Tasks in the Project

The main tasks that have come out of the discussion are:[4]

(1) planning the project,
(2) finding information and analysing,
(3) setting up experiments,
(4) setting up (theoretical) models,
(5) preparing and making the presentation.

---

[4] Another team might come up with a different list: there is no 'correct' answer.

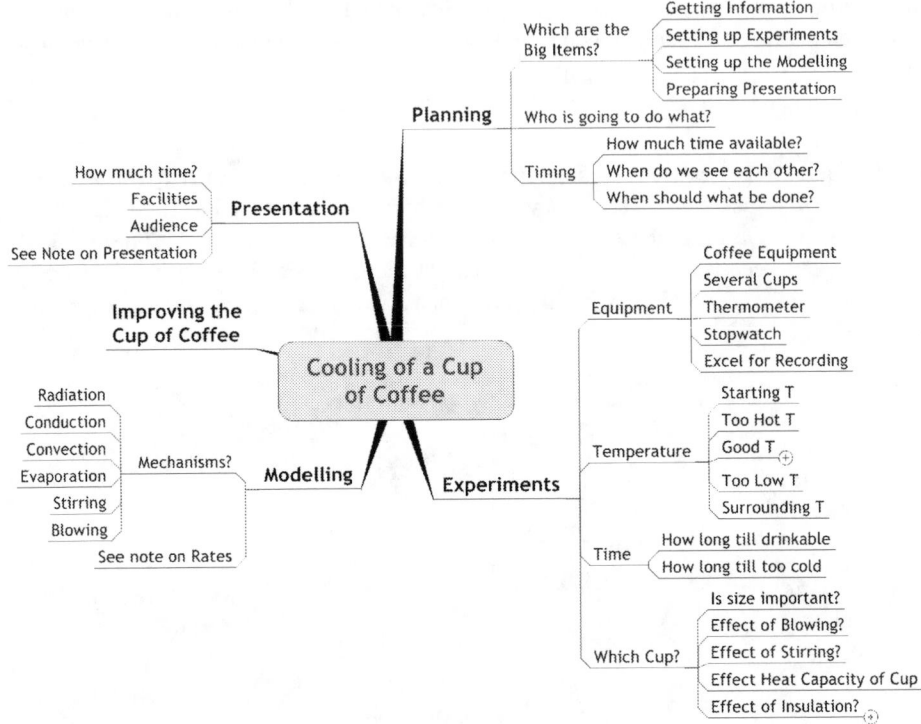

Figure N2-4 Mind map version 3

The points suggest giving one task to each person. However, it is often best to have difficult tasks (you think 3 and 4 will be the most difficult) done by two people simultaneously, and you cannot do that if everybody gets one task.

In project work, you can expect either of two situations:

(1) you have to estimate the time (or money) required to attain a goal, or
(2) you have a certain time (or budget) and have to do with that.

The second situation is just as common as the first: it is the one you are dealing with here. You have 14 work days. Team members expect to be able to put about 2 hours a day into the project. You have five team members. So the maximum amount of work is estimated as 140 hours. In a moment you will be guessing times required for your activities. A useful rule here is the first law of Hofstadter: it tells you that any activity will take longer than you expect (Figure N2-5). It suggests that you should include a wide safety margin for activities in which you have little experience.

Further clues to planning can be found when you consider the sequence of the tasks. Planning will be mostly done in the beginning, with updates and adjustments until just before the end. You are already 'planning'. Finding information and analysing will also be done early.

> **It always takes longer than you expect**

Figure N2-5 The first law of Hofstadter[5]

Experiments can be set up *in parallel* with finding of information. Setting up theories is probably best done when you already know something about the problem, and have done some experiments, but it can be partly in parallel with those activities. Putting the presentation together will be done when you have most of the ideas and data, so towards the end. A rough plan along these lines is shown in Figure N2-6.

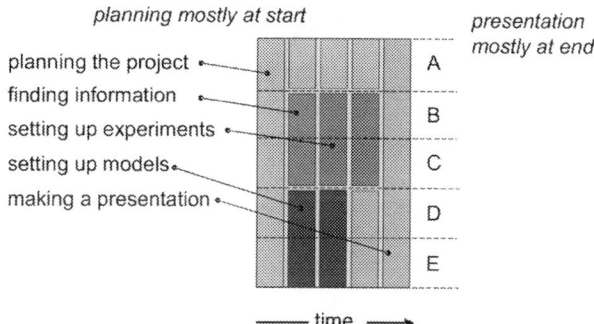

Figure N2-6 A first idea of the timing of the tasks

In the previous figure, you had already assigned tasks to the team members. In reality, getting this done can be quite difficult, and it is part of the task of the chair to see that it happens smoothly. Several conflicting ideas play a role:

(1) You may wish to use the capabilities (experience and personality) of the team members in an optimal fashion.
(2) Certain team members may have certain interests, and may want to learn new things.
(3) There may be tasks that nobody wants to do.

We can only say one thing about this: good teams do not waste their time bickering about this. All members just take their share after a little consultation by the chair.

Timing and Scheduling

We now consider the timing in a bit more detail. Here is a *time line* of the period we are considering (Figure N2-7). It is plotted in Excel, but you could also draw it by hand. We have left out the days of the two weekends, assuming that they will not be available. The days with lectures are coloured; these are natural meeting points for the team. For simplicity you might assume that everybody works 2 hours per day on the project.

---

[5] The second law of Hofstadter reads: 'It always takes longer than you expect, even when you take into account Hofstadter's law'. Very helpful, indeed!

Tasks	30	31	01	02	03	06	07	08	09	10	13	14	15	16
Plan														
Inform														
Experiment														
Model														
Present														

Tasks														
Plan														
Inform														
Experiment														
Model														
Present	30	31	01	02	03	06	07	08	09	10	13	14	15	16

Figure N2-7 The project time line with tasks

A natural point for ending the 'blocks' of activities would be the meeting times scheduled in the course.[6] The plan would then look like Figure N2-8. The two charts show the hours spent on the activities and the people who are to do them. Note that all time in the first day has already gone into the first meeting – into planning. You realize that you have to minimize the time spent on meetings. You have little experience both with the experiments and with setting up models. According to Hofstadter you should assign more time to these activities.

Tasks	30	31	01	02	03	06	07	08	09	10	13	14	15	16	
Plan	10	2	2	2	2	2	2	2	2	2					28
Inform		4	4												8
Experiment		4	4	4	4	4	4	4							28
Model				4	4	4	4	4	4	4					28
Present									4	4	10	10	10	10	48
	10	10	10	10	10	10	10	10	10	10	10	10	10	10	140

Tasks	30	31	01	02	03	06	07	08	09	10	13	14	15	16
Plan	All	A	A	A	A	A	A	A	A	A				
Inform		DE	DE											
Experiment		BC	BC	BC	BC	BC	BC	BC						
Model				DE	DE	DE	DE	DE	DE	DE				
Present									BC	BC	All	All	All	All

Figure N2-8 Times (top) and people (bottom)

A possible solution is shown in Figure N2-9. You don't think the chair needs all her time for planning, and shift the job of looking for information elsewhere to her. You also reduce the time for preparing the presentation as you know how to do that. This frees up time for experiments and for modelling. There may still be a bit of spare time in 'presentation', but you leave it like this for the moment.

In projects it is usually a good idea to get working as soon as you can. Then you try to get something acceptable, be it possibly a bit simple and not quite enough, so that you have

---

[6] Some people regard all meetings as a waste of time. However, in a team they are necessary for coordination. The trick is to keep them short by following an agenda. However, that will not be possible when a free flow of ideas is required, such as in the beginning of a project. The chair can then better fix the time beforehand.

Tasks	30	31	01	02	03	06	07	08	09	10	13	14	15	16	
Plan	10	1	1	1	1	1	1	1	1	1					19
Inform		1	1	1	1	1	1	1	1	1					9
Experiment		4	4	4	4	4	4	4	4	4					36
Model		4	4	4	4	4	4	4	4	4					36
Present											10	10	10	10	40
	10	10	10	10	10	10	10	10	10	10	10	10	10	10	140
Tasks	30	31	01	02	03	06	07	08	09	10	13	14	15	16	
Plan	All	A	A	A	A	A	A	A	A	A					
Inform		A	A	A	A	A	A	A	A	A					
Experiment		BC	BC	BC	BC	BC	BC	BC	BC	BC					
Model		DE	DE	DE	DE	DE	DE	DE	DE	DE					
Present											All	All	All	All	

Figure N2-9 Revision of the former figure

something to present at any moment. You can improve if there is time left. Being early is essential in Project Planning.

The 'temperature' usually rises towards the end of a project, as the deadline approaches (Figure N2-10). This seems natural and unavoidable. However, if you start early, and try to have some result at any moment, the problems will be less acute. What would the ideal profile be like? We suggest that it would have the highest degree of activity (temperature) *in the beginning*. As a result, you would have time to perfect things at the end, and to feel comfortable at the final presentation. Do you remember the time that you had prepared that examination early enough?

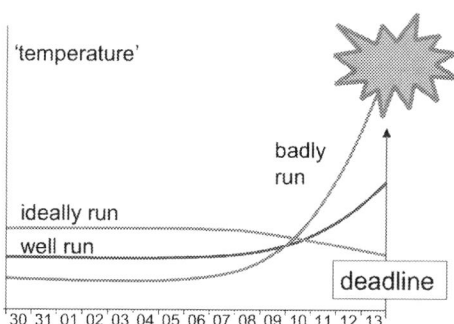

Figure N2-10 The temperature in a project

Summary

The summary shows the steps that we have considered (Figure N2-11). Here we repeat: every project is different, and so is every team. This is not a prescription, only a suggestion. Feel free to do things differently.

Further Reading

Most literature and software on project planning concerns problems that are well-defined to start with. In development much of the work goes into *defining* the problem, into that part

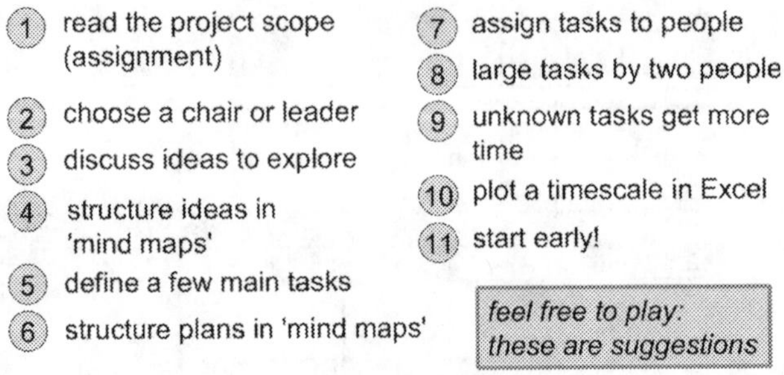

1. read the project scope (assignment)
2. choose a chair or leader
3. discuss ideas to explore
4. structure ideas in 'mind maps'
5. define a few main tasks
6. structure plans in 'mind maps'

7. assign tasks to people
8. large tasks by two people
9. unknown tasks get more time
10. plot a timescale in Excel
11. start early!

feel free to play: these are suggestions

Figure N2-11 The summary

where formal planning methods are not only irrelevant, but even a nuisance. This is because they hold back the free flow of ideas that are necessary to define a problem. A very readable book which avoids this pitfall is:

Gary R. Heerkens *Project Planning*, McGraw-Hill 2002.

Note 3: Present Your Results

Before Reading this Note

Your teachers find all of this rather obvious ... It seems that it is not so to all speakers. We see them sinning against presentation rules time and again, in student projects but also in large international symposia.

Have a look at the summary first. If you apply all guidelines already, you can skip this note!

Content

When you are setting up a presentation, begin with the four W's:

What?

Who?

hoW?

When?

What?

In most lectures you want to get something over to your public. In a short lecture, you cannot manage more than one point (Figure N3-1). So choose this carefully. Ideally, you would know your 'point' beforehand. However, we often find that we only start getting a clear idea while we are constructing the lecture.

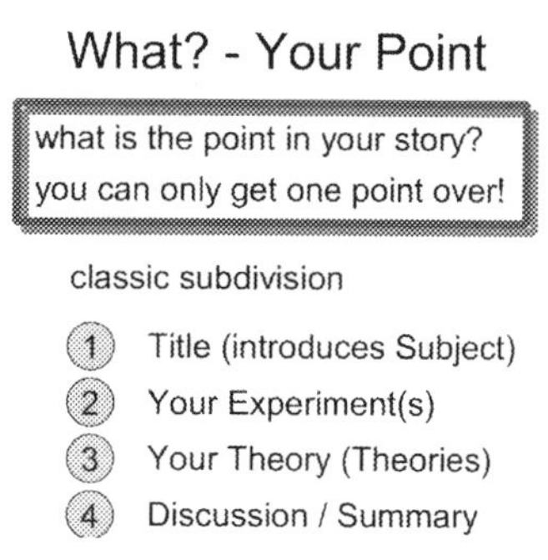

What? - Your Point

what is the point in your story?
you can only get one point over!

classic subdivision

1. Title (introduces Subject)
2. Your Experiment(s)
3. Your Theory (Theories)
4. Discussion / Summary

Figure N3-1 Setting up your lecture

Design and Development of Biological, Chemical, Food and Pharmaceutical Products   J.A. Wesselingh, S. Kiil and M.E. Vigild
© 2007 John Wiley & Sons, Ltd

In 8 minutes, you cannot tell what five people have done in 30 hours. Don't try, make a choice. You can use the title of the lecture as the shortest possible summary. However, you do not have to. In your presentation, we expect you to tell about your experiments and the theory that you have constructed. This is to lead to a short discussion. You can do this under the headings above, but can also try something more adventurous.

Who?

Who will form your audience? In your case there are two groups:

> your fellow students, say 20 of them, and
> one or two teachers.

You may think that your teachers are the most important because they give marks. However, realize that it is the 20 students who largely determine the atmosphere. Aim at them. Try to think what they would like to hear. It is improbable that you will be able to impress them, but they certainly will like to hear what went wrong . . . A short story and a joke may do wonders, but realize that they take time.

hoW?

'W' number three: hoW? You can use several techniques. Almost certainly you will be talking. If your audience is larger than about 40, you need a microphone. It is quite possible to give an excellent lecture only using your voice. You do not need PowerPoint! Some of the best lectures we have heard were without any visual aids. However, for your kind of subject you do need 'visuals'.

In educational institutes you can use the blackboard (which is usually green . . .). Clean it beforehand – even if you do not use it. Text and equations from a previous lecture can be quite distracting, and you don't want that. Clean with *sponge and water* – in two steps. It takes about 5 minutes for a blackboard to dry – unless you have a towel. If you want to put more than one word or equation on the blackboard: plan that beforehand. Begin at the top left corner, not in the middle!

Overhead projector and beamer have much in common. Focus them beforehand and try them out by looking at the projection from poor places in the room. A good overhead projector gives ten times the light flow of a beamer. However, it also distorts the projection and has a low contrast. Beamers are getting more reliable, but we always try them out before the presentation; *before* the public is in the room.

With some beamers you can project a video film – if lighting in the room can be turned down sufficiently. Try this out: even the tiniest bit of sunlight in the room can ruin your video presentation. For small audiences (as in your case) an experiment is well possible. However, do organize and time it properly.

When

The last 'W' is for 'When?' Or to put it bluntly: how much time do you have? In your case that is 8 minutes (plus two for the discussion). You *must* manage in the time allocated, otherwise you will be hammered off by any good chairperson.[1]

Keep in mind that text-only slides take half a minute to one minute. A slide with graphs, and especially with one or more equations, may take several minutes. So does a joke or a story. For a lecture of 8 minutes you probably will not need more than five slides. If you use PowerPoint, you can time your lecture with 'Slide Show' – 'Rehearse Timings'. Do that with a separately saved file; we have never been able to get rid of the timing markings! You may feel a bit ridiculous talking loudly to your computer screen, but that does not matter if there is nobody else around . . .

Plan which item(s) you might leave out if time turns out to be shorter than you thought. It is seldom a problem if you finish too early.

Slide Layout

Now some guidelines on the layout of your slides.

Letter Size

Slides that cannot be read are worse than no slides. We use 24 point letters as standard: they are readable in nearly all situations (Figure N3-2). Letters of 20 points are marginal – *never* use letters below that size. If you cannot get by with 24 point letters, you have too much information on your slide. Remember that the public has to pick up everything in – say – 1 minute.

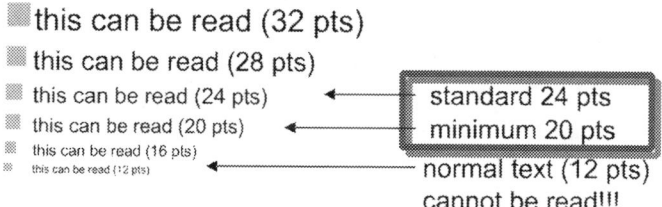

Figure N3-2 Don't use letters smaller than 20 pts

In Figure N3-3 we are using scanned text to show you that you should *never* use text scanned from an article or a textbook. This kind of material is good for reading, but it will only *annoy* your audience when it is projected. Also be careful with scanned figures and graphs. We usually redraw them: they are never formatted properly for projection.

---

[1] If you are the only speaker you may go over your time by perhaps ten percent.

Never

The best such guide uses solubility parameters. This guide, originally suggested by Hildebrand and effectively extended to polymers by Hansen, assumes that all solutions are nonideal, and are described by a relation of the following form:

$$\mu_2 = \mu_2^0 + RT\,ln x_2 + \omega x_1^2. \tag{4.1-1}$$

where μ_2 is the chemical potential of the product solute; μ_2^0 is its value in a reference state (pure 2 at the specified T and p), the "standard state"; ω is an activity parameter with the dimensions of energy per mole; and x_1 and x_2 are the mole fractions of the solvent and the product, respectively. The logarithmic term in this equation represents the free energy change of ideal mixing, and is related to entropy changes. The term with ω includes any heat of mixing. This simplest nonideal relation is known as the Margules equation.

> **never use scanned text**

Figure N3-3 Never use scanned text

Fonts

Which font you use is not terribly important. For projection we prefer 'non-serif' fonts such as Arial (Figure N3-4). The serif fonts – such as Times – are better for ordinary text, but they are a bit weak for projection. If you use fancy fonts with a beamer, check that you have them on the computer used for projecting. You can also embed all fonts in your PowerPoint presentation.

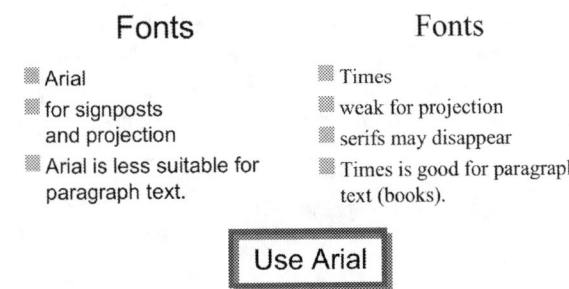

Figure N3-4 Arial is not a bad choice for a font

Pictures

Pictures ('graphics' for professionals) are often necessary to show and explain things. Figure N3-5 shows one from a lecture that describes the wetting of a strip of tissue paper with its lower end placed in water. The water rises in the tissue due to changes in the interfacial energy when the cellulose fibres in the tissue are wetted. Making pictures can take some time. The fibre structure in the middle took us 20 minutes – and we are experienced amateur artists. We only spend so much time if we will be able to reuse the graphic.

If you stick to simple forms (as in Figure N3-6) you can work more quickly. This only took us a few minutes, once we had decided what to do. If you lecture often, make a collection

Picture 1

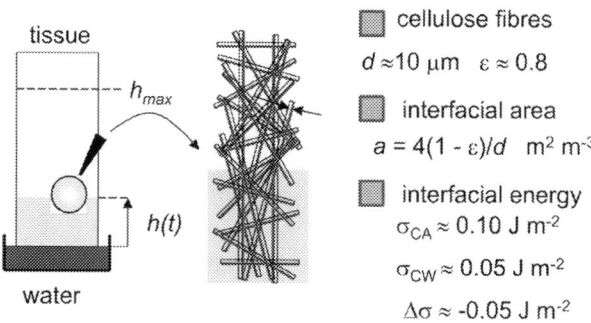

Figure N3-5 Making pictures takes a lot of time

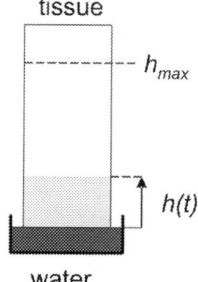

Figure N3-6 ... unless you keep them simple, or recycle

of drawings. We have thousands of them, brought together in over 15 years. There is any amount of clipart on the Internet. Surprisingly, you seldom find exactly what you need ...

When water rises in the tissue the gravitational energy *increases* quadratically with height. At the same time the interfacial energy *decreases* linearly. Both these affect the Gibbs energy of the system. The system will come to equilibrium when the Gibbs energy has reached a minimum, and the height is largest. You can show all this clearly in a graph (Figure N3-7).

When using graphs in a presentation, try to keep them simple (Figure N3-8). Use simple legends (with units if required). Keep the legends horizontal; vertical text is difficult to read! Minimize the use of numbers along the axes and avoid 'embellishments'. Make lines and points stand out by using thicker lines than for the axes.[2] You *can* make decent graphs in Excel, but *the standard format is not acceptable* for presentation. Check why this is using our remarks above.

---

[2] Use points only for measured values, not for calculated ones.

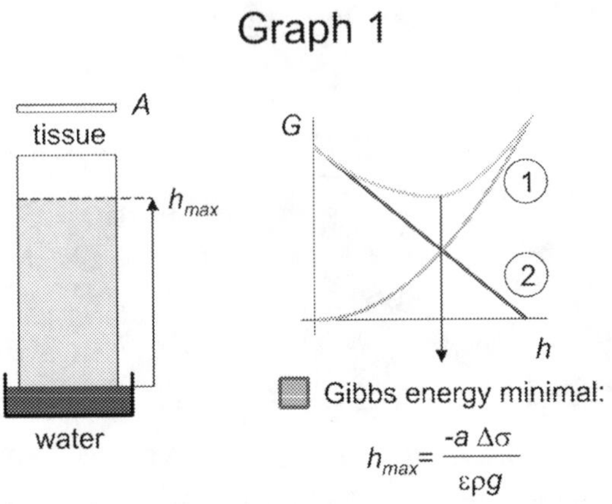

Graph 1

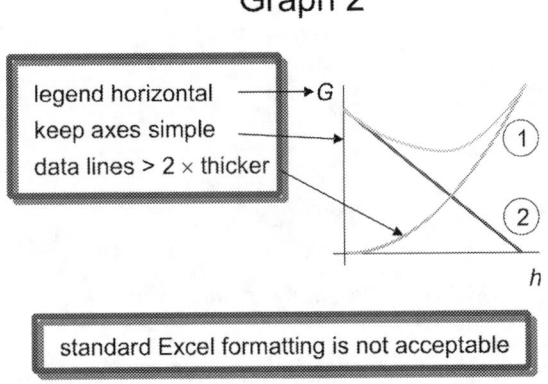

Figure N3-7 Make graphs specially for a presentation

Graph 2

standard Excel formatting is not acceptable

Figure N3-8 Rules for presentation graphs

Equations

Whether you use equations depends strongly on your audience. In most audiences you can better not use them at all. In technical and scientific lectures you can use them sparingly – we would say not more than one per 5 minutes. In theoretical discussions you may need derivations, but these are better done on a blackboard than via projection!

Figure N3-9 contains two equations: one for the change of the gravitational energy of water rising in the tissue, and one for the change in the interfacial energy as the tissue fibres are wetted. During your lecture you will have to *explain every symbol*. This takes time; an equation easily takes a few minutes.

When using equations, explain them, both in your slide and by talking about them. Note that we have included titles to the equations, and have sub-divided one of them. If possible, keep the equations simple. And do not overdo them. As said, one equation per 5 minutes is probably the maximum, even in an audience like yours.

Equations 1

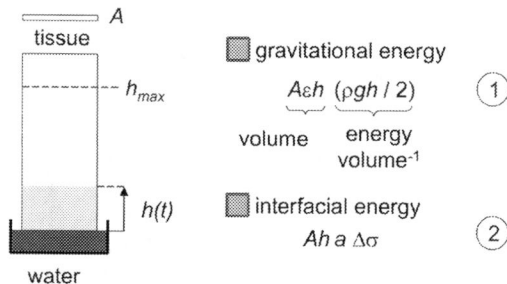

Figure N3-9 You must explain equations

Contrast

To distinguish two areas, one needs a difference in lighting intensity of about a factor of two (Figure N3-10). With an overhead projector, the white (transparent) areas are roughly ten times lighter than the dark (black) areas. Check that black on a screen is not dark at all! This means that the number of gradations available is only four (for a contrast of 8) or five (for a contrast of 16). You might think that you could increase this by using colour differences. However, human eyes have different responses to colour differences: you are best off using the rule 'Get it Right in Black and White'. As a result, overhead projection is not good for colour photographs. You have more leeway with a beamer – at least if the lighting conditions in the lecture room are optimal. (They seldom are.) A good beamer can attain a high contrast, *but only when there is no stray light.* The standard choices of colours in PowerPoint are not bad – we often use them.

Contrast 1

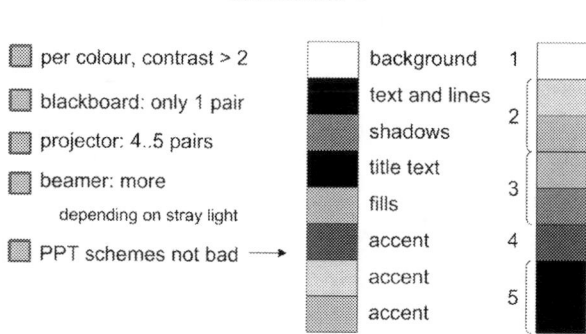

Figure N3-10 You need a contrast of a factor of 2 for every colour pair used

You will undoubtedly want to play with coloured backgrounds at some point (Figure N3-11). They look so attractive! However, do realize that any background reduces the contrast that you have available. Only use coloured backgrounds if you know that projection is going to be very good. Don't use them with an overhead projector. (They not only give poor projection, but also require huge amounts of very expensive ink.)

Contrast 2

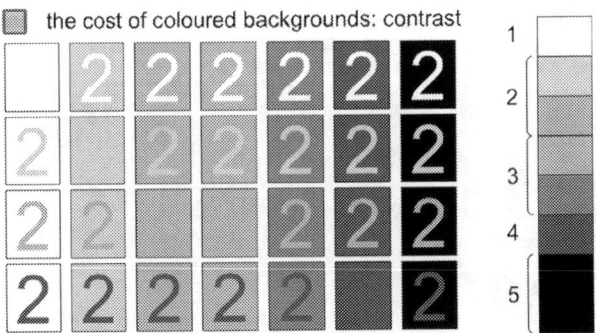

Figure N3-11 A background reduces contrast

The Presentation

Only two points on this final act:

Be on time to check that the beamer or projector is working (and to clean the blackboard if necessary).
Look at your audience while you are speaking! You may occasionally have to look back to see whether the projection is in order, or to point at something. Otherwise you should be facing your audience, and looking at them. There is hardly a worse way of ruining a presentation than by talking to the projection screen! When you look at the audience, don't keep staring at a single person, but let your eyes wander around.

Summary

Every presentation must have an end: you have to plan this beforehand. For a lesson, or a report of work done, a summary is not a bad end. In other cases you may wish to end with something flashier. Anyhow, have something ready. Here we use the summary to end (Figure N3-12).

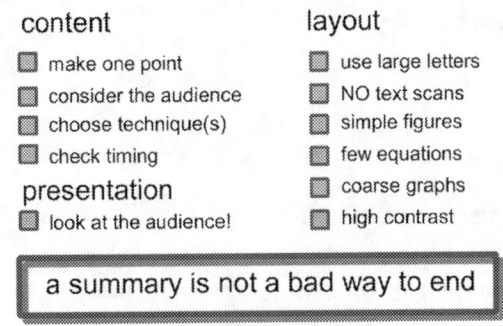

Figure N3-12 Ending with a summary

Note 4:
Interview Your Customer

You want to know the needs of your customer. The best way to find out is to interview her. It can make a big difference how you do that. As an engineer, you may never have been trained professionally in talking with other people. Other professions, such as journalism, psychology, law and nowadays even the medical profession, *do* train their students in communicating. We regularly find out that they are better at it than we are. This little introduction cannot fully remedy your possible disadvantage, but we hope it will help a bit.

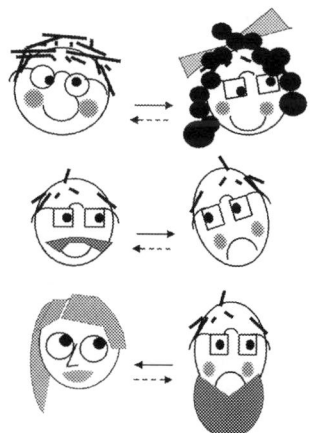

Communicating

Interviewing is a common method of communication. You do it all the time, although you may not realize. You are continually trying to find out things from other people. Communication begins with a speaker (or sender) giving a message that is picked up by a listener (receiver) (Figure N4-1). At the beginning of an interview, the speaker will be the interviewer, but during most of the time this should be the interviewed person ('interviewed' for short).

The speaker has to put the message in the form of words (to *code* the message). The listener has to *decode* the message to understand it. Problems in communication may occur in either coding or decoding. This is especially so when there are differences in background between the two people. Language is an obvious source of problems, but differences in profession and position can also cause them. The listener seldom gets *exactly* the same message as the speaker thinks he has sent.

Design and Development of Biological, Chemical, Food and Pharmaceutical Products   J.A. Wesselingh, S. Kiil and M.E. Vigild

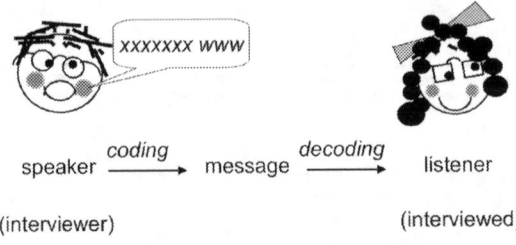

Figure N4-1 Speaker and listener

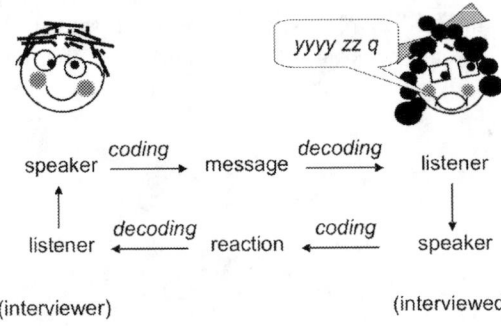

Figure N4-2 The message and the reaction

Even a simple communication requires a reaction to show that the message has been received (Figure N4-2). More complicated communications are *cyclic*. An important use of this cycle is to check whether a message has come across correctly. The interviewer can do this by giving a summary of the answer. In interviews the cycle has many more uses. Switching of roles is essential: the interviewer and the interviewed should have their turns.

Communication can be disturbed by *noise* (Figure N4-3). This can be the noise of drilling in the building, but also that of a telephone, or some outsider getting in between. Personal problems of the participants can also disturb communication, because one or both may not listen or speak. So can feelings of antipathy or anger. For a good communication, you must arrange such that there is not too much noise.

Even with a simple sentence, you convey many different things – although possibly not consciously (Figure N4-4). When you say something to somebody else, you are not only conferring facts. You are also telling the other who you are. For example, you may be trying to impress. You are trying to find some common ground such as interest for the products you want to discuss. Nearly always you are trying to get something done by the other, if only that she will tell you what she thinks about a product.

It is often useful to consider these four aspects of any communication:

(1) the facts,
(2) the personal ('I am ...'),

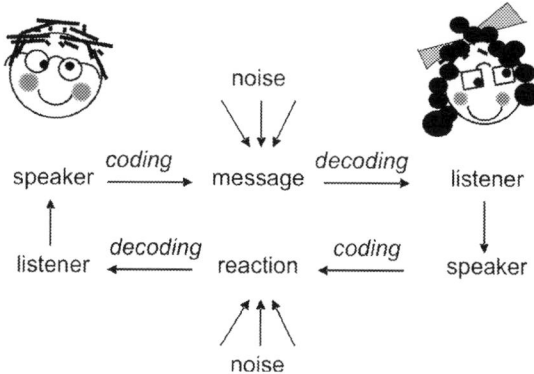

Figure N4-3 Disturbance by 'noise'

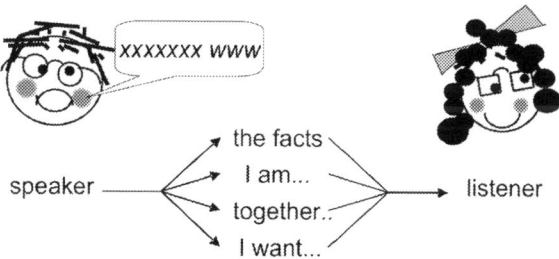

Figure N4-4 Four groups of things conveyed

(3) the communal ('together . . .') and
(4) the asking for ('I want . . .').

You must expect problems when the listener misinterprets any of these four aspects, not only the facts!

You might think that the content of words would be all in communication. This would be a big mistake; there are many studies showing that more than half of communication occurs in other ways. One important method of conveying information is in the *way* you say things. Whether you deliberately speak quickly or slowly, the intonation you use, the loudness, whether your sentences are strongly articulated or not, and whether you appear to waver by using *ummm*'s and *eheh*'s. The way you say things may not change the factual content of your message, but it does have important effects on the personal, communal and asking aspects of communication.

Just as important are the non-spoken (non-verbal) signs that people give (Figure N4-5). The gestures, the way they stand or sit, whether the mouth is sagging or turned up, whether people look at you, just gaze, or close their eyes, how they move their head and bodies. Telephone and Internet are not suitable for communicating difficult subjects, because they do not transfer the non-spoken signs.

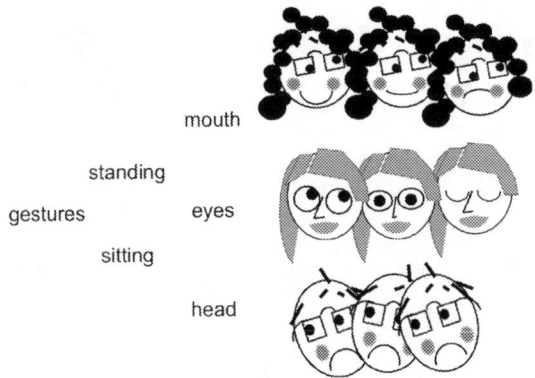

Figure N4-5 Non-verbal signs

The important non-speaking signs in interviewing are those that show that the interviewer is *interested*. This means looking at (but not staring at) the speaker, nodding, giving stimulating hints such as 'ah, yes . . .'. Be aware that there is as much difference in the non-spoken part of language as in the spoken part. In the Western world, nodding the head signifies agreement; in many parts of the world it means the opposite!

The important part of interviewing is *listening*! (Figure N4-6) It is not the interviewer who should have the last word. However, listening usually starts with a question from the interviewer. You may be tempted to use 'closed questions': questions on which the answer might be yes or no, or one out of a small choice, or questions where you force the interviewed to agree or not. However, you may then only get the answer to your question; the interviewed may not go on. Closed questions can be useful to get simple facts such as the name of the interviewed, and you can use them to prod the interviewed person, but do not only use closed questions.

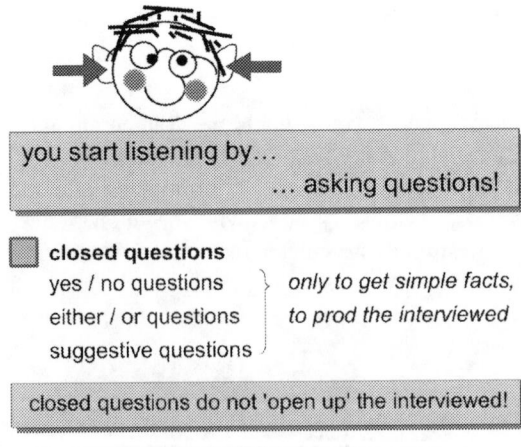

Figure N4-6 How to listen (1)

More useful are 'open' questions: questions to which the answer is not programmed (Figure N4-7). What is an open question? Well, the previous sentence is a nice example! It is question

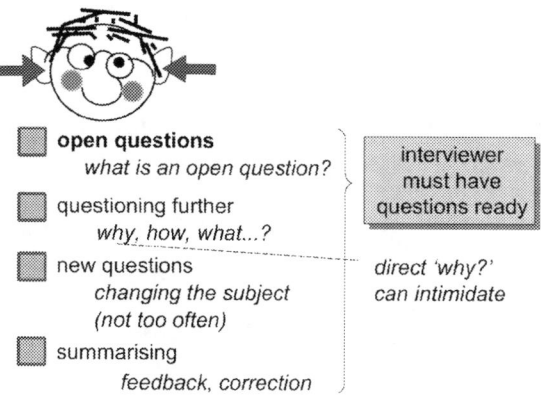

Figure N4-7 How to listen (2)

that allows many answers. Open questions allow the interviewed to say what she wishes, and to give more information. You may get a lot of information that you do not want, but that is the price to pay . . .

A skilful interviewer will question further; he will ask the interviewed *why* she thinks certain things, *how* she has done them, *what* is needed . . . However, a direct 'why?' can be intimidating. It may be better to ask whether the customer has considered alternatives, how the alternatives compare, and so on. The interviewer can get further with new questions which do change the subject, and should not be used too often. It helps to make summaries: these show that the interviewer has listened, allow corrections to be made, and help deciding which details are relevant.

Preparing

It will be getting clear that a good interview requires preparation (Figure N4-8). You must have thought about which information you want to get out of it. At the same time, realize that you never know that exactly beforehand. It is important to keep an open ear for information that you had not expected. It may happen that this will force you to change track. You should

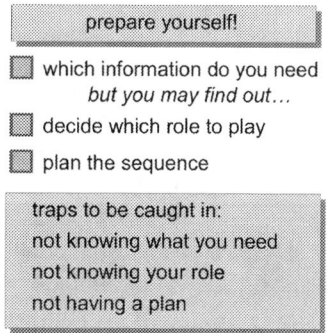

Figure N4-8 Prepare yourself!

also decide beforehand which role you wish to play, and have some plan for the sequence of subjects. We come back to these points in a moment.

It takes two for an interview. The interviewed person spends some time and effort; she must get something back out of the interview. Otherwise you can forget any next meeting. Try to find out who the person is you are to interview; you must know her name and position in the company or organization where she is working. You must try to find out points where you might help each other (Figure N4-9).

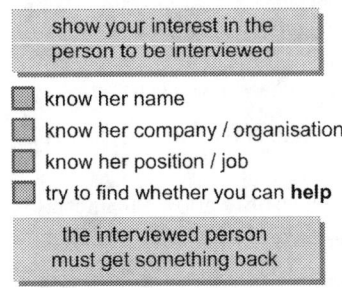

Figure N4-9 Interacting with the interviewed

Information from interviews is often divided into facts, opinions and feelings (also called emotions). You will need both facts and opinions about products (Figure N4-10). In product interviews, feelings or emotions (which are difficult to handle) are usually not important. Remember that you are mainly interested in *what* products do or should do. While you are trying to find this out, you should *not* focus on *how* this should be done. If the interviewed has ideas on how a product might work, jot them down, but do not pursue them. That comes later.

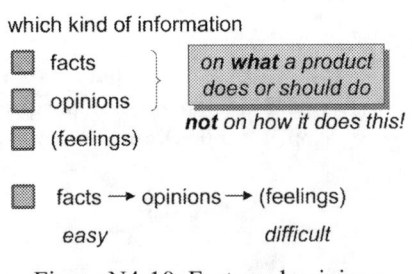

Figure N4-10 Facts and opinions

Whether you manage to get an open atmosphere depends on how strongly you try to structure the interview (Figure N4-11). If you determine the sequence and all questions in detail beforehand, as is often done with marketing enquiries, you leave no room for the interviewed. You only get answers to the question that you ask, but no other information. This is alright if you know exactly what you want, but then you could just as well let the interviewed fill in a list, which takes a lot less time. If you want to get information that you have not thought about before, at least part of the interview must be unstructured, and you should have some open questions to keep this going.

structured	many closed questions
interviewer determines questions and sequence	*you get answers to what you ask, but no other information.*
unstructured	*few open questions*
interviewed determines subjects and sequence	*can open new routes, but can become chaotic*

you need both in a good interview

Figure N4-11 Part of the interview has to unstructured

As the interviewer you can choose to play your role in different ways. In an accepting role, you let the interviewed determine what happens. This role combines well with open questions and little structuring of the interview. If you are new in a field, (and 'groping') you can probably best take an accepting role. If you know the customer, and have a reasonable idea of the field, you will get more out of the interview if you are bit more critical, and use more structure. This mildly critical form is the most used one.

You will often have seen interviews on television that use the confrontational mode. Here the interviewed is provoked to react sharply and to give direct answers. This mode *is not suitable* for product interviews!

You should plan a sequence for the subjects (Figure N4-12). You need to begin an interview by introducing and getting used to each other, with 'why' you are conducting the interview, and 'what' is going to happen with the information. The most common sequence is to begin with the simpler items (facts), and to go the more difficult ones (opinions or even emotions) after you have warmed up. After each item, you summarize before going on to the next.

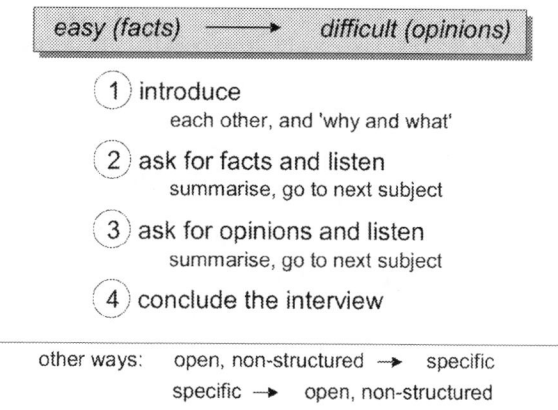

easy (facts) ⟶ *difficult (opinions)*

1. introduce
   each other, and 'why and what'
2. ask for facts and listen
   summarise, go to next subject
3. ask for opinions and listen
   summarise, go to next subject
4. conclude the interview

other ways: open, non-structured → specific
specific → open, non-structured

Figure N4-12 The sequence in an interview

There are other ways of sequencing. For example, you can work from open questions to specific ones or the other way around. Both allow the interview to be partly open. We will not pursue these further, but you may wish to try one of them. You always need a little time for concluding the interview, allowing questions or final remarks from the interviewed, and for thanking.

Ideally you should have enough time to discuss all your questions. In practice, the length of most interviews is limited to perhaps 1 hour and it can be less. It is then useful to have a rough idea of the timing (Figure N4-13). If you have an hour, you might lose 5 minutes for the introduction and the same time for the conclusion. That leaves 50 minutes for the questions. A closed question takes little time, perhaps 1 minute. The time required for an open question is longer, and variable. For a rough plan of your interview you might assume 5 minutes. Do not plan rigidly; that leads to a strongly structured interview with a closed atmosphere. Keep time open for unexpected things, but also have spare questions. You will find that you are quite limited in what you can ask in one hour.

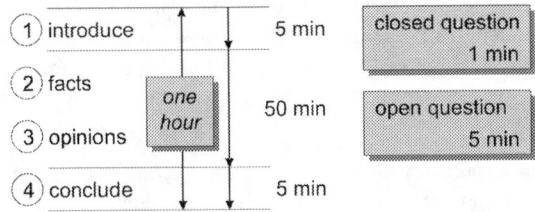

do not plan rigidly!

Figure N4-13 Timing

Interviewing

Figure N4-14 shows some of the things you might do and ask during a product interview. If you have the product, and related or competing products, you may be able to take something along with you to show. You may be able to let the interviewed use it. Watch carefully: this can lead to product improvement ideas. The questions in the figure should be clear, but you should have other ones yourself.

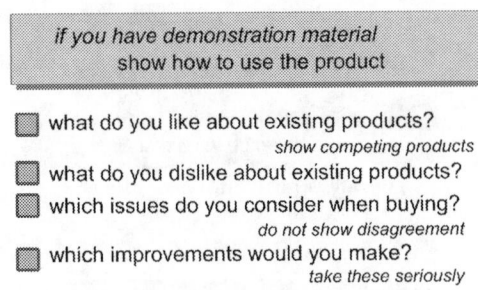

Figure N4-14 Things to do and ask

During the interview you register what is said (Figure N4-15). There are two ways: (1) taking notes, and (2) using a recorder. We recommend that you *always* take notes *on paper*. Using

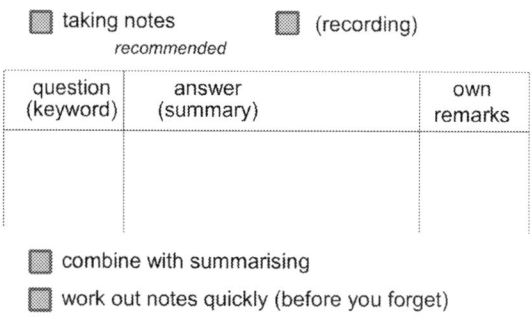

Figure N4-15 Recording the interview

a computer keyboard interferes with the interview, and working out an audio record takes a long time. You cannot write down answers literally – that takes too much time. So you must shorten them. We use a piece of paper with three columns. In the first we put the question number (for prepared questions), or the question itself (short or via a keyword); in the second column a short form of the answer; in the third any remark of our own (for example on the reactions of the interviewed). A good reporter combines part of the note-taking with summarizing; this also gives the chance of checking whether you have got things right. Taking a little time for making notes is allowable, but too much disturbs the interview.

You should work out your notes as soon as possible; they may be cryptic, and after a few days you will have forgotten many details. If possible let the interviewed check your notes.

Summary

We summarize with a checklist for your preparations (Figure N4-16). Good Luck!

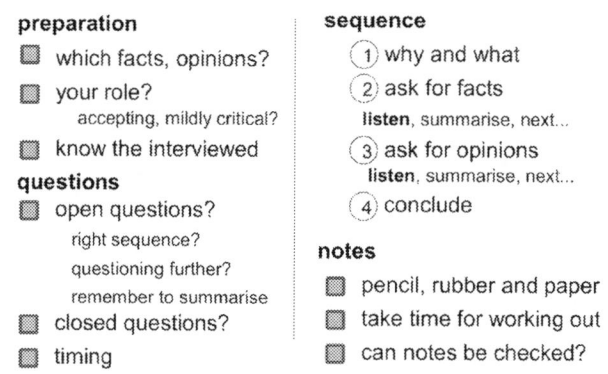

Figure N4-16 A check list

Acknowledgment

This Note owes much to the work of F. Schultz von Thun, which is in German and not accessible to most of our readers.

Colloids

Contents

Colloids 1: Product Structure

In this lesson we look at some common aspects of formulated products. We first consider their micro- and nano-structures.

Terminology of Structures

Most formulated products are not homogeneous: they consist of two or more phases. Together these form a structure: a more-or-less regular arrangement of parts. This structure or morphology largely determines the properties of a product, often more than the chemical composition.

We use structure to make a solid out of a liquid (in ice-cream, shaving foam, a sponge and in tissue), to make a liquid out of a solid (in fluids for polishing), or to adsorb impurities (in activated carbon). We use structure to change optical properties (in paint), to make food digestible (in bread), and to make a thermal insulator out of a heat conductor (in a blanket). We use structure to mix liquids that cannot be mixed (such as in mayonnaise), and to make composites that can handle large forces with little material. You find structures almost everywhere. Getting to understand the structure is one of the best points to start improving a product.

Figure C1-1 shows a few examples of structures. The first column shows a microphoto of shaving cream at the top, with a schematic model below. This is a foam: a dispersion of gas bubbles in a liquid. The photo shows about 2 mm across, so most bubbles are roughly 0.1 mm in diameter.

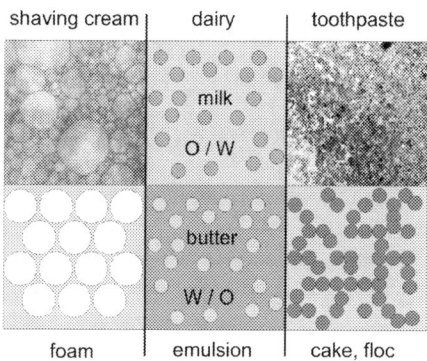

Figure C1-1 Some structures

Design and Development of Biological, Chemical, Food and Pharmaceutical Products   J.A. Wesselingh,
S. Kiil and M.E. Vigild
© 2007 John Wiley & Sons, Ltd

The second column shows models of two dairy products: milk and molten butter. Milk consists mainly of a watery solution with about 4% by volume of fat (oil). This is dispersed in the form of droplets with a diameter of a few micrometres. This is an example of an oil-in-water or O/W emulsion. Molten butter is a mirror of this system, with water dispersed as droplets of a few micrometres. Molten butter is a water-in-oil or W/O emulsion. When it is cooled the fat crystallizes partly, and we get a three-phase structure: butter.

The third column shows toothpaste. This is a dispersion of fine abrasive particles. The photograph shows about 0.7 mm across and the particles seen are about 20 μm in diameter. The particles stick to each other where they touch, and this causes them to form a weak open solid structure. Such a structure is called a cake or floc.

Structures can also contain solids in the form of struts or fibres (Figure C1-2). The first column here shows a sponge: a structure with open walls between cells. Not all walls are open, as you can see in the photo, but most are. The model with cubic cells may not seem to describe reality very well, but it is easily drawn and does show most of the character of a real sponge. The cells are about 0.2 mm in diameter and the struts have a thickness of about 20 μm.

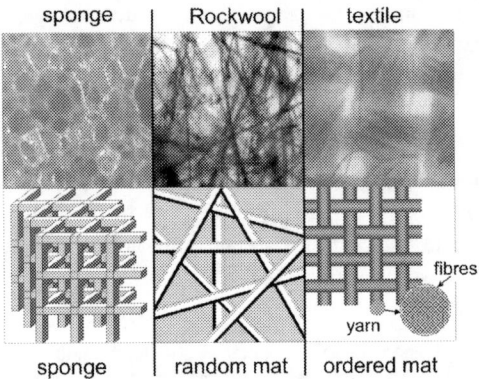

Figure C1-2 Structures with struts and fibres

Rockwool is an example of a structure consisting of fibres arranged more or less randomly in space. They are glued together at their contact points. The fibres have diameters a little below 10 μm. The air in between occupies about 95% of the volume, making this material a good thermal insulator. It is also fireproof. Such a structure is known as a random mat. The structure of paper tissue is similar.

Textile is an ordered mat. It is more complicated in that it consists of yarns which in turn are formed by spinning of fibres. The cotton fibres have a diameter of around 10 μm; the yarns are perhaps 20 fibres thick. This gives textile a large internal volume and surface, which allow it to adsorb moisture and dirt.

In structures you can often distinguish a continuous phase (Figure C1-3). In milk, water is a continuous phase. In molten butter the continuous phase is oil. You can move around over

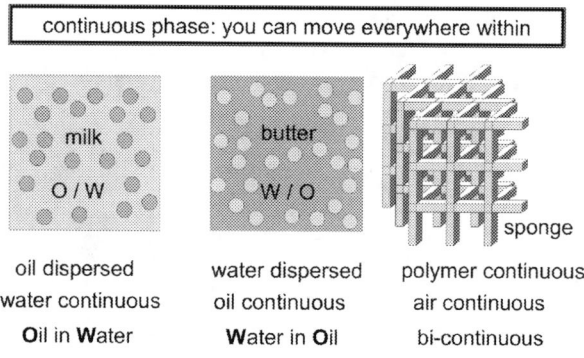

Figure C1-3 Dispersed and continuous phases

large distances through a continuous phase without leaving that phase (at least in your mind). A dispersed phase consists of parts that are not connected. The oil droplets in milk and the water droplets in butter are examples. In a sponge both phases are continuous: a sponge is bi-continuous. Bi-continuous structures are important both in life and technology, but they are not easy to make.

Stabilization of Structures

Making a structure usually requires work (Figure C1-4). For example you can make a foam by beating air into a liquid. If you stop working the structure tends to revert: the air and liquid separate. So structures need to be stabilized. Whipped cream is strongly stabilized.

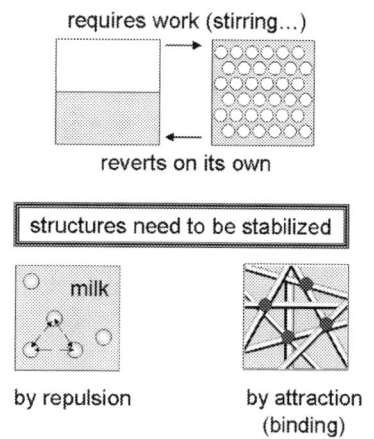

Figure C1-4 Structures need stabilization

The confusing thing is that structures can be stabilized both by repulsion between parts and by attraction (binding). The fat droplets in milk are stabilized by repulsive forces between the droplets – these are mainly due to a negative electrical charge on the droplets. Rockwool is stabilized by binding of the fibres at their contact points.

So structures need small amounts of stabilizers (Figure C1-5). There are many kinds of these; some important ones are shown. Fine particles that do not like either phase in a dispersion, tend to stay on interfaces. They work against the disappearance of the interface and so stabilize a structure.

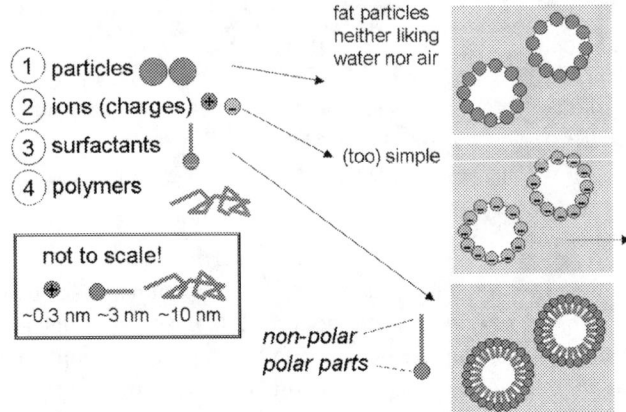

Figure C1-5 Four kinds of stabilizers

Ions can selectively occupy part of an interface and so cause an electrical charge. This can stabilize a dispersion as we have seen in milk. The mechanism of stabilization is more complicated than simple electrostatic repulsion; we discuss this further on.

A third group of stabilizers are the surfactants (or amphiphiles). These consist of a non-polar part such as a hydrocarbon chain, and a polar part such as an ion or hydroxyl group. Such molecules also tend to accumulate on interfaces, with the polar part in a polar phase and the apolar part in the less polar phase. A fourth group are the polymers, which we also discuss separately. Structures are often stabilized by several mechanisms.

Drawings of colloidal structures are usually not to scale. The parts (bubbles, drops, fibres and so on) of a structure typically have dimensions in the range of a micrometre; the stabilizing species mostly have dimensions in the range of a nanometre, so a thousand times smaller. Stabilizers only occupy a thin layer near an interface.

Materials in solution tend to adsorb on interfaces: we discuss this further in lesson 3. This also applies to ions, and the adsorption of positive and negative ions is usually different. As a result, interfaces are charged electrically (Figure C1-6).

Adsorbed ions attract oppositely charged ions from the solution and so form an electrical double-layer. The outer part of the double layer is diffuse as the counterions are held by a dynamical balance between diffusion and the electrical force. The thickness of the double layer is of the order of nanometres, but it gets thinner when the concentration of ions in the bulk solution is increased.

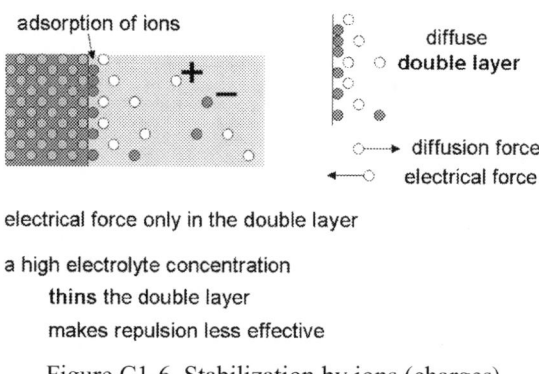

electrical force only in the double layer

a high electrolyte concentration
thins the double layer
makes repulsion less effective

Figure C1-6 Stabilization by ions (charges)

The complete double-layer is electrically neutral, so electrical interactions between particles only occur when the double layers overlap. As a result, an increased concentration of ions reduces the range and effect of electrical stabilization. It is this effect that causes milk to flocculate if you add an acid such as vinegar.

Polymers may cause either attraction or repulsion between parts. A few important mechanisms are shown in Figure C1-7. If the polymer does not adsorb on the interface, but has a high concentration in the bulk fluid, it will pull water away from points where particles touch. This gives a lower pressure (often quite negative!) near these touching points and forces the particles together. This depletion binding is important in toothpaste.

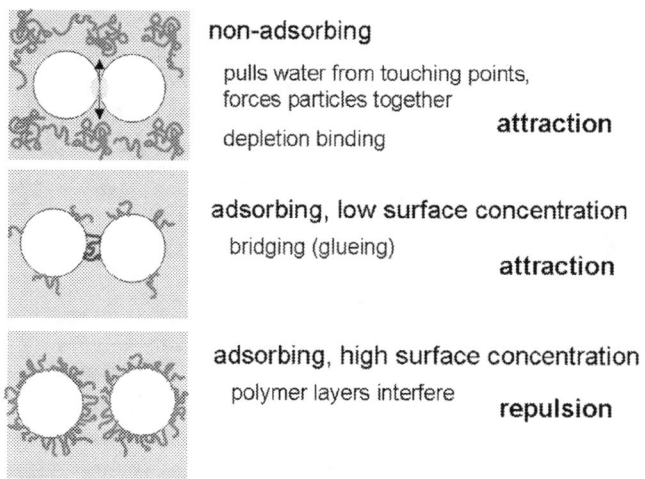

Figure C1-7 Stabilization by polymers

Small amounts of polymer may cause bridges between particles. This mechanism of flocculation is used on a large scale for removing fine particles from water.

Finally, polymers may have a high surface concentration on the particles. The diffuse outer part of the polymer layers can then interfere and keep particles apart. This method of stabilizing is used in many products.

Modelling of Structures

As you can see from Figures C1-1 and C1-2, structures are seldom completely regular and neither are their parts. Even so, we often describe them using simple model parts. Figure C1-8 shows three of these which are characterized by a single dimension.

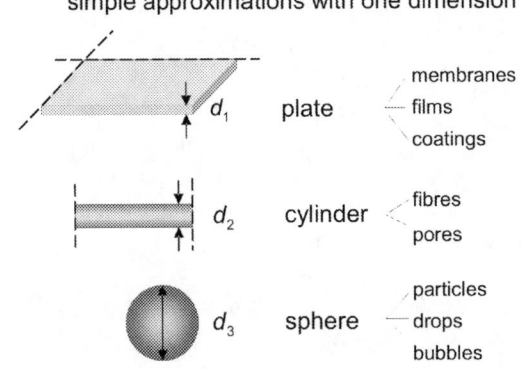

Figure C1-8 Model elements

A plate is a model for membranes, films and coatings. Cylinders can be models for fibres, but also for pores. We often regard particles, drops and bubbles as if they are little spheres.

Parts seldom all have the same dimension (Figure C1-9). A glance on the microphoto of this shaving foam shows bubbles with diameters from about 0.05 mm up to 0.7 mm: a range of a factor of 14. Even so, we often regard structures as if they consist of parts of a single size. Before you do this, think about which size might best characterize your problem.

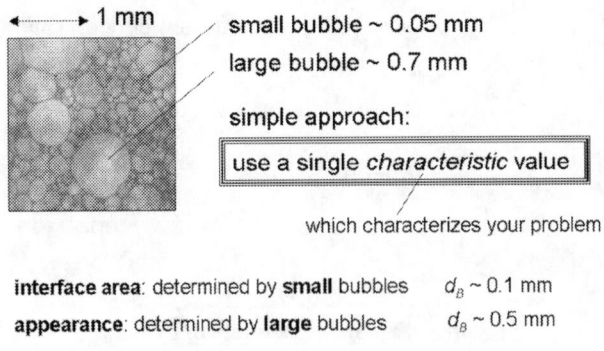

Figure C1-9 Parts have different dimensions

In the shaving foam you might be interested in the interface area of the bubbles to understand how much stabilizer is necessary to occupy the interface. The interface area is largely determined by the smaller bubbles, so you would choose a diameter in the lower part of the range – perhaps 0.1 mm. On the other hand, if you are considering the appearance of the foam, you would be interested in the larger bubbles – perhaps you would characterize this foam with bubble diameter of 0.5 mm.

There are more complete ways of describing systems with a distribution of sizes; you will find these in texts on particle technology. They are outside the scope of this introduction.

You should develop an idea of orders of magnitude of sizes of parts in structures. As an exercise try to position each example in Figure C1-10 on the logarithmic scale shown. Our answer is given further on, but try yourself. An important group of parts is those larger than small molecules, but small enough that they cannot be seen. These are known as colloids. Their dimensions range from a little above 1 nm, to about 10 µm. They are the subject of colloid science.

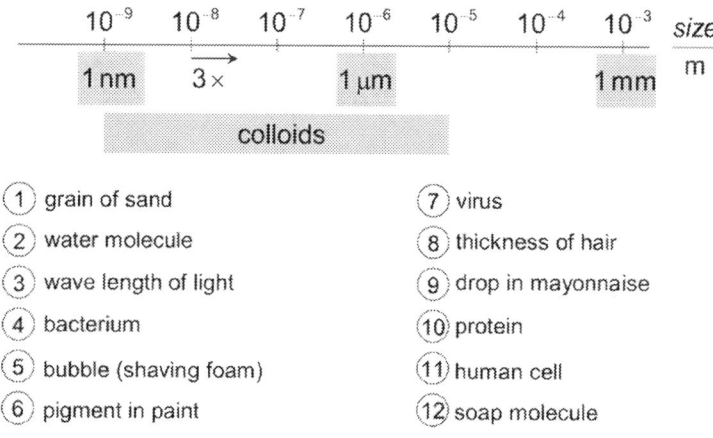

Figure C1-10 A size exercise

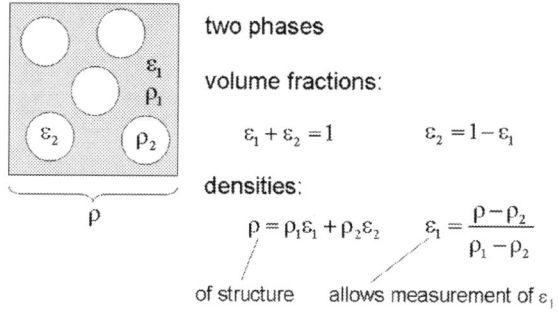

Figure C1-11 Volume fractions in a two-phase mixture

The volume fractions of phases in a structure can be very important (Figure C1-11). In a system with two phases the two volume fractions add up to one. The density of the structure is equal to the sum of the products of (volume fraction times density) of the pure phases. If you know these pure densities, you can determine the volume fractions from a measurement of the density of the structure.

The procedure here does assume that a phase has the same density as its pure counterpart. This may not be accurate in fine dispersions or if the phases partly dissolve in each other.

Colloids 2: Interfaces

In this second lesson we look at the interfaces between parts – at their size and thickness, and at what happens there. This has important effects on the behaviour of fine structures. This lesson considers only interactions of a pure gas or liquid with an interface – mixtures will come later.

Interface Properties

If you assume a simple geometry for the parts in a structure and take them to all have the same size, you can easily calculate the interface area. Figure C2-1 shows this for spherical particles. (Try cylinders and plates yourself.) As you see in the Figure C2-1 the interface area may be as high as 10^8 m^2 per m^3 of dispersion. This is 10 km $\times$ 10 km, an area of 100 km^2 packed into 1 m^3. Such areas are often given in square metres per gram of dispersion: 10^8 m^2 per m^3 is about 10^2 m^2 per g.

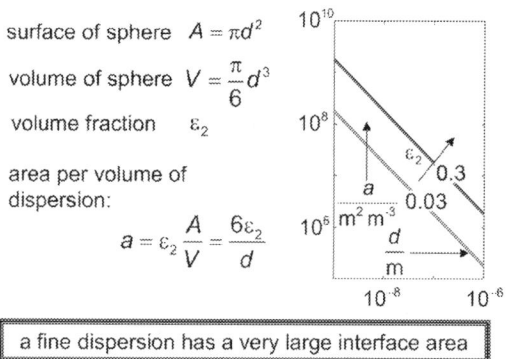

surface of sphere $A = \pi d^2$

volume of sphere $V = \dfrac{\pi}{6} d^3$

volume fraction ε_2

area per volume of dispersion:

$$a = \varepsilon_2 \frac{A}{V} = \frac{6\varepsilon_2}{d}$$

a fine dispersion has a very large interface area

Figure C2-1 Interface area of a swarm of spheres

Near interfaces properties change rapidly, but not abruptly. The distance over which they change depends on the interface and the stabilizers used. This thickness is not sharply defined, but typically a few nanometres. For a given interface thickness it is not difficult to estimate the volume fraction occupied by the interface. As you see from Figure C2-2 this becomes substantial for structures with parts smaller than about 100 nm. In fine suspensions a large part consists of 'interface'.

The simplest interfaces are those between liquids and gases. In the experiment in Figure C2-3, we have a thin liquid film supported by a wire frame. The film can be stretched by a 'travelling wire': to do this you need to exert a small force. This force is independent of how

Design and Development of Biological, Chemical, Food and Pharmaceutical Products J.A. Wesselingh, S. Kiil and M.E. Vigild
© 2007 John Wiley & Sons, Ltd

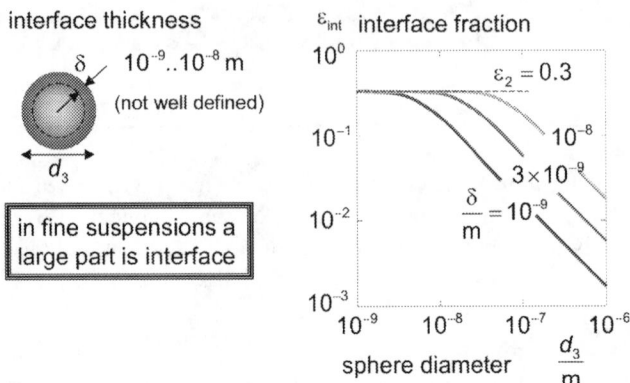

Figure C2-2 The volume of the interface

far you stretch the film; it is as if the film exerts a constant tension at its two interfaces. This is the surface tension. It is a property of the interface, and it has dimensions of N m^{-1}. You can only do this experiment with strongly stabilized soap films. A film of a pure liquid such as water breaks spontaneously.

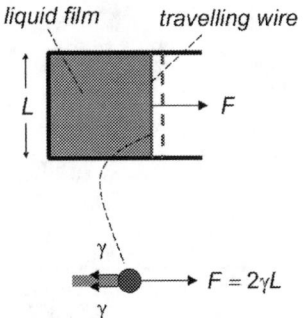

each surface has a 'surface tension' γ

Figure C2-3 Surface tension

Solids also have a surface tension (although this cannot be determined by simple methods). Figure C2-4 shows surface tensions of some liquids and solids under their own vapour pressure. The values differ only slightly from what they would be under vacuum. There are two groups: small liquid molecules and non-polar solids with low surface tensions (less than 0.1 N m^{-1}) and ionic and metallic surfaces with high tensions. Surface tensions of solids are not as well defined as those of liquids. Solid surfaces are usually inhomogeneous, and they can be rough. As a result, their surface tension varies with position.

The interface between two fluids, or a fluid and a solid, also has an interface tension. The value is related to the values of the surface tensions of the two components: if the difference in surface tensions is large, you may also expect the interface tension to be large. The interface tension is not fully predictable from surface values. The formula in Figure C2-5

$\gamma \times 10^3 / (N\ m^{-1})$ ambient conditions

liquids		solids		
n-Hexane	18	Teflon	20	*low tension interfaces*
Toluene	28	Polystyrene	40	
Water	72	NaCl	110	
Mercury	480	Tungsten	>1000	*high tension interfaces*

not so well defined ↑

Figure C2-4 Some surface tension values

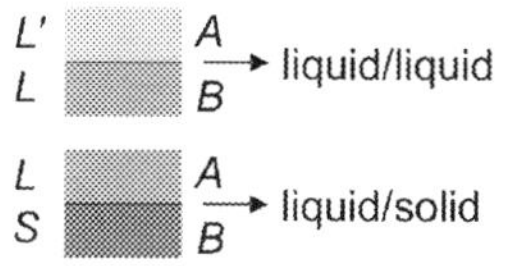

$$\begin{array}{l} L' \\ L \end{array} \quad \begin{array}{l} A \\ B \end{array} \rightarrow \text{liquid/liquid} \qquad \gamma_{AB} \approx \gamma_A + \gamma_B - 2\sqrt{\gamma_A^{nh}\gamma_B^{nh}}$$

'no hydrogen bonds'

$$\begin{array}{l} L \\ S \end{array} \quad \begin{array}{l} A \\ B \end{array} \rightarrow \text{liquid/solid}$$

	$\dfrac{\gamma \times 10^3}{N\,m^{-1}}$	$\dfrac{\gamma^{nh} \times 10^3}{N\,m^{-1}}$
n-Hexane	18	18
Water	72	22
Hex/Water	51	

ambient conditions

Figure C2-5 Surface and interface tensions

gives approximate values for the common situation where one liquid is water. In the last term you need a value of the 'surface tension with no hydrogen bonds'. For water this has a value of 22 N m^{-1}; in non-polar solvents there are no hydrogen bonds and the two interface tensions are equal.

Consequences of Interface Tension

The pressure inside a drop or bubble is a little higher than outside. You can calculate the amount from the surface tension (Figure C2-6). Imagine the drop split in two equal parts. The two parts are held together by the surface tension along the circumference. The result is balanced by the pressure force working on the cross-section. The smaller the drop, the larger the pressure difference becomes. Because of the higher pressure inside, very small drops and bubbles tend to dissolve and disappear. For a bubble in air there are two gas–liquid interfaces. As a result the pressure difference is twice that in a drop. Such bubbles are very unstable: they can only exist if they are strongly stabilized.

With a drop of liquid in contact with a solid (Figure C2-7), there are three interfaces: the solid/liquid; the solid/vapour and the liquid/vapour interfaces. Each of these has its own interface tension. For a drop that partially wets a solid, the horizontal components of the interface tensions must be in equilibrium. This determines the value of the contact angle θ

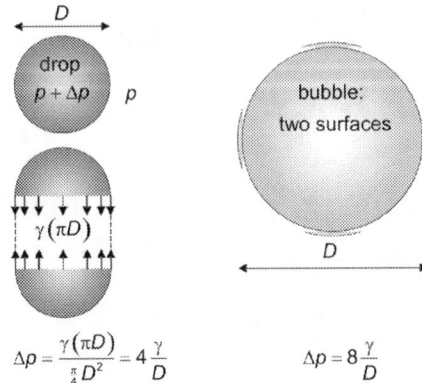

$$\Delta p = \frac{\gamma (\pi D)}{\frac{\pi}{4} D^2} = 4 \frac{\gamma}{D} \qquad \qquad \Delta p = 8 \frac{\gamma}{D}$$

Figure C2-6 Pressure in drops and bubbles

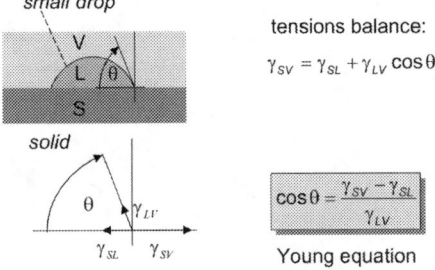

tensions balance:

$$\gamma_{SV} = \gamma_{SL} + \gamma_{LV} \cos \theta$$

$$\cos \theta = \frac{\gamma_{SV} - \gamma_{SL}}{\gamma_{LV}}$$

Young equation

Figure C2-7 The contact[1] angle

between liquid and solid. This is an important property of three-phase systems. The relation between the tensions is known as the Young equation.

A small contact angle implies that the drop spreads over the surface: if the contact angle is zero, the surface will be wetted completely (Figure C2-8). This happens when the solid/vapour tension is much larger than the solid/liquid tension: the system then avoids any solid/vapour interface. If the contact angle is equal to π, there is no wetting. This happens when the solid/liquid tension is much higher than the solid/vapour tension. The system then minimizes the liquid/vapour interface, as with a drop of mercury on paper.

You can measure the contact angle by determining the spreading of a small drop of known volume, for example under a microscope. Figure C2-9 shows the diameter of the drop as you see it from above. For a non-wetting system, you see the diameter of the sphere, not that of the contact disk. Results from this part of the graph are not accurate.

A liquid usually rises in a narrow capillary (Figure C2-10). The liquid is pulled upwards by the vertical component of the surface tension at the liquid top or meniscus. It rises until this

---

[1] The Young equation can predict imaginary values of the contact angle, or values larger than π. These have no geometrical meaning: if the value is imaginary the surface wets completely; if it is larger than π there is no wetting.

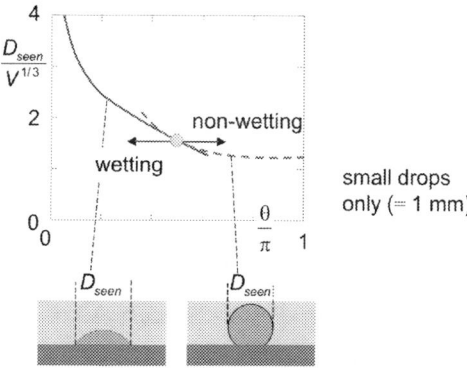

$$\cos\theta = \frac{\gamma_{SV} - \gamma_{SL}}{\gamma_{LV}}$$

$\theta \leq 0$	$\theta = \pi/2$	$\theta \geq \pi$

wetting   no wetting

$\gamma_{SV} \gg \gamma_{SL}$ $\gamma_{SL} \gg \gamma_{SV}$

low tension   low tension
solid/liquid   solid/vapour

Figure C2-8 Wetting

Figure C2-9 Measuring the contact angle

force is balanced by the weight of the column of liquid. If the liquid does not wet the solid, it will be pushed down or depressed in the capillary. You can use a capillary rise experiment to determine the product of surface tension and cosine of the contact angle. If you determine the contact angle separately, for example from photographs of a small drop, you can get hold of the surface tension.

In sufficiently fine porous media the effect of gravity is not important (Figure C2-11). You would then expect the solid either not to wet at all (the left figure) or to wet completely (the right figure).

Some Complications

In reality things are not so clear cut. The solid surface is heterogeneous and dirty, and it is usually rough on a molecular level. As a result air can get trapped when the structure fills up and liquid can be retained when it is drained. Nevertheless it is usually quite clear whether a porous material wets (such as with kitchen tissue) or does not (such as with a Goretex raincoat).

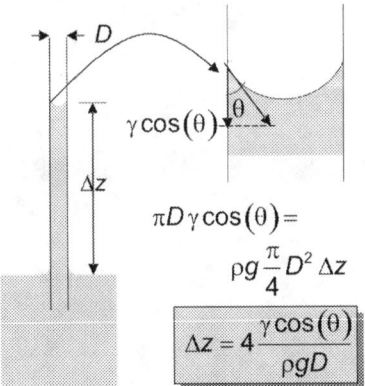

Figure C2-10 Capillary rise

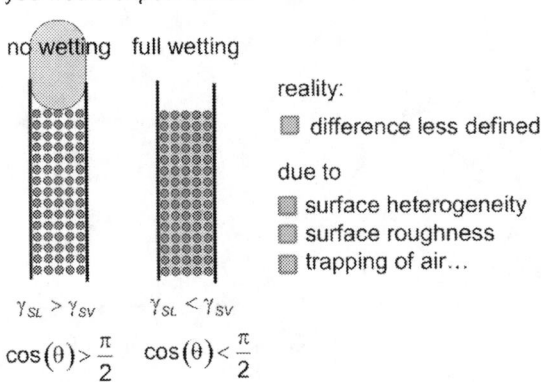

Figure C2-11 Wetting in porous media

The Young equation predicts that contact angles only depend on the three interface tensions. These might be thought to be only properties of the binary combinations S/L, S/V and L/V. However, there are complications. Especially on high tension surfaces, part of the vapour of the liquid will adsorb on the solid (Figure C2-12). This lowers the tension of the S/G interface. On a rough solid, the actual interface area is larger than the one that we see: this causes the effective tensions of the solid interfaces to be larger than those of a flat surface. If there are contaminants (dirt) in the system, these will adsorb on the solid and lower the effective interface tension of the solid. We discuss this further when we consider surfactants. As a result, simple calculations using 'pure' interface tensions are often inaccurate. Even so, they can be quite useful for a first understanding.

If the solid surface is rough, dirty, or just heterogeneous, then the contact angle depends on how the liquid is applied (Figure C2-13). The surface has spots with a high effective tension, and spots with a low effective tension. A liquid advancing along the surface will be retarded by spots with a low interface tension. A liquid retreating from the surface will be kept back by spots with a high interface tension. As a result, the advancing and retreating contact

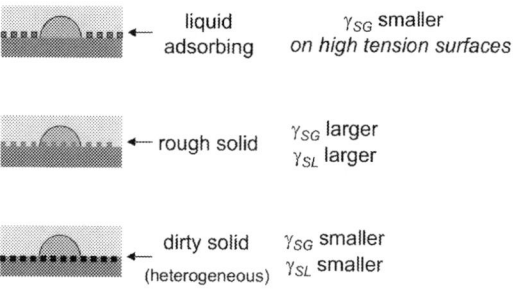

Figure C2-12 Complications on wetting

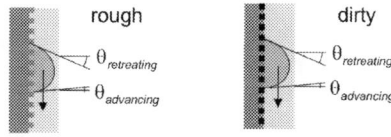

at solid interfaces there is often no equilibrium

Figure C2-13 Advancing and retreating wetting angles

angles differ. The advancing value is always the largest. Drops with different advancing and retreating contact angles are in a metastable state: they are not in true equilibrium. You can see this effect with drops of rain on a window pane.

Clean, flat, homogeneous surfaces can be obtained in the laboratory, but only with difficulty. You must expect all surfaces around you to be rough and contaminated. So don't expect accurate results from amateur experiments on surface phenomena. The cleanest surfaces around tend to be those of low surface-tension materials such as Teflon and polyethylene films. High-tension surfaces are always contaminated, if only by water adsorbed from air. Clean aluminium foil is perhaps as close as you can get. You often get best results with a little tapping or vibration as this reduces the difference between the two angles.

Colloids 3: Adsorption

An interface in contact with a mixture shows all sorts of interesting things. The layer next to the interface can have a composition very different from that of the bulk fluid; this lowers the interfacial tension and can greatly enhance the stability of foams, emulsions and suspensions.

Adsorption Terminology[1]

Consider a solvent A with a low concentration of a solute B (Figure C3-1). If the solute does not like the solvent it may concentrate strongly on an interface. This can be any interface: with a gas, with another liquid or with a solid. This accumulation on an interface is known as adsorption. The phase on the other side of the interface is the adsorbent. Adsorption can be characterized by the fraction of the surface that is occupied by the solute – this can usually only be determined indirectly. This surface fraction is often much larger than the fraction of the solute in the bulk of the liquid. Here we consider only a solute that dissolves in a phase to one side of the interface; dissolution in both phases is also possible.

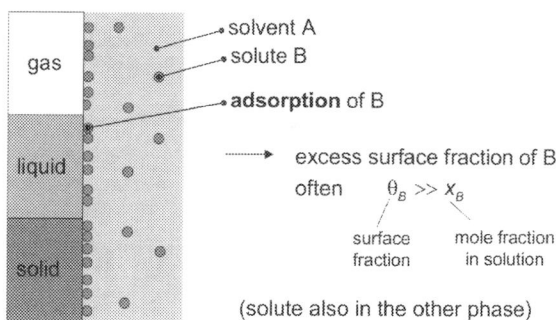

Figure C3-1 Terms describing adsorption

Adsorption Mechanisms

A handy concept to understand much of adsorption is that of polarity (Figure C3-2). Heptane is an apolar molecule: it has no electrical poles. Water is a polar molecule: the two protons are positive and the oxygen atom is negative. Polar molecules bind more strongly than do similar apolar molecules. This is because the charges cause hydrogen bonding between the molecules. Ethanol is less polar than water, but still quite polar. The aromatics are less polar again, but not completely apolar. This is because double bond electrons can be slightly

---

[1] Adsorption is not to be confused with absorption, which is dissolution of a gas in a liquid.

Design and Development of Biological, Chemical, Food and Pharmaceutical Products   J.A. Wesselingh, S. Kiil and M.E. Vigild
© 2007 John Wiley & Sons, Ltd

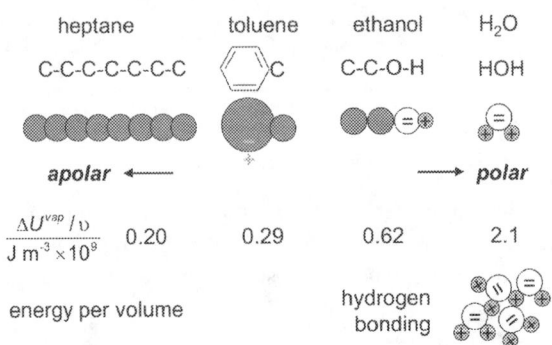

Figure C3-2 Polarity of solvents

polarized by other charged molecules. A simple quantitative measure of polarity is the energy of vaporization per volume. That of heptane is low; that of water high. Polarities of polymers cannot be determined in this way, but they are similar to those of corresponding smaller molecules. Polyethylene is like heptane, polystyrene like toluene, and poly-ethylene-glycol (PEG) like methanol. Carbon is a fairly apolar adsorbent, but its surface can be modified to increase polarity; silica gel is highly polar.

Two examples of adsorption are given in Figure C3-3. Hexane (apolar) dissolves only slightly in the polar solvent water. In contact with carbon (apolar) hexane then adsorbs strongly.

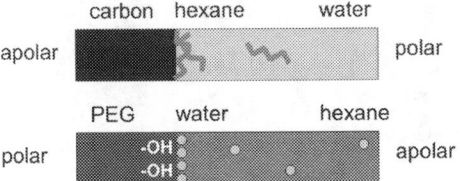

Figure C3-3 Hexane in water adsorbs on carbon, water in hexane adsorbs on PEG

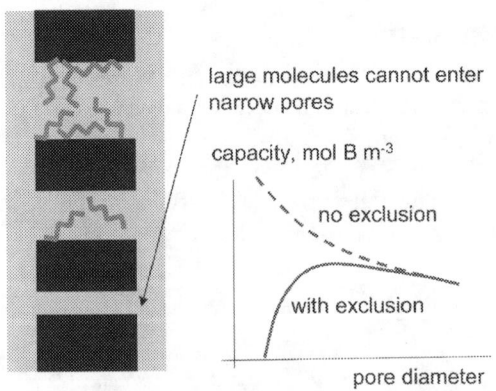

Figure C3-4 Large molecules can be excluded by small pores

Similarly, when hexane is the solvent, water adsorbs on a polar sorbent such as poly-ethylene-glycol (PEG), a polymer with many – OH groups. Small pores in an adsorbent increase the interfacial area, but large molecules can be excluded (Figure C3-4). So adsorbents not only select on polarity, but also on the size of molecules.

Adsorption can also be affected by electrical charges (Figure C3-5). This is used in ion exchange. Here certain charges are anchored to a matrix (in the example here these are sulfonic acid groups). Counter ions are strongly adsorbed, but can be exchanged with other ions that are equally (or more strongly) adsorbed. The example here is a cation exchanger. The opposite type with fixed positive charges exchanges anions.

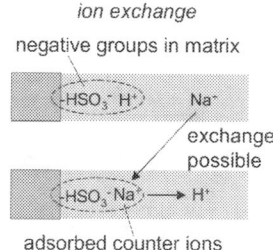

Figure C3-5 Counter charges adsorb on a charged matrix

Surfactants

Surfactants have a particularly large effect on interfacial properties (Figure C3-6). They consist of molecules with a polar head (that tends to dissolve in water) and an apolar tail (that tends to dissolve in oil or stick out into air, but does not like water). Such molecules adsorb strongly on interfaces. Figure C3-6 shows a few properties of surfactants. The polar head can consist of an ion (either a cation or an anion), or it may contain a number of – OH groups (as in 'non-ionic' surfactants). The tail is a hydrocarbon, with a length of about 12 carbon atoms. There are many different surfactants; Figure C3-6 only gives a rough idea of the dimensions.

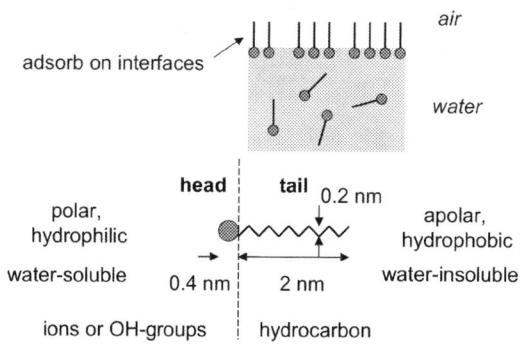

Figure C3-6 Properties of surfactants (soaps)

Adsorbing species lower the interfacial tension. In Figure C3-7 you see how this happens with the common surfactant SDS (sodium dodecyl sulphate). Note that the concentration

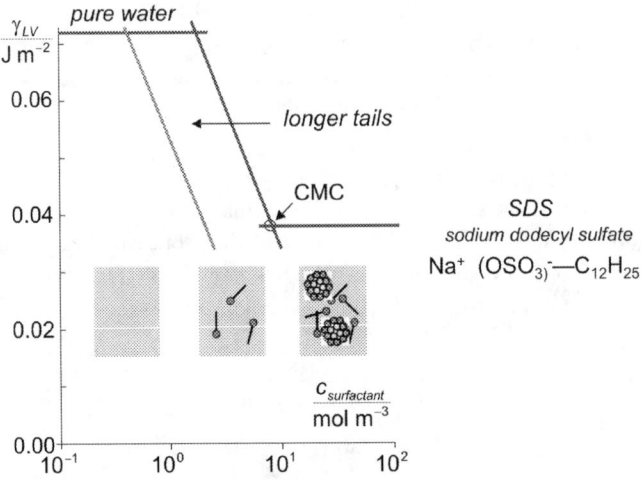

Figure C3-7 How a surfactant lowers the interfacial tension

scale along the bottom axis is logarithmic. At very low SDS concentrations in water, the surface tension is equal to that of water. Above a certain threshold value it starts falling rapidly in an exponential fashion to about one half of the original value. This stops abruptly at the CMC (critical micelle concentration) where the surfactant molecules form micelles consisting of about 50 SDS molecules each. The CMC depends greatly on the length of the hydrocarbon tail of the surfactant; the longer the tail the less surfactant is needed to lower the surface tension.

One of the mechanisms for stabilizing an interface is shown in Figure C3-8. It concerns the film around a bubble from soapy water. Any stretching of the film causes a local depletion of surfactant so that the surface tension rises. This opposes further thinning and so stabilizes the film.

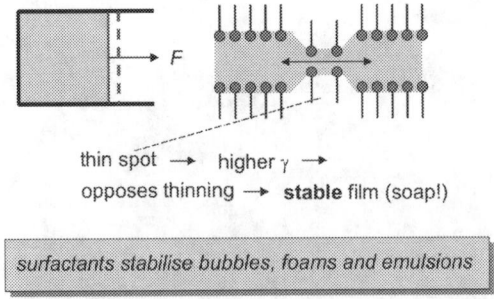

Figure C3-8 Stabilization of a film by a surfactant

Polymers

Polymers follow the same rules as other species, but more strongly so (Figure C3-9). This is because they can have multiple adsorption bonds on interfaces. An apolar polymer in a polar solvent will adsorb strongly on an apolar interface and vice versa. Such adsorption can get

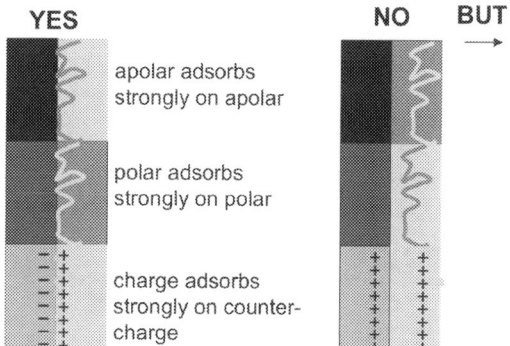

Figure C3-9 Adsorption rules for polymers

stronger in time as the polymer configures itself along the surface. Adsorption of a polymer is sometimes irreversible: it can be forced to be so by chemical linking of the polymer with the surface or with other polymer molecules. This is often required for coatings and adhesives. Also polymers can be charged and can then adsorb on a counter charge. Polymers are of course sensitive to size exclusion. The right side of Figure C3-9 shows situations where the polymer will not adsorb. There are further complications, of which we discuss a few on the next figure.

Polymers may consist of different parts with different adsorption properties (Figure C3-10). This gives an almost unlimited number of possibilities that we cannot explore here. You have already seen some of them in the lesson on Structures.

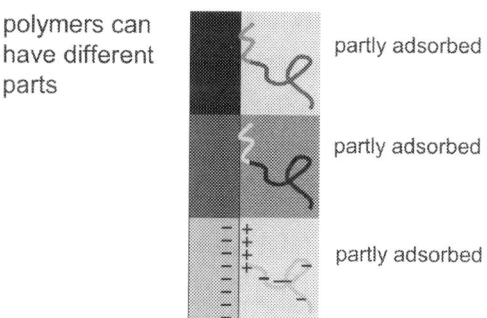

Figure C3-10 Adsorption of block co-polymers

Adsorption Equilibrium

Adsorption is often roughly described by what is known as the Langmuir isotherm (Figure C3-11). This tells us that the fraction of the surface occupied by the solute (at equilibrium) increases with increasing solute concentration, but to a limiting value. The initial slope of the isotherm is a measure of the affinity of the solute for the surface (how much it likes the surface). The higher the affinity, the higher the slope. As you can easily check, the inverse of the constant K is the concentration at which one half of the surface is occupied by the solute.

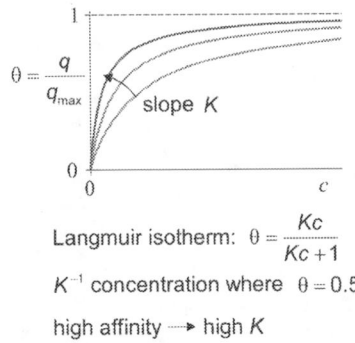

$$\theta = \frac{q}{q_{max}}$$

slope K

Langmuir isotherm: $\theta = \dfrac{Kc}{Kc+1}$

K^{-1} concentration where $\theta = 0.5$

high affinity $\longrightarrow$ high K

Figure C3-11 Adsorption equilibria

The second parameter in the isotherm is the capacity: the amount that will be adsorbed when the solute concentration becomes high. Then the surface will be (almost) completely covered with solute. The surface occupied by a solute molecule is usually in the range of 10^{-19} to 10^{-18} m^2. If you know both this value and the interface area of the adsorbent you can calculate the capacity of the adsorbent. This can be given in many units: in kilograms or moles per cubic metre, or per kilogram of adsorbent, or in other ways.

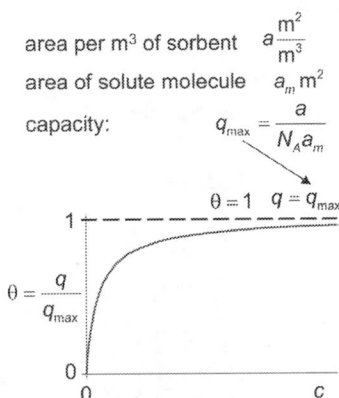

area per m^3 of sorbent $\quad a\,\dfrac{m^2}{m^3}$

area of solute molecule $\quad a_m\,m^2$

capacity: $\qquad q_{max} = \dfrac{a}{N_A a_m}$

$\theta = 1 \quad q = q_{max}$

$$\theta = \frac{q}{q_{max}}$$

Figure C3-12 The capacity of the adsorbent

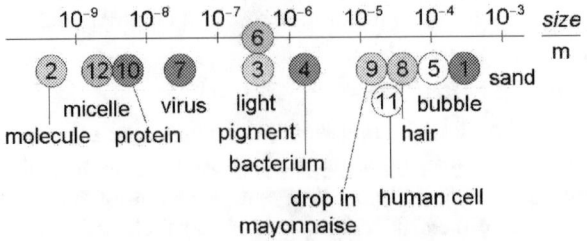

Figure C3-12 The answer to the size exercise

Size Exercise (Lesson 1)

This is the answer to the size exercise in Colloids 1 (Figure C1-10). Your answers may differ perhaps by a factor of three from ours – most sizes are not that accurately defined.

Colloids 4: Rheology

This lesson is an introduction to the flow behaviour (rheology) of pastes and gels. Examples of such 'non-Newtonian' liquids are:

1. rubber solutions such as used to repair bicycle tyres or to paste photographs: these are elastic solids when they are stretched quickly,
2. liquids like sauces and custard, which become less viscous ('thinner') when stirred, but then can thicken again,
3. peanut butter and mud, which are solid when the stresses are below a certain minimum value (the 'yield stress').

Before introducing these complicated liquids, we first discuss the simpler kind: the 'Newtonian' liquids.

Viscosities and Shear Rates

The flow of gases and simple liquids can be described by a single property: the shear viscosity or viscosity for short. You can measure the viscosity by shearing the liquid between two parallel plates (as in Figure C4-1). This causes a velocity gradient normal to the direction of the motion (also known as the shear rate). The viscosity is the ratio of the shear stress to the shear rate.

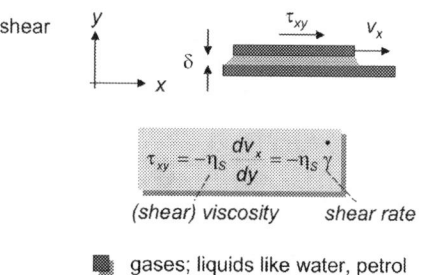

$$\tau_{xy} = -\eta_s \frac{dv_x}{dy} = -\eta_s \dot{\gamma}$$

(shear) viscosity   *shear rate*

■ gases; liquids like water, petrol

Figure C4-1 (Shear) Viscosity

The shear rate is an important concept, also for non-Newtonian liquids. It is defined as the rate of change of the shear angle γ, as shown in the left part of Figure C4-2. You can also interpret the shear rate as the velocity gradient, as is done in the middle part. That the two concepts are identical is shown at the bottom of the figure. Finally, you can regard the inverse of the shear rate as the time required to shear the fluid through an angle of 1 radian.

Design and Development of Biological, Chemical, Food and Pharmaceutical Products J.A. Wesselingh, S. Kiil and M.E. Vigild
© 2007 John Wiley & Sons, Ltd

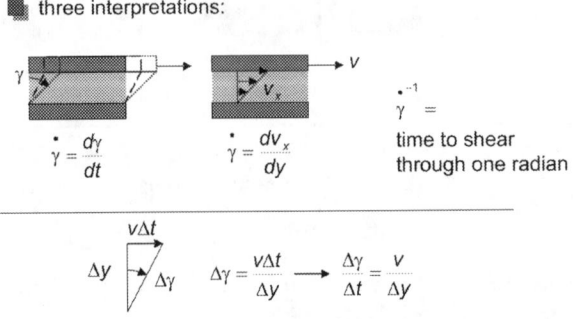

Figure C4-2 Shear rate

In non-Newtonian liquids, you will often encounter a second viscosity parameter: the elongational viscosity (Figure C4-3). Elongational viscosity plays a role when a fluid is stretched, such as when a filament is drawn out of a viscous liquid. It causes a stress in the same direction as the stretching, proportional to the elongation rate. For a Newtonian fluid, the elongational viscosity has a value of three times the shear viscosity, so it is not an independent parameter. A filament of a Newtonian fluid is unstable. A thin spot in the filament will undergo a higher stress than the surroundings and will thin more quickly until the filament breaks.

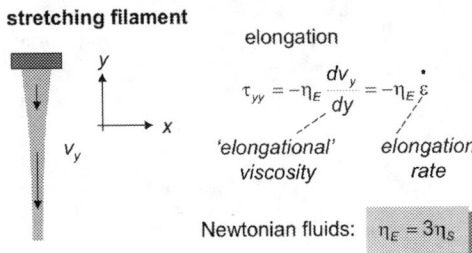

Figure C4-3 Elongational viscosity

Polymers

Our first non-Newtonian liquids are solutions or melts of a polymer (Figure C4-4). In equilibrium the polymer strands tend to form more or less spherical coils. However, when the liquid is sheared, the coils are stretched and tend to become aligned. This stretching increases their energy, and when the shear is removed, they 'rebound'. So the fluid has elastic properties in addition to viscous ones. An important property of the polymer in solution is its relaxation time. This is a measure for the time that it takes to rebound. It is of the order of nanoseconds for small molecules, of seconds for polymers in processing equipment, and of centuries in construction materials. Yes, these last ones also flow or 'creep'.

A simple equation that shows much of viscoelastic behaviour is due to Maxwell (Figure C4-5). You see that it is the same as the Newtonian equation, but with one additional stress term containing the relaxation time. We can see two extreme cases:

1. for small values of the relaxation time (or long times) the new term disappears. The stress is proportional to the shear rate. We regain a Newtonian fluid.
2. for large values of the relaxation time (or short times) we see that the stress is proportional to the shear angle or deformation. Our substance now behaves as a solid.

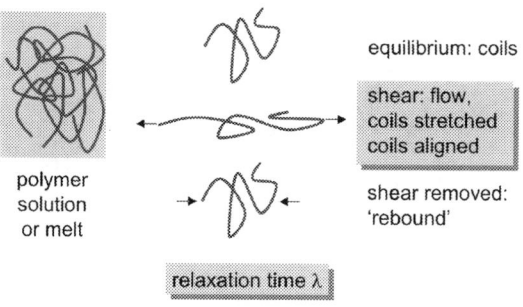

equilibrium: coils

shear: flow, coils stretched coils aligned

polymer solution or melt

shear removed: 'rebound'

relaxation time λ

Figure C4-4 Viscoelasticity

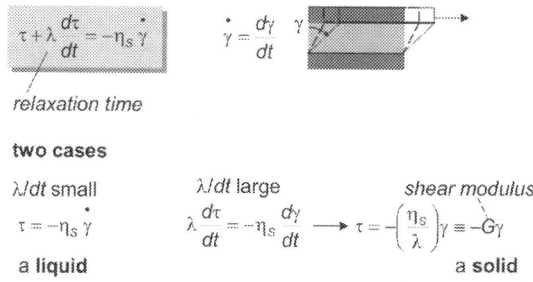

$$\tau + \lambda \frac{d\tau}{dt} = -\eta_s \dot{\gamma}$$

$$\dot{\gamma} = \frac{d\gamma}{dt}$$

relaxation time

two cases

λ/dt small

$$\tau = -\eta_s \dot{\gamma}$$

a liquid

λ/dt large

$$\lambda \frac{d\tau}{dt} = -\eta_s \frac{d\gamma}{dt}$$

shear modulus

$$\tau = -\left(\frac{\eta_s}{\lambda}\right)\gamma = -G\gamma$$

a solid

Figure C4-5 The Maxwell equation

Whether we have a liquid or a solid, is governed by the Deborah number (Figure C4-6). This is a ratio of the relaxation time to the time used to shear the fluid over one radian. If the Deborah number is very small, we are dealing with a Newtonian liquid. If it has a value around unity, we have a viscoelastic fluid; if the value is very large, a creeping solid.

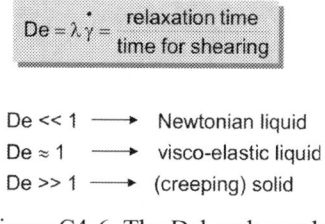

$$De = \lambda \dot{\gamma} = \frac{\text{relaxation time}}{\text{time for shearing}}$$

De << 1 ⟶ Newtonian liquid

De ≈ 1 ⟶ visco-elastic liquid

De >> 1 ⟶ (creeping) solid

Figure C4-6 The Deborah number

Stretching of polymer coils (Figure C4-7) in the liquid causes two effects:

1. it increases the resistance to elongation (and so the elongational viscosity) and
2. it decreases the resistance to shear (as the polymer molecules become more aligned).

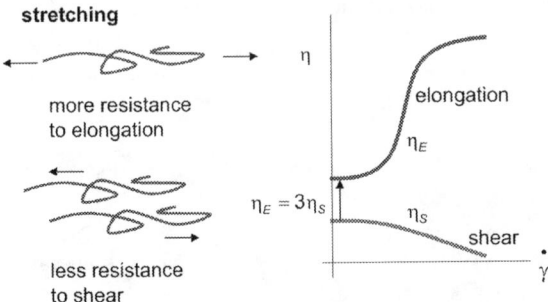

Figure C4-7 Behaviour of the two viscosities

Both effects have important consequences for processing of polymers. The 'thickening' of the elongational viscosity stabilizes filaments and films of polymers. The 'thinning' of the shear viscosity causes many problems in mixing and dispersion in polymer products, because flow then mainly occurs in high shear regions and not elsewhere.

Stretched polymer coils 'want' to expand. So they exert a stress normal to their direction of elongation (Figure C4-8). The normal stress is often (roughly) proportional to the square of the shear rate. The normal stress coefficient is again another property that we need to describe the rheology of mixtures with polymers. We note that the Maxwell model does predict elongational thickening, but neither shear thinning nor normal stresses.

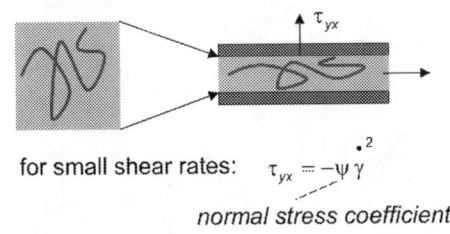

for small shear rates: $\tau_{yx} = -\psi \, \dot{\gamma}^2$

normal stress coefficient

Figure C4-8 Normal stresses

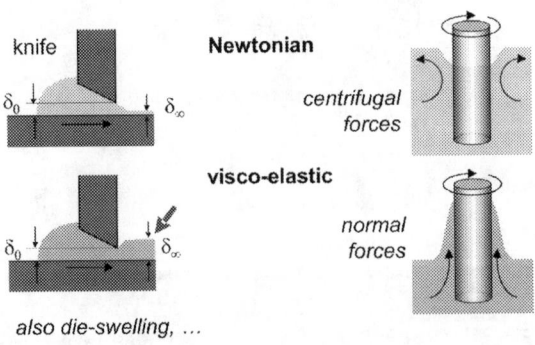

also die-swelling, ...

Figure C4-9 Rebound and rod-climbing

Normal stresses cause effects that can be rather surprising. Sometimes they are useful, sometimes a nuisance. Two of them are shown in Figure C4-9. A coating formed by a knife and a Newtonian liquid is always thinner than the slit; a coating formed by a viscoelastic fluid can be thicker. Profiles extruded, or films blown, can be thicker than the die-opening in the extruder. In rotating equipment (such as mixers) Newtonian liquids are thrown outwards by centrifugal forces. In viscoelastic fluids normal forces can cause the fluid to move normal to the main flow, and to give what is known as 'rod climbing'. You can recognize a viscoelastic fluid quite easily by spinning a rod in it; you may be surprised to find that many fluids in the kitchen are viscoelastic.

Dispersions

Our second kind of non-Newtonian liquids are dispersions (Figure C4-10): suspensions (small solid particles in a liquid), emulsions (small drops of an immiscible liquid in another liquid) and foams (small bubbles of a gas in a liquid). At equilibrium, the particles, drops and bubbles will attain a configuration at which their Gibbs energy is minimal: the drops and bubbles will be spherical, and particles, drops and bubbles will be randomly distributed over space. Extension causes the particles, drops or bubbles to deform and to align. This usually results in shear thinning: the shear viscosity decreases with increasing shear rate. Occasionally, interparticle forces cause a structuring of particles. This can be disturbed by the flow, and can lead to 'particle locking' which increases the shear viscosity: this is shear thickening.

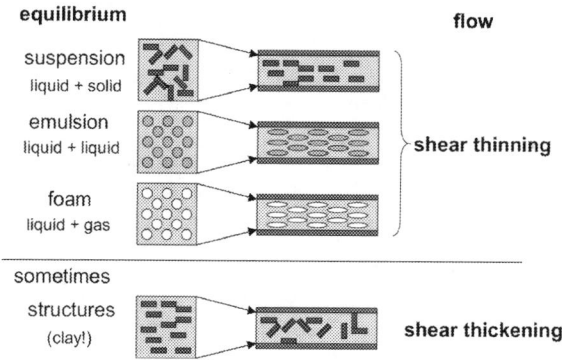

Figure C4-10 Flow of dispersions

All these fluids can show the other non-Newtonian properties that we have already discussed: elastic properties, normal stresses, and thickening or thinning of the elongational viscosity. In addition, they can also have a yield stress or a time-dependent viscosity.

Figure C4-11 shows a few examples of what the shear stress/shear rate diagram (or rheogram) of different dispersions can look like. We have only shown the shape: the values along the axes can vary by many orders of magnitude for different liquids.

Power-law Fluids

The rheograms can often be described over a fairly wide range by a power-law function (Figure C4-12). This means that you get a straight line in a logarithmic graph. The slope

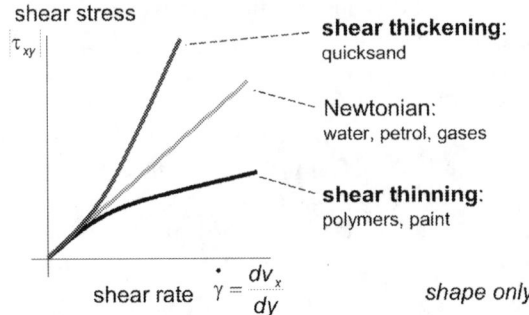

Figure C4-11 Rheogram shapes

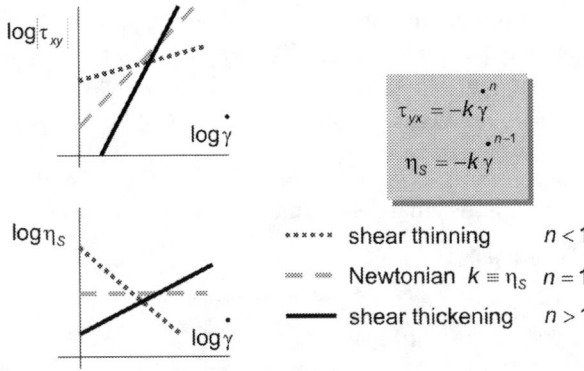

Figure C4-12 Power-law fluids

is smaller than unity for a shear thinning liquid, equal to unity for a Newtonian liquid, and larger than unity for a shear thickening liquid. For a power law liquid the shear viscosity is also a simple function of the shear rate, except that the exponent is now lower by one. Of course a Newtonian liquid has a constant viscosity.

Shear thinning and thickening have substantial effects on flow. Figure C4-13 shows what you can expect in pressure driven flow in a tube or slit. The middle diagram shows the Newtonian case with which you will be familiar. The velocity profile is parabolic, both in slits (Couette flow) and in tubes (Poiseuille flow). Shear thinning liquids have a low viscosity near the wall (where the shear rate is high), but a high viscosity in the middle. As a result, the velocity profile is flat, and the liquid flows like a plug. The opposite is true for shear thickening fluids.

Bingham Fluids

In concentrated suspensions, the particles touch each other. If there is also an attraction between the particles, the suspension may not flow when the shear stress is small: it is a solid (Figure C4-14). The stress at which the liquid starts moving is known as the yield stress. Once the liquid yields, it often behaves like a Newtonian liquid with a constant differential viscosity. The behaviour of such 'Bingham' fluids is similar to that of shear thinning fluids:

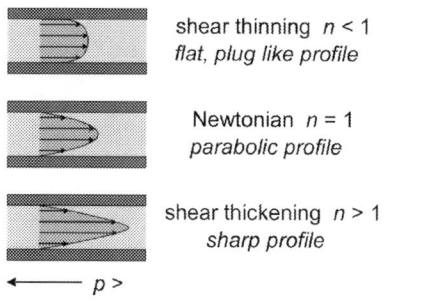

shear thinning $n < 1$
flat, plug like profile

Newtonian $n = 1$
parabolic profile

shear thickening $n > 1$
sharp profile

$\longleftarrow p >$

Figure C4-13 Flow profiles

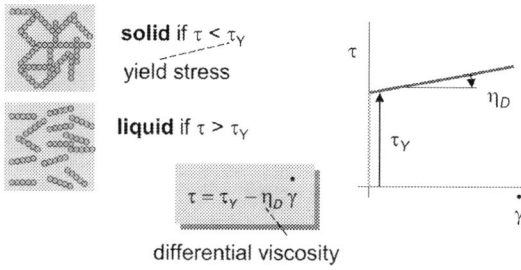

solid if $\tau < \tau_Y$
yield stress

liquid if $\tau > \tau_Y$

$\tau = \tau_Y - \eta_D \dot{\gamma}$

differential viscosity

Figure C4-14 Bingham fluids

often the two models are equally good. The Bingham model is simple to understand, but not as easy to implement as the power-law fluid. Examples of Bingham fluids are toothpaste and ketchup.

Time-dependent Fluids

Many suspensions, and also some polymer solutions, change in time (Figure C4-15). This is usually because structures are broken or formed by shearing. The result can be that the viscosity decreases in time (a thixotropic liquid) or increases (a rheopectic liquid). Yoghurt is a good example of a thixotropic liquid; rheopectic fluids are rare. The changes in viscosity are often, but not always, reversible. Note that these time effects are not the same that we saw in viscoelastic liquids.

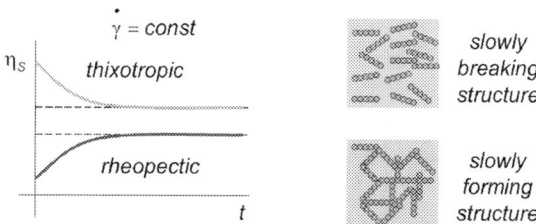

$\dot{\gamma} = const$

η_S thixotropic

rheopectic

t

slowly breaking structure

slowly forming structure

Figure C4-15 Time-dependent fluids

Rheology Measurements

Measuring rheological parameters is not easy. There are a large number of instruments available, but none can be used for every property. A few of the more important types are shown in Figure C4-16. The Couette (or rotating) cylinder instruments give parallel shear with a constant shear stress: they measure the shear viscosity. The elongational viscosity can be measured by drawing a thread, but only for viscous liquids. A cone and plate viscometer can measure the normal stress, from the vertical force exerted by the fluid. Also in this instrument, the shear rate and stress are independent of position. The simplest looking instrument uses a capillary with a given pressure drop or liquid height to drive the liquid. The shear stress varies across the diameter, so the flow in this instrument is not really simple.

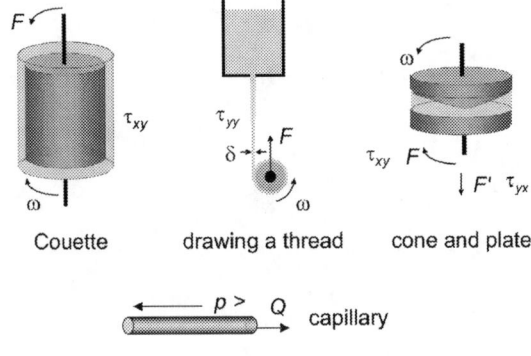

Figure C4-16 Rheometers

Going Further

This was an introduction to rheology. If you want to go further, you will find that it is a difficult subject. For three-dimensional problems you need sophisticated mathematics to get anywhere. You will need tensor equations: the three stresses τ_{xy}, τ_{yx} and τ_{yy} that you have seen are three of the nine components of the stress tensor (Figure C4-17). And that is just

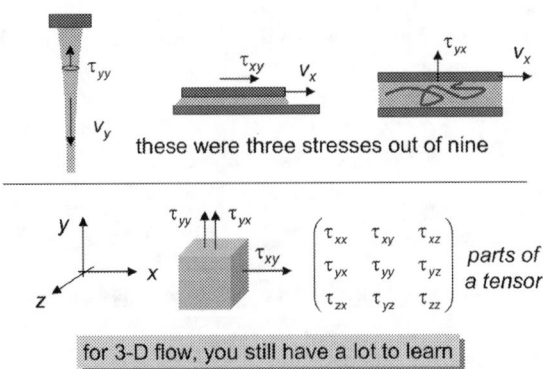

Figure C4-17 Complications to expect

one of several tensors that you will need to write down the transport equations ... Even so, you can get a feeling for rheology from these notes, and from estimating the different parameters with simple experiments with liquids around you.

Further Reading

There are many books on Colloid Science. A good starting point is Paul C. Hiemenz and Raj Rajagopalan, *Principles of Colloid and Surface Chemistry*, 3rd edition, Marcel Dekker 1997.

Index

Design and Development of Biological, Chemical, Food and Pharmaceutical Products   J.A. Wesselingh,
S. Kiil and M.E. Vigild
© 2007 John Wiley & Sons, Ltd